# Life Expectancy in Africa

# Life Expectancy in Africa

## Improving Public Health Policy

Augustine Adu Frimpong

Foreword by
Onyumbe B. Lukongo

LEXINGTON BOOKS
*Lanham • Boulder • New York • London*

Published by Lexington Books
An imprint of The Rowman & Littlefield Publishing Group, Inc.
4501 Forbes Boulevard, Suite 200, Lanham, Maryland 20706
www.rowman.com

6 Tinworth Street, London SE11 5AL, United Kingdom



British Library Cataloguing in Publication Information Available

Library of Congress Control Number:2019949928

ISBN: 978-1-7936-0356-2 (cloth : alk. paper)
ISBN: 978-1-7936-0357-9 (electronic)

*I dedicate this book to my supportive uncle and his spouse (Dr. Akwasi Bretuo, formerly deputy editor of* Pioneer *newspaper of Ghana and Editor-in-Chief of Liberia-based newspapers* Daily Listener, Saturday Chronicle, *and* Sunday Digest, *and Dr. Yvette M. Alex of Breaux Bridge, Louisiana, USA), respectively, whose unflinching/active support and many sacrifices ensured the fulfillment of my apparent higher educational dream as well as ambition and labor; therefore, today, I have succeeded in earning the Ph.D. degree, as I followed their earlier shining academic*-cum-*intellectual footsteps. Furthermore, this work is dedicated to my dear wife, Mrs. Theresah Kye Adu Frimpong (nee Kye), as well as my dear mother (Elizabeth Nana Yaa Agyeman), and my beloved maternal grandmother, Nana Hannah Abena Amoatemah, all of Ghana; they have blessed me with their love, prayers, and indeed, abundant patience. Above all, you are the beat of my heart, the pulse of my veins, and the energy of my soul, as I say to all of you: Thank you very much for the support and for believing in my abilities! I am eternally grateful to all of you!!*

# Contents

# Foreword

## LEARNING FROM DEVELOPMENT LITERATURE, SPATIOTEMPORAL AND SPATIAL REGRESSION ANALYSES AS WELL AS EXPLORATORY RESEARCH

For this foreword to be very reminiscent I made it a point to familiarize myself with several facets of the research and the author's expressed thematic interests in his five-chapter book. I am, therefore, happy to write to endorse positively this very imperative book, which essentially deals with various vital aspects of *Life Expectancy in Africa: Improving Public Health Policy*. In this crucial book, the author looked at the overview of half century of Africans' life expectancy at birth spanning from 1960 to present from the context of spatial spillover of civil war, terrorism, and minor and major wars across the African continent. In the context of validity and reliability of data, what Dr. Augustine Adu Frimpong has expertly written to constitute this admirable policy, development, and healthcare book solicited data from reputable agencies such as International Monetary Fund, World Bank, Barro and Lee, which date back from 1960 to 2015. Indeed, the author's specific emphasis is on both exploratory spatial temporal and spatial regression analyses.

As an econometrician, with expert knowledge in spatial analytics and policy analysis, writing my foreword has, therefore, provided me with the singular opportunity to reinforce certain spatial econometrics-*cum*-public policy as well as development nuances that have been admirably explored by Dr. Adu Frimpong in his work, which he explained that the Genesis of this particular manuscript stems from his doctoral research, which he later revamped to the current book length, with multidisciplinary values and dimensions.

According to the author, as an expert in his field of endeavor for this publication, the overall information gathered during his expanded study resulted from utilizing exploratory spatial temporal and spatial regression analyses and, in the final analysis, also an in-depth analysis of decades of maps of life expectancy at birth across regions and time, maps of hotspot and coldspot zones across regions and time, and finally maps of spatial spillover of civil war, and minor and major conflicts in the three vignettes of African countries (Demographic Republic of Congo (DRC), Liberia, and Burundi). Apart from these exploratory spatial temporal and spatial regression analyses of life expectancy at birth, I expect readers to benefit tremendously from the publication, which is purposefully filled with very rich archival-source materials. Other included information for the benefit of researchers, in general, and students, in particular, are the groupings of the various development indicators over decades—African Renaissance Period, African Political Cycle, contemporary independence phases I and II, Cold War era, and post-Cold War era. Indeed, it is admirable that Dr. Adu Frimpong has amply discussed the Genesis, the past, and the current situation of life expectancy in Africa, by centering on the literature of life expectancy, health care theories, geospatial analytics, and war/conflict theories. The author further demonstrated how the spatial spillover of war and conflict/terrorism has affected or impacted Africans' life expectancy at birth across regions and time.

It is also very imperative that Dr. Adu Frimpong goes further in a variety of ways to document his sources very well. Very usefully, his overall work is supported by evidence of exploratory spatial data analysis, which included spatiotemporal and spatial regression procedures. In the book, he has underscored through the exploratory spatial data analysis that the spatial error model was provided as the best fit for the data after the evaluation of the alternative specifications, including the standard regression model and the spatial lag model in explaining life expectancy at birth across regions and time in Africa. Furthermore, Dr. Adu Frimpong demonstrated in his book that the major armed-wars' spillover not only affects a country's life expectancy at birth, but also affects the life expectancy at birth of other neighboring countries. Additionally, as part of his contribution to development and health care policy literature, the African continent suffers substantial losses in the life expectancy at birth when certain countries experience major armed conflict or terrorism attacks.

It is certainly important to underscore the fact that, upon very carefully perusing the completed manuscript for this majestic and timely book, I can mention the unequivocal fact that Dr. Adu Frimpong's research for the publication will contribute greatly to development literature, public policy literature, public health literature, and conflict and terrorism literature across the globe.

Above all, it is both wonderful and timely that this very well-researched manuscript will soon be published as part of The Rowman & Littlefield

Publishing Group, indeed as a Lexington book! I am, therefore, very thrilled to be part of this important work, which deals extensively with several aspects of spatial analytics of *Life Expectancy in Africa: Improving Public Health Policy* across the region and overtime.

Onyumbe B. Lukongo, PhD
Associate Professor, Public
Policy Department
Southern University and A &
M College, Baton Rouge

# Preface

It is never an exaggeration to conclude unequivocally that policymakers in the developing world, which includes Africa, have key developmental goals of improving the peoples' economic well-being and health conditions. In the process, I also learn without equivocation that, indeed, life expectancy, from birth, is one of the outcome indicators of development. In the year 2000, for example, the World Health Organization (WHO) reported that children growing up in Sierra Leone and other war-torn African country zones can expect to live healthily for fewer years than in any other country in the world. Despite the numerous factors, which have been suggested in the literature to explain life expectancy at birth, little or no attempt has been made to investigate either issues or other factors that determine the spatial and temporal components of life expectancy at birth and the spatial spillover of major conflicts frequently recorded in Africa.

Indeed, my book thematically deals with *Life Expectancy in Africa: Improving Public Health Policy* on the African continent, which has been studied for the period between 1960 and 2015. To a large extent, the research for the monograph aims at offering an understanding of the changes in life expectancy at birth across regions and time in Africa, mostly in order to inform public policy. The research for the book used secondary and extant sources of data from World Bank, Barro and Lee, WHO, and the International Monetary Fund (IMF), which span from 1960 to 2015. As part of the quantitative design, the publication adopted the exploratory spatial data analysis, which included spatiotemporal and spatial regression procedures. The spatial error model was provided as the best fit for the data after the evaluation of the alternative specifications, including the standard regression model and the spatial lag model. Furthermore, the book revealed that the major armed-wars' spillover not only affects a country's life expectancy at birth, but also affects the life expectancy at birth of other neighboring countries.

Additionally, as part of the findings, the African continent suffers substantial losses in the overall life expectancy of its citizenry, from birth, when certain countries on the continent experience major armed conflicts—often in the form of civil wars—unabated. Finally, the monograph makes several substantive policy recommendations, including the fact that it recommends that the governments of the various African countries as well as their policymakers, international peace-making advocates, and such crucial organizations as the United Nations (UN) and the African Union (AU) are to ensure effective constitutional arrangement of peaceful transfer of power among leaders of the various African countries. When that continues to happen in meaningful ways, the younger generation will be prompted to follow suit to make sure that, instead of power flowing from the barrel of a gun through a *coup d'etat*, the ballot box will be used a lot more, just as major democracies in the United States, the United Kingdom (or Great Britain), France, Germany and others do in their efforts to either perpetuate or promote meaningful democracy.

Of course, there is such a democratic country as Sweden, which has enshrined social democracy as its way of political life, whereby the citizenry also live comfortably with a way of life that is imbued with social upliftment based on a national social contract for the citizenry from cradle to grave. Leading economists and other scholars have confirmed unequivocally that the Swedish model of social democracy is as viable as other national ideologies practiced in both capitalist and socialist nations of the world, indeed having in mind such thriving nations as the United States, the United Kingdom, Russia, Germany, France, Italy, Spain, Portugal, as well as such other Scandinavian nations as Norway, Finland, Denmark and, to some extent, Iceland. Most certainly, the Scandinavian nations, as combined geographical entities, have been known to play very meaningful roles, sometimes through award of developmental aid assistance and other forms of grantsmanship to sponsor various activities on the African continent, including carrying out population census and in running educational institutions.

For example, in the 2004 monograph titled *Sweden Versus Apartheid: Putting Morality Ahead of Profit, former Howard University* Professor Abdul Karim Bangura, born in the African nation of Sierra Leone, has provided a very useful analysis of the extent of the material assistance that Sweden, as a Scandinavian nation, provided the anti-apartheid freedom fighters of Africa, including future president Nelson Mandela's African National Congress (ANC). The 157-page publication was published by the United Kingdom-based Ashgate Publishers.

# Acknowledgments

My profound gratitude and appreciation go to many people, who made it possible for me to reach this stage, whereby I have advanced my initial research from a short doctoral study at Southern University and A&M College in Louisiana, USA, to a revamped and *bona fide* book manuscript, with the main intellectual purpose of shedding ample light on several aspects of life expectancy on the second largest continent, Africa, between 1960—the year my home country, Ghana, attained a republican status to do away with the British Queen as the titular Head of State and, in the process, to become Republic of Ghana on July 1—and 2015, a year before a real estate mogul called Mr. Donald Trump surprised American voters and the world to win the November 2016 presidential elections to be crowned the Leader (or President) of the United States of America, where I had decided to study and earn a doctoral (Ph.D.) degree on Friday, December 14, 2018. The many people I have in mind to thank effusively, with my deepest appreciation, include all of my current and past teachers, lecturers as well as professors, and my many mentors, whose guidance as well as instructions have impacted on my expedition to research and, in the end, to complete this book manuscript, which is being eventually published as my second book. Indeed, my first book-length manuscript, which was published in the year 2016 as a monograph, is titled "*Theory and Practice of Health Economics*," *International Institute for Science, Technology & Education.*

Without mincing words, I sincerely wish to convey my unlimited thanks and appreciation to my hard-working Southern University and A&M College professors and advisors, who have now become also great mentors for me: Dr. Damien Ejigiri, Dr. Kingsley Esedo, Dr. Onyumbe Lukongo, Dr. James Larson, and Dr. Chanika R. Jones. I am very deeply grateful for their pieces of profound advice, insight, direction, and constructive criticisms, all of which aided the completion of my initial research and, in the end, the completion of this manuscript. While I am grateful to several of my classroom professors at Southern University and A&M College, I wish to single out Ghana-born professor Vladimir Appeaning, who also taught me but also checked on me on several occasions to make sure that everything is going well for me, especially since I was very new in Louisiana, and my sponsors were living out of town in the State of Oregon. Also, very helpful to me were Dr. Allison Anadi, Professor and Chairperson of Department of Criminal Justice; Dr. Sunday Anadi, Professor of Department of Criminal Justice; fellow doctoral student Ucheoma Nwagbara; and former SUBR law professor Evelyn Wilson, who was introduced to me by my uncle and auntie. In varied ways, their support helped in making my graduate student life very smooth and, in the end, successful.

Indeed, I cannot express enough words of thanks to all those who believed in me when I did not have the courage to believe in myself, especially my dear wife (Mrs. Theresah Kye Adu Frimpong; nee Kye), my siblings (Stephen, Mary, and Noah) and my various cousins as well as all of my extended family members in the USA and Ghana.

Above all, I also owe a debt of unlimited gratitude to my inspirational uncle (Dr. Akwasi Bretuo) and aunt (Dr. Yvette M. Alex) for their sincere love, overall active and material support, and many prayers. I also wish to reiterate the debt of gratitude that I owe to my dear mother back in Ghana (Elizabeth Nana Yaa Agyeman), who sacrificed a lot for my own upbringing as well as the upbringing and training of my siblings (Stephen, Mary, and Noah).

Most certainly, as I earned my doctoral (Ph.D.) degree on Friday (December 14, 2018), I also remembered some academic mentors and intellectual colleagues back in Ghana, who are far too many to name each of them individually here, especially as I encountered them in high school (or secondary school) as well as on campuses of my country's premier University of Ghana as well as the Kumasi-based Kwame Nkrumah University of Science and Technology (KNUST), from where I earned my undergraduate and postgraduate academic degrees.

I still remember some crucial mentors as I was preparing to embark on the application processes that would, in 2017, allow for me to travel to America for graduate (and postgraduate) studies. Needed written recommendation letters were promptly dispatched on my behalf to the United States by such scholars as Dr. Yusif Hadrat; Dr. (sis) Eugenia Amporfu; and Dr. George Adu, all of KNUST, Kumasi. Also, campus leaders of Ghana-based Valley View University deserve thanks and appreciation for their unflinching belief in my abilities to pursue doctoral studies and, eventually, for their active support in a variety of ways. They include Rector of Valley View University, Techiman Campus; Dr. Peter Agyekum Boateng; and Dr. Robert Osei-Bonsu, Pro-vice Chancellor of Valley View University, Oyibi, Accra.

Above all, several campus staff employees played diverse roles for the promotion of my academic interests. I am particularly grateful to Mrs. Juliet Williams in Dean Ejigiri's office; Ms. Gloria Underwood, Ms. Patricia Smith, and Mrs. Alberta Robertson in the Department of Public Administration, Department of Social work, and Department of Criminal Justice, respectively.

Finally, to God Almighty be the Glory, as I unlimitedly acknowledge Thee!

# *Chapter 1*

# The Genesis, the Past, and the Current Situation of Life Expectancy in Africa

This chapter of the book provides the overview of life expectancy, coupled with utilizing the opportunity to present the statement of the overall researched problem that prompted the writing of the book in the first place. Other crucial aspects of the publication, which have been discussed in this chapter, are the logic model, the objectives and, above all, the questions I undertook, as an author, to research for its completion. Furthermore, chapter 1 also delimits the scope of the research, while serving as the mirror, which presents the way the book is organized.

Still, it is pertinent to reiterate the fact that one of the key policy initiatives in overall developmental policy is, indeed, to improve the ultimate quality of life in any given situation or society through the provision of quality health care. In this context, policymakers in the developing world have key developmental goals of improving the economic well-being and health conditions of the citizenry (World Bank, 2000; World Health Organization, WHO, 2000). Toward the foregoing end, the overall life expectancy, at birth, is one of the outcome indicators of development (World Bank, 2000).

According to Brett (2015), the idea of development emerged to describe two distinct processes, namely (1) incremental improvements in organizational and technological capacities generated by the normal operation of liberal capitalist institutions in developed countries (DCs) and (2) processes of structural change in either late-comers or less developed countries (LDCs) in the South and East, which are still attempting to build them. Furthermore, Brett (2015) has argued that development theory, as a distinct academic tradition, deals with the latter problem, but it is heavily influenced by the coexistence of advanced societies with well-established institutions.

Consequently, Brett (2015) and Malinowski (1945) were of the respective view that the orthodox social sciences go a long way to provide the models needed to understand the processes that enable well-established institutions to survive and adapt in developing countries. Also, they were similarly invoked to enable LDCs to construct them in their own societies. However, they do not provide LDCs with all the requisite knowledge that they needed to manage the disruptive structural changes, by which the existing order of particular society can be transformed from one type into another. Additionally, Malinowski (1945, 1961) further argued that development theory is an inherently prescriptive discipline that requires a full understanding of not only the orthodox theory, but also the even more complex problems involved in using models and several indicators, which are often derived from the West, to reconstruct the institutional arrangements of late-comers.

Nonetheless, scholars and policymakers like Inglehart (1997), Fukuyama (2010), Birdstall and, again, Fukuyama (2011) as well as many others have also used such models as modernization and neo-liberalization theories—coupled with indicators like life expectancy, mortality rate, economic growth, cultural, values, and political changes—to measure and subsequently to explain the global development across countries. Notwithstanding, Inglehart (1997) has argued that economic development, cultural change, and political change go together in coherent and even, to some extent, predictable patterns.

More so, the Global Policy Forum (2015) indicates that several developing countries are endowed with immense natural and human resources as well as great cultural, ecological, and economic diversity. Yet, the African continent remains underdeveloped (or it is still only a developing society). According to the Global Policy Forum (2015), most of the African nations have suffered from military dictatorships (Wangome, 1985; Ayittey, 2017), corruption (Jean-François, 1993; Broadman and Recanatini, 2000; Bedirhanoglu, 2007; Becker and Becker, 1993; Baldauf, 2013; Hope and Ronald, 2017), civil unrests (Lauritsen, 2016; Ali and Matthews, 1999; Elbadawi and Sambanis, 2000; Annan, 2014; Jeffrey, 2010), very destructive civil wars (Ali and Matthews, 1999; Lauritsen, 2016; Elbadawi and Sambanis, 2000; Annan, 2014; Jeffrey, 2010), underdevelopment (Lauritsen, 2016, and Rodney, 1972), and deep-seated poverty (World Bank, 2016; Lauritsen, 2016; Wangwe, 1998). Additionally, most or the majority of the countries, which are classified by the United Nations (UN) as least developed or Third World countries, are located in sub-Saharan Africa, where numerous development strategies have failed to yield the expected results. Although some experts believe that the African continent, as a whole, is doomed to perpetual poverty and economic slavery, Africa is still deemed to have immense potential (Global Policy Forum, 2015; World Bank, 2016; Lauritsen, 2016; Wangwe, 1998).

According to Roser (2015), global life expectancy has increased rapidly since the Enlightenment. Therefore, the author suggests that, in a pre-modern, poor world, life expectancy was around 30 years in all regions of the world.

Life expectancy at birth (LEB), in each region of the world, also stayed fairly at the same level for most of history until the onset of the "health transition," which is thus the period when life expectancy began to increase. The chart below shows that the health transition began at different times in different regions (Roser, 2015; Riley, 1990); for example, Oceania began to see increases in life expectancy around 1870, while Africa did not see any measure of increases until around 1920 (Roser, 2015; Riley, 1990).

Meanwhile, in the early nineteenth century, life expectancy started to increase in the rising industrialized countries, while it stayed low in the rest of the world (Roser, 2015; Riley, 1990). Since 1900, for example, the global average life expectancy has more than doubled and it is now approaching 70 years (Roser, 2015; Riley, 1990).

As observed in figure 1.1, the life expectancy and economic growth in Africa remain very low as compared to other continents (World Bank, 2014). It is, however, not surprising that World Bank (2014) reported that health is a fundamental dimension of the well-being of all citizens as well as is a key component of human capital development. Furthermore, the wealth of every nation can be measured by the health status of its citizens, which is expected to include rural and urban populations (World Bank, 2014). The scenario confirms the popular adage that "Health is Wealth." However, the World Bank

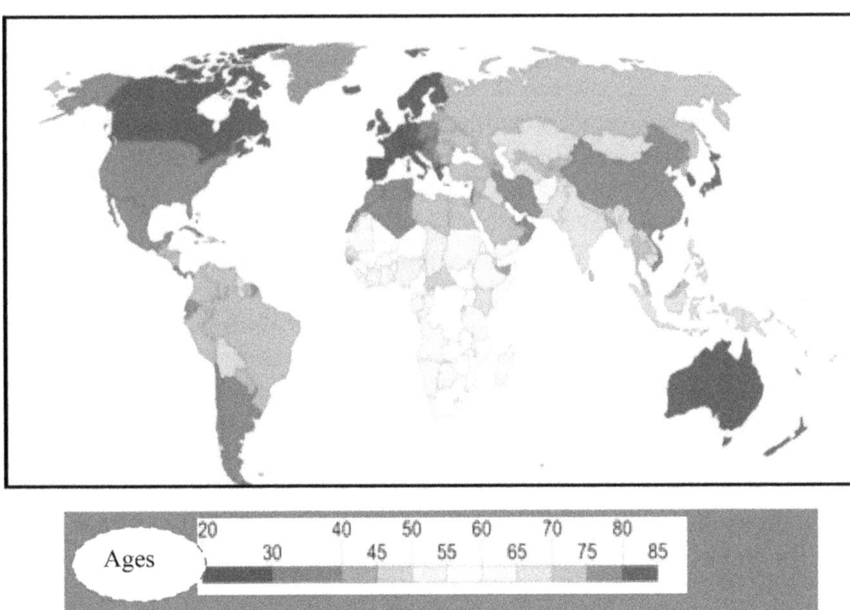


**Figure 1.1 Showing the Downward Spiral of African Countries' Life Expectancy.**
*Source*: Author's modification.

(2014) reports that 5% of economic growth differentials between developed and developing nations are perhaps associated with ill health and low life expectancy. Since little is known about life expectancy and its determinants on the African continent. This publication tries to fill this gap in the literature.

In a pertinent report of the United Nations Development Program, UNDP (2008), we learn that most of the countries of Africa are very much endowed with fertile land, with food crops for cultivation on the soil, mineral deposits, and several herbal medicines that are essential to the improvement in the quality of life of the people. Also, all of the foregoing resources are expected to provide food security and a healthy African society for the people to live longer (or ensure improvement in LEB). Despite the continent being rich in both natural and human resources, economies of many of the African countries are still underperforming when compared to other regions. Several reasons have been discussed in the existing literature, including corruption (Global Policy Forum, 2015; World Bank, 2016; Lauritsen, 2016; Wangwe, 1998), lack of proper medical (WHO, 2000) and education facilities (World Bank, 2014), underdeveloped infrastructure (Lauritsen, 2016; Rodney, 1972), low life expectancy (Roser, 2015; Riley, 1990), civil wars (Ali and Matthews, 1999; Lauritsen, 2016), political unrest (Ali and Matthews, 1999; Lauritsen, 2016), and other problems not listed here are impeding Africa's economic progress, human development, and social mobility.

While the rest of the world's economy grew at an annual rate of close to 2% from 1960 to 2002, growth performance in Africa has been dismal (National Bureau of Economic Research, 2018). For example, between 1974 and the mid-1990s, overall growth was negative, as it reached negative 1.5% in 1990–1994 (National Bureau of Economic Research, 2018). Then, in 2015, available data showed that the region experienced its slowest growth since 1998 (International Monetary Fund, 2016). According to the October 2016 edition of the IMF Regional Economic Outlook for Africa, the growth rate fell from 5.1% in 2014 to 3.4%. However, in 2016, the continent's GDP growth rate continues to decline, as the International Monetary Fund (IMF) predicts a drop to 1.4%, 2.9 percentage points below the initially predicted growth rate. As a consequence of the foregoing, hundreds of millions of African citizens have become poor; therefore, one half of the African continent lives below the poverty line (UNDP, 2017). In sub-Saharan Africa, for example, per capita GDP is now less than it was in the 1970s, having declined drastically (see National Bureau of Economic Research, 2018; World Bank, 2016 for more details). The three poorest African countries over the last five decades have been involved, to some degree, in wars. The GDP per capita has declined from its initial levels in DRC, Burundi, and Liberia. Table 1.1 provides more evidence.

Besides, the WHO Epidemiology and Burden of Disease Team underscored, among other details, that healthy life expectancy in some African

**Table 1.1 Comparison of GDP Per Capita, Life Expectancy, and War-Torn Zones (Conflict/War) of Poorest African Countries over Decades**

| *Countries (Poorest Countries)* | *1960s* | *1970s* | *1980s* | *1990s* | *2000s* |
|---|---|---|---|---|---|
| Democratic Republic of the Congo (DRC) | 988.1 | 969 | 782.3 | 429.7 | 310 |
| Burundi | 210.9 | 270 | 308.4 | 280.8 | 229 |
| Liberia | 1363.2 | 1598 | 1184.5 | 236.8 | 337 |
| Life Expectancy over Decades for the Poorest Countries in Africa | | | | | |
| Democratic Republic of the Congo (DRC) | 42.1 | 45 | 47.5 | 49.2 | 55.0 |
| Burundi | 42.6 | 45 | 48.3 | 49.0 | 53.9 |
| Liberia | 36.5 | 42 | 47 | 49.7 | 57.2 |
| Comparison of War-Torn Zones (Conflict/War) of Poorest African Countries over Decades | | | | | |
| Democratic Republic of the Congo (DRC) | 1 | 1 | 0 | 1 | 1 |
| Burundi | 1 | 0 | 0 | 1 | 1 |
| Liberia | 0 | 0 | 1 | 1 | 1 |

*Note*: Zero (0) means no war/conflict was recorded during the decades, while one (1) means at least one war/conflict was recorded during the decades.
*Source*: World Bank, 2015 and Author's modification.

countries is dropping back to levels that have not been seen in advanced countries since medieval times. According to the 2000 WHO report, war (or conflict) is also a major source of low life expectancy and economic growth in Africa (see Table 1.1 above).

Additionally, the World Health Organization (W.H.O., 2000) also reported that the average health LEB, in a war-torn West African country, is only 25.9 years. Moreover, many of the African countries are considered to be poor (Chia-Wei, 2009). There are, so many of them, which are classified as highly indebted poor countries (HIPC), whereby they owe huge sums of money to the IMF and the World Bank (Chia-Wei, 2009; Rwegasira, 1998). In 2000, the WHO reported that children growing up in the West African nation of Sierra Leone, for example, expect to live healthily for fewer years than in any other country in the world. Despite the numerous factors, which have been suggested in the literature, little or no attempt has been made to investigate factors that determine the spatial and temporal components of life expectancy among African countries. That is, indeed, part of the reason why the research for the book conducted the spatiotemporal analyses for a better understanding of the dynamics in life expectancy in Africa in order to inform public policy with enlightenment.

Indeed, the overall purpose of the research for the book was, indeed, to provide an understanding of the changes of life expectancy across regions and time in Africa, mostly in order to inform public policy in Africa. Therefore, the spatiotemporal analyses, which have been employed, are also to offer additional understanding of the changes in life expectancy in Africa over the last five decades. The research for the book was driven by the following objectives: (a) to conduct the spatiotemporal analyses for a better understanding of the crucial changes in life expectancy in Africa; (b) to identify the best spatial econometric model that is suitable for life expectancy in Africa; and above all (c) to employ results from spatial analysis to inform public policy on the continent. The research for the manuscript was conducted with the following very pertinent research questions in mind: (a) to what extent can spatiotemporal analyses be used to comprehend better life expectancy in Africa?; (b) what is the best spatial econometric model that is suitable for explaining life expectancy in Africa?; and (c) to what extent can I, as a researcher or author of the book, apply geospatial and econometric models to inform public policy in Africa?

The research for the book, in its entirety, covered geographical scope of Africa as the second largest continent of the world. It was, however, restricted to the examination of LEB of African countries. In relation to this particular research for the publication, LEB is defined as the mean number of years still to be lived by a person at birth (World Health Organization, 2000). The study utilizes the World Bank, WHO, Barro and Lee (2010), and IMF datasets on life expectancy, education, war, and conflict in Africa. Also, the research for the publication was specifically directed to the examination of life expectancy in Africa by using geospatial analytics, health system theory, spatiotemporal analysis, economic growth theories, development theories, and conflict theories. The life expectancy is examined over decades (from 1960 to 2015), divisions of political cycles, and before-and-after cold war implications.

Meanwhile, in totality, the research for the monograph is made up of five chapters, the first of which is the introduction; the second chapter reviews the relevant literature, while chapter 3 discusses the methodology and hypothesis. Indeed, chapter 4 presents the analysis, results, and discussion. Then, finally, chapter 5 provides the book's readers with the cumulative summary as well as the conclusion and the implications of my research for the publication.

# *Chapter 2*

# Life Expectancy, Health, Geospatial Analytics, and War/Conflict Theories

This section of the book (chapter 2) is divided into three sub-topics, namely (i) Health Indicators' Framework (or Model), (ii) major theories, and (iii) life expectancy, spatial analytics, conflict, economic growth and development of the literature review.

## HEALTH INDICATORS' FRAMEWORK (OR MODEL)

Figure 2.1 represents the health model. Health care is, therefore, defined as medical care plus public health. In this model by Arah et al. (2006), medical care is divided into somatic and mental medical care services that can span the primary, secondary, and tertiary levels of the health care system. However, the "response" in the model also refers to the individual—mostly biological, psychological, or social—reaction to the constellation of health determinants, acting singularly or in combination. These authors defined "health care" as the combined functioning of public health and personal health care services. They further explain that Africa's health system includes all activities and structures, whose primary purpose is to influence health in its broadest sense. This notion is, indeed, in keeping with the use of the term health system by the WHO: that "all the activities whose primary purpose is to promote, restore or maintain health" (World Health Organization, 2000; Adu-Frimpong, 2016).

According to Arah et al. (2006), health is determined by many inter-dependent variables or factors, one of which is health care. This multi-determinant approach to health was principally advanced by the Lalonde "White Paper" in Canada in 1974, and subsequently expanded on in many publications,

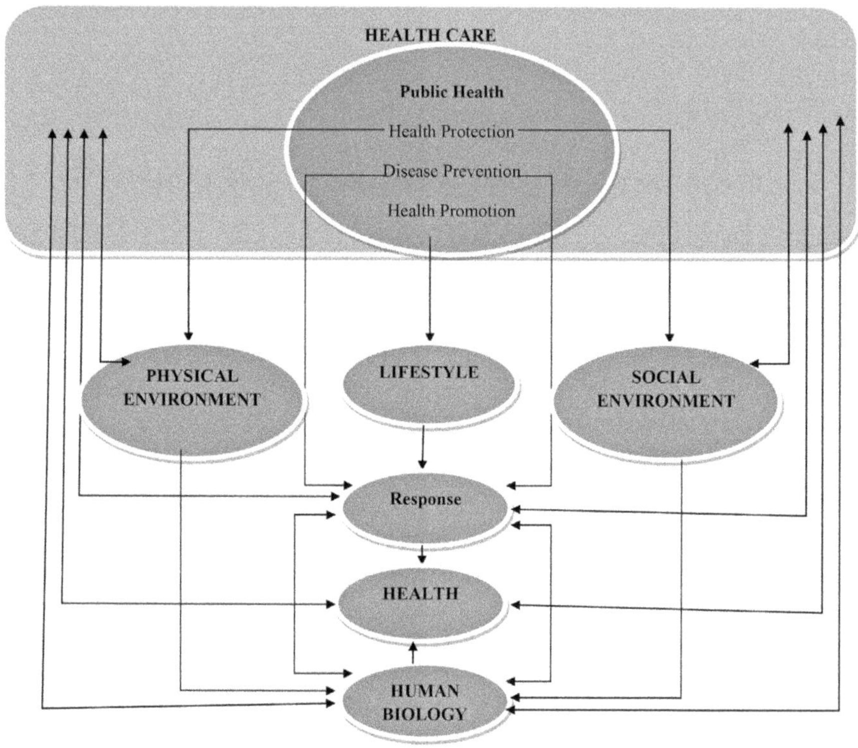


**Figure 2.1 Determinants of Health Care and Health.** *Source*: Author's Modification of Health and Health Care Determinants designed for OECD by Arah et al. (2006).

including the seminal paper by Evans and Stoddart in 1990. However, the non-health care determinants were largely grouped into such three main fields as environment, lifestyle, and human biology (Lalonde, 1974). Interestingly, Arah et al. (2006) defined the concept of environment to include both physical and social (living) circumstances of human existence, and how these go a long way to shape or disrupt health. Additionally, lifestyle was also defined as the behavioral or such choice-related issues as nutritional styles, drinking, smoking, and other habits, as well as education or knowledge-based activities that influence health and illness.

Furthermore, Arah et al. (2006) explained human biology to bring about a reference to either the biological or genetic constitution that determines how the human body primarily functions to maintain a healthy state, and also how it responds to others, mainly exogenous, determinants of health. In addition to its direct effects on health and illness, health care may act indirectly on the other determinants to maintain or improve health. For instance, public health—through its classical health prevention, promotion, and protection strategies—influences the host constitution, lifestyle, and environment, respectively.

Meanwhile, Arah et al. (2006) also posited that the response factor represents the final common pathway to health; its final manifestation is seen as health change, illness, or disease. They further theorized that the interrelationships among the health care system and other determinants of health can be of at least three types, namely:

- Linkages exist between health care and health (seen in Figure 2.1 by the arrows running between health care and health fields, including those running through the "response" box);
- Linkages exist between health care and non-health care determinants (seen in Figure 2.1 by the arrows running from the health care space to lifestyle, environment, and host constitution and by arrows running between the latter non-health care determinants); and
- Linkages exist between non-health care determinants and health (seen in Figure 2.1 by the arrows running from lifestyle, environment, and host constitution to the health field, mainly through the "response" box).

Subsequently, Arah et al. (2016) further theorized that in trying to measure performance, policymakers and researchers need to form a clearer image of what it is they want to measure and the key goals of health policy. In view of that they make a distinction between conceptual frameworks for health care system performance (or health care performance) as shown in figure 2.1 and those for health system performance (or health performance) as shown in figure 2.2.

As very well explained by WHO (2000) and Arah et al. (2006) in their respective publications, health care performance refers to the maintenance of an efficient and equitable system of health care without emphasizing an assessment of the non-health care determinants. That is, in an assessment of health care performance, the direct functioning of the delivery system of health care is evaluated in comparison with its established public goals for the level and distribution of the benefits and costs of personal and public health care.

Then, in accordance with the work of Arah et al. (2006), a health care performance evaluation is, therefore, concerned with linkages between health care and health, pointed out in the health care and other determinants of health model. They further explained that health performance is a much broader conceptual approach for measuring performance by explicitly using non-health care determinants, health care, and contextual information to give a clearer picture of population health. In the quest of Arah et al. (2006) conceptualizing health and health care performance, they postulated that

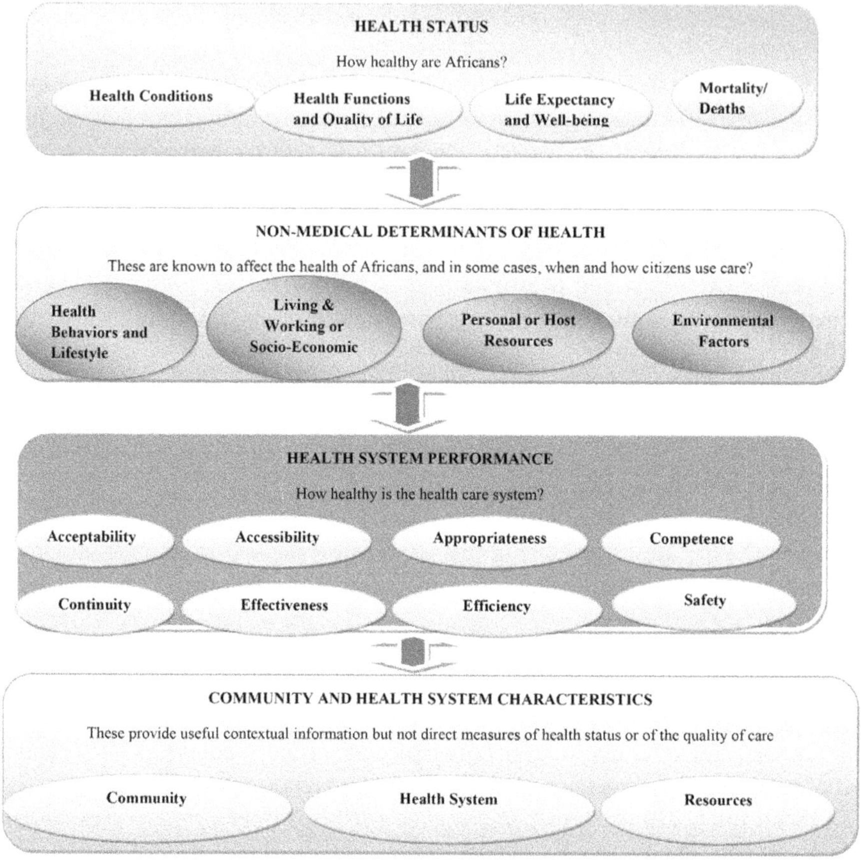


**Figure 2.2 Conceptual Frameworks for Health Status.** *Source*: Author's Modification of Canada's Health Indicators Framework Espoused by Arah et al.

the main policy goals for health care assessment should be efficiency and equity, but a much wider view of the determinants of health and their costs must be adopted. Furthermore, they explained that equitable distribution of health status itself is an important concern, and responsiveness to consumers is amplified by the concern to persuade lifestyles. Given that a health performance framework is largely concerned with all the interrelationships among health, health care, and non-health care factors, as well as health performance or health care performance (see figure 2.2).

The research for the monograph has subsequently proposed this particular framework, which was built on the common dimensions of performance model, which was borrowed heavily from the Institute of Medicine's national health care quality indicator framework, developed for the United States. What was later modified to conceptualize the Canadian Health Indicator

Framework and its adaptations has been seen in Australia and within the European Community Health Indicators (ECHI) Project and on the WHO and Organization for Co-Operation and Development (OECD) proposals for identifying key economic and social goals for health policy. The result is, in fact, a health performance framework that interconnects well with the one suggested by the International Organization for Standardization (ISO), mainly for its health informatics network (ISO, 2003) and Arah et al. (2006).

Based on the foregoing framework, the OECD on the HCQI project has suggested that the health performance indicators should be developed in the following priority areas: (1) cardiac care, (2) mental health, (3) diabetes mellitus, (4) patient safety, and (5) primary care and prevention/health promotion. The foregoing five areas were, in fact, chosen on the basis of the high impact of Africa's three health areas on the burden of disease, an informal survey of member countries' priorities for indicator development in different health service areas, and a discussion about priorities at the first meeting of the Health Care Quality Indicators (HCQI) Expert Group in January 2003. The HCQI framework has four interconnected tiers, which represented the following:

- Health—to capture the broader measures of the health of the society that may be influenced by health care and non-health care factors using LEB;
- Non-health care determinants of health—to delineate mostly society-wide, non-health care factors that also influence health such as lifestyle, income, governance, political instability, civil war, conflicts, food insecurity and many others (as suggested in figure 2.1 earlier);
- Health care system performance—to capture the processes, inputs, and outcomes of the health care system and its efficiency and equity and to recognize that these may sometimes influence non-health care determinants; and
- Health system design and context—to give pertinent country and health system policy and delivery characteristics which affect costs, expenditure, and utilization patterns and which are necessary for appreciating and contextualizing the findings of the health care performance tier.

Figure 2.2 represents dimensions of effectiveness, safety, responsiveness/patient centeredness, access, and cost/expenditure. These dimensions map approximately into the structure, process, and outcome (from right to left). Meanwhile, the effectiveness, safety, and responsiveness of patient centeredness are taken to be the core quality dimensions.

In addition to the core quality dimensions, the effectiveness covers the Health Care Quality Indicators (HCQI) priority areas of cardiac care, mental health, diabetes, and primary care and prevention/health promotion. However, the link between the third tier (health care performance) and the second (non-health care determinants) is captured by the priority area primary care and prevention/health promotion. These dimensions are, in essence, those core attributes of health care, which increase the likelihood of desired outcomes. Similarly, the cost/expenditure is a dimension that is included in the framework, although it is explicitly linked on a performance level to questions of efficiency. Respectively, macroeconomic efficiency and microeconomic efficiency are concerned with finding the right level of health expenditure and maximizing the value for money (or the ratio of quality to costs). Equity, for example, is also concerned with the fairness of the distribution of health care across populations and also with the fairness of payment for health care. The term "equity" can also be estimated for non-health care determinants of health and for health status. Within the fourth tier ("health system design and context") will be located the levers that countries try to pull to influence the performance of the health system for the better.

However, such non-represented dimensions as appropriateness, continuity, timeliness, and acceptability can easily be accommodated within other dimensions, as was partly done within the Commonwealth Fund's International Quality Indicators Project (2004). For example, appropriateness based on its conceptual definition could be mapped into effectiveness, whereas continuity and acceptability could be absorbed into patient-centeredness. Patients' health care needs are represented by the rows in the health care performance tier of figure 2.2 and are defined to reflect evolving needs over the life cycle (Hurtado, 2001).

It is for the foregoing stated reason that the research for the monograph has adopted the conceptual frameworks for health status and health care performance, which were first used by the United States, followed by Canada, Australia and many other OECD countries to be utilized as a framework for examining their health indicators (or LEB and its determinants).

## MAJOR THEORIES

### System Theory

The system theory was developed by the biologist Ludwig von Bertalanffy in the 1930s (Bertalanffy, 1962). The development of the theory resulted from the author's perceived need for a theory to guide this research in multiple fields. The theory provides a common framework, which created shared and common language that scientists from different disciplines can use to communicate their findings. Specifically, systems' theory is used to understand how things around us work. Systems theory looks at the world as a system composed of smaller subsystems. Systems as a representation of life phenomena are used by humanity in everyday life to describe the functioning of these phenomena. For example, a hospital is a system with inputs, processes, and outputs. The hospital itself is a component of a larger system—health care system. The health care system, banking system, educational system, and judicial system, are emblematic examples of the socio-economic-political system within which we live (Bertalanffy, 1962). According to Bertalanffy (1962), a system is a collection of independent but interrelated elements or components organized in a meaningful way to accomplish an overall goal. The function of any system is to convert or process materials, energy, and/or information (inputs) into a product or outcome for use within the system or outside of the system (the environment) or both.

### *Analyses of Systems' Theory*

Systems' theory has been widely used for a clear and concise understanding of health care structures, processes as well as outcomes processes and their interactions within a health care system. Again, systems' theory has been used as a framework to describe the components of systems and the relationships between the components, the boundaries of the system, the goals of the system, and system's ability to change and adapt in response to internal and external forces. Furthermore, systems theory and thinking have helped researchers and health care practitioners to understand how health care organizations and systems behave. The theory has allowed researchers and health care practitioners, with clarity, to assess, visualize, analyze as well as to understand the structure, processes, and feedback loops that make up the organization. This correct and clear understanding of the organization, as a system, is a necessity to be able to manage organizations effectively and efficiently in order to achieve the organization's goals.

### *Key Concepts: Definitions of Systems' Theory*

Inputs include raw material, energy, and resources processed to produce the outputs of the organization. Examples include information, money, nurses' effort, physician's time, fuel, energy, time, individual effort, and any raw material of some kind. Elements or components are the things, parts, or substances that make up the system. These parts may be humans, material, equipment, and so forth. Elements have attributes or characteristics that can be measured or described such as size, color, volume, quantity, temperature, and mass.

Black-box/processing/throughput is the process used by the system to convert raw materials or energy (inputs) from the environment into products or services that are usable by either the system itself or the environment. Examples include, thinking, physical examination of patients, diagnosing, planning, decision-making, writing prescription, taking vital signs, operating on a patient, constructing, sorting, making a speech, sharing information, meeting in groups, discussing, melting, shaping, hammering, and so forth. Output is the product or service that results from the system's throughput or processing of technical, social, financial, and human inputs. Examples include health services, better health, software programs, documents, decisions, laws, rules, money, assistance, cars, clothing, bills, and so forth.

Feedback is information about some aspect of data or energy processing that can be used to evaluate and monitor the system and to guide it to more effective performance. How many patients were seen in two hours in the clinic? How many medical errors were committed in a hospital? Why were mistakes made? HealthCareReportCard.com is an example of how hospitals are doing with certain diagnoses. Hospital accreditation reports are an example as are patient satisfaction surveys, sales reports, and test results. Subsystem is a system, which is a part of a larger system. They can work parallel to each other or in a series with each other. Information system is an example of a subsystem in a hospital. Also, a medical staff in an organization is an emblematic example of a subsystem of the hospital.

### *Health Care Facility or Hospitals as Systems' Theory*

The applicability of the systems' theory concepts and principles can be applied to help us understand as well as explain hospitals and their operation. According to Pan American Health Organization (2004) the concept of a hospital is defined as any medical facility with an organized medical and professional staff and beds available for continuous hospitalization of patients formally admitted to it for medical observation, care, diagnosis, or surgical and non-surgical treatment. Alternately, Miller (1997) further defined hospital as an institution, which provides beds, meals, and constant nursing care for its patients while they undergo medical therapy at the hands of professional physicians. In carrying out these services, the hospital is striving to restore its patients to health. Nonetheless, perhaps, in observing health care facility or hospital as a system, then hospitals or health care facilities are open systems that interact with the environment to complete necessary trades for survival of the system, growth, and fulfillment of the systems' goal.

A hospital is a subsystem that exists within a hierarchy of other systems. Adding to that, hospitals are complex systems, which contain large number of subsystems such as the radiology department, nursing services, housekeeping, food services, laundry, laboratory department, and so forth. Each of these subsystems can be looked at as a system of its own. Furthermore, hospital systems consist of a pattern of organized relations whereby different components of the system are related to each other in a particular way. Organizational structures and charts constitute a graphical representation of these relationships. Interestingly, the hospital by laws, rules, policies, and procedures regulate these relationships. Toward this end, it is very important to note that hospitals are subsystems of overall health care system of a nation.

## Spatial Theory

Spatial theory discusses concepts like spatial data analysis, spatial autocorrelation, spatial stratified heterogeneity, spatial interpolation, spatial regression, spatial interaction, and geographic information systems (Haining, 2003, p.4). Over the years, scholars have tried to explain the general theory of geographical space that could be a theory of concentrations, of spacing, of spatial structures and of evolution of spatial systems, relying on knowledge of behaviors in space and of spatial representations (Upton and Fingelton, 1985). Most of these theories, attempt to explain location and distribution of human activities. Two major roles were played by distance, that is, (1) slows down interactions and (2) makes value of places vary in function of their relative geographical situation (Upton and Fingelton, 1985). Several studies have been conducted, namely, the center/periphery theory (Amin, 1976; Frank, 1978), the central places theory (Galtung, 1971; Appadurai, 1986; Law, 1992), and the theory of spatial diffusion of innovations (Blaikie, 1978; Hedstrom, 1994; Kota and Jokipii, 2000; regional 1928; Weber, 1909; Palander, 1935; Hoover, 2008; Moses, 2008). However, the general theoretical position of spatial analysis consists in proposing a partial explanation as well as prediction possibilities about the state and probable evolution of geographical objects/entities, on the basis of knowledge of their situation with respect to other geographical objects (Upton and Fingelton, 1985). Interestingly, spatial data come in many varieties, and it is not easy to arrive at a system of classification that is simultaneously exclusive, exhaustive, imaginative, and satisfying (Upton and Fingelton, 1985).

### *Spatial Analysis*

According to Harman (1960) and Rummel (1970), urban and regional studies have a great deal with large tables of spatial data obtained from censuses and surveys. They argued that it is vital to simplify the huge amount of detailed information in order to be able to extract the main trends. Multivariable analysis (or factor analysis (FA)) allows a change of variables, transforming the many variables of the census, usually correlated between themselves, into fewer independent "factors" or "principal components" which are, actually, the eigenvectors of the data correlation matrix weighted by the inverse of their Eigen values. They further theorized that factor analysis depends on measuring distances between observations: the choice of a significant metric is crucial. The Euclidean metric (principal component analysis), the chi-square distance (correspondence analysis) or the generalized Mahalanobis distance (discriminant analysis) was among the more widely used (Harman, 1960). More complicated models, using communalities or rotations have been proposed (Rummel, 1970).

### *Spatial Autocorrelation*

Spatial autocorrelation statistics, by definition, measures and analyzes the degree of dependency among observations in a geographic space (Knegt et al., 2010). Meanwhile, the standard spatial autocorrelation statistics include Moran's I, Geary's C, Getis's G, and the standard deviational ellipse (Knegt et al., 2010). These statistics require creating a spatial weights matrix that reflects the intensity of the geographic relationship between observations in a neighborhood, for example, the distances between neighbors, the lengths of shared border, or whether they fall into a specified directional class such as "west" or "east" (Knegt et al., 2010).

The classic/standard spatial autocorrelation statistics compare the spatial weights to the covariance relationship at pairs of locations (Knegt et al., 2010; Anselin and Rey, 2014; Lukongo and Miller, 2017). Regarding interpretation, Anselin and Rey (2014) and Knegt et al. (2010) postulated that the spatial autocorrelation value that is more positive than expected from random indicate the clustering of similar values across geographic space, while significant negative spatial autocorrelation indicates that neighboring values are more dissimilar than expected by chance, suggesting a spatial pattern similar to a chess board (Anselin and Rey, 2014; Knegt et al., 2010; Lukongo and Miller, 2017). In fact, these authors pointed out clearly that such spatial autocorrelation statistics as Moran's I and Geary's C are global in the sense that they estimate the overall degree of spatial autocorrelation for a dataset. The possibility of spatial heterogeneity suggests that the estimated degree of autocorrelation may vary significantly across geographic space. Local Indicators of Spatial Association (LISA) can also be mapped and tested for significance of spatial heterogeneity to provide an indication of clustering patterns within the study region (Knegt et al., 2010; Anselin, 1995).

### *Spatial Stratified Heterogeneity*

According to Wang, Zhang, and Fu (2016), spatial stratified heterogeneity is referred to the within-strata variance less than the between-strata variance, which is ubiquitous in ecological phenomena, such as ecological zones and many ecological variables. They further explained that spatial stratified heterogeneity reflects the essence of nature, implies potential distinct mechanisms by strata, suggests possible determinants of the observed process, allows the representativeness of observations of the earth, and enforces the applicability of statistical inferences. Finally, it was theorized and underscored that spatial stratified heterogeneity of an attribute can be measured by geographical detector q-statistic (Wang, Zhang, and Fu, 2016).

### *Spatial Regression*

Spatial regression methods capture spatial dependency in regression analysis, avoiding statistical problems such as unstable parameters and unreliable significance tests, as well as providing information on spatial relationships among the variables involved. The estimated spatial relationships can be used on spatial and spatiotemporal predictions (Song and Yong, 2016; Lesage and Pace, 2009, p. 8; Getis and Aldstadt, 2004, pp. 135–145). Depending on the specific technique, spatial dependency can enter the regression model as relationships between the independent variables and the dependent, between the dependent variables, and a spatial lag of itself or in the error terms.

## The "Conflict Theory"

The conflict theory, suggested by Karl Marx, claims society is in a state of perpetual conflict because of competition for limited resources (Crossman, 2018; David, 1977; Randall, 1994; Roseel, 2017). It holds that social order is maintained by domination and power, rather than consensus and conformity (David, 1977; Randall, 1994). According to conflict theory, those with wealth and power try to hold on to it by any means possible, chiefly by suppressing the poor and powerless (Crossman, 2018; David, 1977; Randall, 1994; Roseel, 2017). Furthermore, the conflict theory explains that tensions and conflicts arise when resources, status, and power are unevenly distributed between groups in society and that these conflicts become the engine for social change (Bartos, and Wehr, 2002; Crossman, 2018; David, 1977; Jolle, 2012; Randall, 1994; Roseel, 2017). In this context, power can be understood as control of material resources and accumulated wealth, control of politics, and the institutions that make up society, and one's social status relative to others (determined not just by class but by race, gender, sexuality, culture, and religion, among other things) (Bartos, and Wehr, 2002; Crossman, 2018; David, 1977; Jolle, 2012; Randall, 1994; Roseel, 2017).

### *Marx's Conflict Theory*

Conflict theory, as briefly noted earlier, was propounded by Karl Max, who focused on the causes and consequences of class conflict between the bourgeoisie (the owners of the means of production and the capitalists) and the proletariat (the working class and the poor) (Crossman, 2018; David, 1977; Jolle, 2012; Randall, 1994; Roseel, 2017). Focusing on the economic, social, and political implications of the rise of capitalism in Europe, Marx theorized that this system, premised on the existence of a powerful minority class (the bourgeoisie) and an oppressed majority class (the proletariat), created class conflict because the interests of the two were at odds, and resources were unjustly distributed among them (Jolle, 2012; Randall, 1994; Roseel, 2017).

Within this system, an unequal social order was maintained through ideological coercion, which created consensus, and acceptance of the values, expectations, and conditions as determined by the bourgeoisie (Bartos and Wehr, 2002; Crossman, 2018; David, 1977). Marx postulated that the work of producing consensus was done in the "superstructure" of society, which is composed of social institutions, political structures, and culture, and what it produced consensus for was the "base," the economic relations of production (Bartos, and Wehr, 2002; Crossman, 2018; David, 1977).

Marx further reasoned that as the socioeconomic conditions worsened for the proletariat, they would develop a class-consciousness that revealed their exploitation at the hands of the wealthy capitalist class of bourgeoisie, and then they would revolt, demanding changes to smooth the conflict production (Bartos and Wehr, 2002; Crossman, 2018; David, 1977). According to Marx, if the changes made to appease conflict maintained a capitalist system, then the cycle of conflict would repeat production (Bartos and Wehr, 2002; Crossman, 2018; David, 1977). However, if the changes made created a new system, as observed in socialism, then peace and stability are likely to be achieved (Crossman, 2018; David, 1977; Jolle, 2012; Randall, 1994; Roseel, 2017).

### *Evolution of Conflict Theory*

Many social theorists have built on Marx's conflict theory to bolster it, grow it, and refine it over the years (Bartos and Wehr, 2002; Crossman, 2018;

David, 1977; Jolle, 2012; Randall, 1994; Roseel, 2017). Explaining why Marx's theory of revolution did not manifest in his lifetime, Italian scholar and activist Antonio Gramsci argued that the power of ideology was stronger than Marx had realized and that more work needed to be done to overcome cultural hegemony or rule through common sense (Gramsci, 1971). Max Horkheimer and Theodor Adorno, critical theorists who were part of Frankfort school of thought, focused their work on how the rise of mass culture—mass produced art, music, and media—contributed to the maintenance of cultural hegemony (Adorno and Horkheimer, 2002). To illustrate, Mills (1956) drew on conflict theory to describe the rise of a tiny "power elite" composed of military, economic, and political figures who have ruled America from the mid-twentieth century

Many others have drawn on conflict theory to develop other types of theory within the social sciences, including feminist theory, critical race theory, postmodern and postcolonial theory, queer theory, post-structural theory, and theories of globalization and world systems (Crossman, 2018; David, 1977; Jolle, 2012; Randall, 1994; Roseel, 2017).

Therefore, while initially conflict theory described class conflicts specifically, it has lent itself over the years to studies of how other kinds of conflicts, like those premised on race, gender, sexuality, religion, culture, and nationality, among others, are a part of contemporary social structures, and how they affect our lives.

## Economic Growth Theory: The Three Vignettes of Contemporary Africa

This particular section discusses three poorest countries in the sub-Saharan Africa as the three vignettes. The three vignettes of contemporary Africa are DRC, Burundi, and Liberia.

### *The DRC Vignette*

Several decades ago, when she was 17 years old, Selina Abdul did something no girl from her village had ever done before. She left her home in a beautiful but poor part of the state of Mai-Ndombe in DRC, where people grow rice in the valleys and tap rubber trees in the nearby hills, and went to work in a rubber factory in the busy city of Inongo, 75 miles away. Selina's family was poor even by the modest standards of her village, and her parents welcomed the opportunity for their daughter to earn her own keep and possibly even send money back to help them feed and clothe the family, deal with recurrent emergencies, and raise their six younger children. With these benefits in mind, they set aside their reservations about their unmarried daughter's unheard-of plan to go off by herself to work in the city.

Selina got a job that entailed manufacturing copper products owned by a Belgian company. Every day, she patiently soldered hundreds of tiny wires onto minute silicon chips. It was tedious, repetitive work that had to be performed at high speed and with flawless accuracy. With a long day of hard work with few breaks, Selina could earn the equivalent of $3.00.

Since their wages were low, Selina and her colleagues welcomed opportunities to work overtime. Often, they put in two or three extra hours in a day, for up to seven days a week. They particularly liked working Sundays and holidays, when double wages were paid. With overtime work and occasional bonuses, Selina was able to earn about $95 a month. She shared a small house in a squatter area with seven other factory workers. By living simply and inexpensively, most of the young women managed to set aside $5 to $20 a month to send to their families in the villages, and generally enjoyed the unfamiliar freedom of living apart from their families.

Five years later, Selina, who had accumulated $475 in savings, decided it was time to return to her village, where she soon married a local man and settled down. She later had three children—fewer than her old friends that had stayed in the village and married earlier. Her savings helped provide for her family and she was able to enroll her children in the local school.

Selina's chance to work in copper industry came about because, in the 1885 scramble for Africa, King Leopold II of Belgium declared himself the dictator and sole proprietor of the new Congo Free State. Leopold garnered public support at home by publicly announcing his intent to Christianize and modernize the Congolese population, all the while planning the forced labor of men, women, and children for the lucrative ivory and rubber business (Callaghy, 1984). When people did not meet the king's quotas, his army killed them or cut off their hands (Aronson, 1998; Ball, 1961). The overall population of the country greatly diminished during the early twentieth century due to such cruelty and to the susceptibility of many Congolese to new European diseases (Ball, 1961; Brittain, 1998; Callaghy, 1984).

Mounting international criticism forced Leopold to sell his colony to Belgium in 1908 (Aronson, 1998; Callaghy, 1984). The Belgians, unfortunately, failed to contain his blood-thirsty troops, who were responsible for managing the rubber trade that caused over five million people to perish (Aronson, 1998; Ball, 1961; Brittain, 1998; Callaghy, 1984). From 1890 to 1910 between 5 and 8 million people perished as a direct result of the rubber trade. By 1903, the economy for rubber in the Congo had collapsed, so the new Belgian colony focused on exploiting the Katanga province for copper, diamonds, and oil (Brittain, 1998; Callaghy, 1984). Both forced labor and high taxes continued the horrors of Leopold. Families were split as many men went far away from their villages to the mines to work, nearly destroying the fabric of traditional society.

During the 1930s and 1940s, the Belgian colonial government tried to enforce mass cultivation standards, but without proper transportation mechanisms in place, large amounts of food lay wasted and unsold (Aronson, 1998; Ball, 1961; Brittain, 1998; Callaghy, 1984). The demand for copper grew during the World War II era, creating peripheral markets for household goods such as soap and sugar (Aronson, 1998; Ball, 1961; Brittain, 1998; Callaghy, 1984). Though economic growth increased and education improved during this time, the Belgians remained staunchly authoritarian (Aronson, 1998; Ball, 1961; Brittain, 1998; Callaghy, 1984). Local chiefs were used as pawns of the government; often they were removed from power if rumored to be anti-colonialist (Aronson, 1998; Ball, 1961; Brittain, 1998; Callaghy, 1984). Finally, the increased poverty and aggravation over colonial rule united this extremely large country, despite its lack of roads, telephones, and newspapers. Under the administration of the Belgians, for example, Congolese were not permitted to travel without a permit and were not allowed to drink hard liquor (Aronson, 1998; Ball, 1961; Brittain, 1998; Callaghy, 1984). Such inequality fed the flames of desire for independence, as did the news of neighboring countries achieving freedom from colonial rule (Aronson, 1998; Ball, 1961; Brittain, 1998; Callaghy, 1984).

Liberation movements from around the country began to cooperate and consolidate their power against the Belgians. Religious movements formed, strongly espousing antiwhite, anticolonialist rule (Aronson, 1998; Ball, 1961; Brittain, 1998; Callaghy, 1984). Massive strikes and retaliatory massacres helped motivate opposition groups in the extremely large and ethnically diverse country. Then the Belgians abruptly left the Congo and independence was declared on June 30, 1960 (Aronson, 1998; Ball, 1961; Brittain, 1998; Callaghy, 1984). After Congolese independence in 1960, income of the average Congolese has fallen over the decades from $ 988.1 in 1960s to $310 in 2000s. Life expectancy has slightly increased over the decade from 42.1 years in 1960s to 55.0 years in 2000s (World Bank, 2014). The region over the decade has recorded a very low literacy rate, but quite a number of conflicts and minor and major wars over the decades from 1960s to 2000s (Aronson, 1998; Ball, 1961; Brittain, 1998; Callaghy, 1984).

### *The Burundi Vignette*

On the same continent and at about the same time, when Selina was on her way to begin working in Inongo, Ahmed Amissi was born in Burundi. Ahmed's family and many of his relatives lived in a rural area outside of Gitega, a day's bus ride from the capital city of Gitega. Meanwhile, Gitega province is one of the seventeen provinces of Burundi. It is the home of the Burundi's National Museum of Gitega and the Archdiocese of Gitega. Several Karyenda royal drum sanctuaries are located in the area, as well as Ibwami (royal court). Ahmed Amissi's family lived in a thatched hut and had few possessions. They owned cooking utensils, some blankets and clothing, radio, and a bicycle. Ahmed's sister spent two hours a day fetching water from a small stream outside their village. The village did not have a paved road or electricity. In addition to growing maize, a cereal crop similar to millet, the family grew vegetables and relied on its own production for most of its consumption needs. The family was especially proud of their livestock, because Burundi's is an agricultural and livestock economy with over 90% of the population engaged in subsistence agriculture. Ahmed's father raised and traded oxen, which earned the family most of their meager income.

Ahmed was the third of five children. He received 5 years of schooling, but the years were not in succession. In some years, he needed to work with his father and brothers tending the family's crops and livestock. In other years, the family did not have enough money to pay for uniforms and other school fees and could afford to send only one or two of their children to school. Priority was given to Ahmed's older brothers. By the time he was 13, Ahmed was able to read and write, although not well.

Ahmed and his family (Mr. Amissi) have known hard times. His mother died shortly after the birth of her last child. This was due, in part, to her weakened state following civil unrest, political instability in 1993, and compounded by multiple births and lack of emergency postpartum care (Forster, 2000; Janzen, 2000; Jennings, 2001). Despite worldwide attention to Burundi's predicaments that year, relief came too late to help them. Since 1993, ethnic tensions and ongoing violence have severely disrupted the economy, bringing the government's economic reforms to a halt (Forster, 2000; Janzen, 2000; Jennings, 2001). International sanctions in 1996 exacerbated the poor economic situation, causing further food shortages and high inflation. There was a 50% increase in the number of people falling below the poverty line (Forster, 2000; Janzen, 2000; Jennings, 2001). That is, from the 1960s to 2000s Gross Domestic Product (GDP) per capita has remained in the two hundreds (i.e., 1960s was $210.9; 1970s was $270; 1990s was $280.8; and 2000s was $ 229) (Forster, 2000; Janzen, 2000; Jennings, 2001).

Although the Arusha Peace Accords had been signed in 2000, violence continued into 2003, as one million people fled their homes. Over 300,000 people since 1993 had been killed in Burundi's civil war. Political instability is also compounded by the HIV/AIDS epidemic. Nearly one in ten adults is infected with HIV/AIDS, and medicines are in short supply (McElrath, 2002). Sanctions imposed by neighboring countries on Burundi have stunted the economy, although a regional trade embargo was lifted in 1999 (Forster,

2000; Janzen, 2000; Jennings, 2001). However, by the end of 2005 fighting had stopped in most parts of the country, and greater internal stability and donor-financed capital expenditure are hoped to aid growth throughout the economy during 2006 and in coming years. This can be seen in the GDP growth for the period 2000–2004. In 2000 GDP grew at a negative growth rate of 0.9% but bounced back in 2001 and 2002 to 3.2% and 3.6% respectively. It declined to a 1.3% in 2003 but strongly bounced back to 5.5% in 2004 (Ould-Abdullah, 2000; Schrerrer, 2002). Lastly, life expectancy over the decades has increased slightly from 42.6 years in 1960s to 53.9 years in 2000s.

### *The Liberia Vignette*

Unlike Selina or Ahmed, Garmuyu and Poady are relatively well educated. Both were born in Arthington, a small town in Montserrado County, Liberia, located along the Saint Paul River northwest of the capital city of Monrovia. It is mainly known as the hometown of former president Charles Taylor, the country's twenty-second president. They graduated from secondary school in 1980 and went on to study for several more years at the local university, which is where they met. Garmuyu studied engineering and Poady architectural drawing. After finishing their studies, they married and Garmuyu began work at the largest timber concession, Oriental Timber Corporation (OTC), owned by an Indonesian. Poady was hired by a municipal agency. As was common during the Soviet era, the couple moved into a one-bedroom apartment where Poady's parents lived. Garmuyu and Poady owned refrigerator and other kitchen appliances, television, furniture, some musical instruments, many books, and a telephone. Garmuyu's and Poady's lifestyle in the 1980s was certainly modest by Western culture standards. They enjoyed few luxuries but most of their everyday needs were met. Often this regards standing on long lines at foreigners' stores for staples such as bread, cooking oil, milk, and sugar. They also had their own garden plot where they grew flowers, fruits, and vegetables. Occasionally they purchased goods in the gray market (technically illegal but not enforced) that came from Lebanese and Indians. Two years after their marriage, Poady got sick and later died due to poor medication and care. Perhaps, the reasons could be due to poor provision of health care facility, poverty level of Liberia, and civil unrest.

Liberia, in West Africa, is one of the poorest countries in the world, and its economy is extremely underdeveloped, largely due to the First Liberian Civil War in 1989–1996. The civil war destroyed much of Liberia's economy, especially the infrastructure in and around Monrovia. The war also caused a brain-drain and the loss of capital, as the civil war involved overthrowing the Americo Liberian minority that ruled the country. Some returned during

1997, but many have not. Liberia is richly endowed with water, mineral resources, forests, and a climate favorable to agriculture, but poor in human capital, infrastructure, and stability. Liberia has a fairly typical profile for sub-Saharan African economies—the majority of the population is reliant on subsistence agriculture, while exports are dominated by raw commodities such as rubber and iron ore. Many of the 1990s' local manufacturing companies were foreign owned.

The democratically elected government, formed in August 1997, inherited massive international debts and currently relies on revenues from its maritime registry to provide the bulk of its foreign exchange earnings (International Monetary Fund, 2011; Government of Liberia, 2011; Toweh, 2011; Konneh, 2010; Schoenurl, 2003). The restoration of the infrastructure and the raising of incomes in this ravaged economy depend on the implementation of sound macro- and microeconomic policies of the new government, including the encouragement of foreign investment (International Monetary Fund, 2011; Government of Liberia, 2011; Toweh, 2011; Konneh, 2010; Schoenurl, 2003).

The Liberian economy had relied heavily on the mining of iron ore prior to the civil war. Liberia was a major exporter of iron ore on the world market. In the 1970s and 1980s, iron mining accounted for more than half of Liberia's export earnings (International Monetary Fund, 2011; Government of Liberia, 2011; Toweh, 2011; Konneh, 2010; Schoenurl, 2003). Since the coup d'état of 1980, the country's economic growth rate has slowed down because of a decline in the demand for iron ore in the world market and political upheavals in Liberia (International Monetary Fund, 2011; Government of Liberia, 2011; Toweh, 2011; Konneh, 2010; Schoenurl, 2003).

Following a peak in growth in 1979, the Liberian economy began a steady decline due to economic mismanagement following the 1980 coup (International Monetary Fund, 2011; Government of Liberia, 2011; Toweh, 2011; Konneh, 2010). This decline was accelerated by the outbreak of civil war in 1989; GDP was reduced by an estimated 90% between 1989 and 1995, one of the fastest declines in history (International Monetary Fund, 2011; Government of Liberia, 2011; Toweh, 2011; Konneh, 2010; Schoenurl, 2003). The United Nations imposed sanctions on Liberia in May 2001 for its support to the rebels of the Revolutionary United Front (RUF) in neighboring Sierra Leone. These sanctions have been lifted following elections in 2005 (Government of Liberia, 2011; Toweh, 2011; Konneh, 2010).

Upon the end of the war in 2003, GDP growth began to accelerate, reaching 9.4% in 2007 (International Monetary Fund, 2011; Government of Liberia, 2011; Toweh, 2011; Konneh, 2010). The global financial crisis slowed GDP growth to 4.6% in 2009 (International Monetary Fund, 2011; Government of Liberia, 2011; Toweh, 2011; Konneh, 2010), though a strengthening agricultural sector led by rubber and timber exports increased growth to 5.1% in 2010 and an expected 7.3% in 2011 (International Monetary Fund, 2011; Government of Liberia, 2011; Toweh, 2011; Konneh, 2010; Schoenurl, 2003). However, over the decades, Liberia's LEB showed a slight increase from 36.5 years in 1960s to 57.2 years in 2000s.

## INSTITUTION, ECONOMIC GROWTH, AND DEVELOPMENT

According to Lukongo (2018), Well (2005) and Perkins, Radelet, and Lindauer (1996) low productivity, low economic growth rate, and low LEB across many of the African countries could be attributed to weather patterns, growing conditions, institutions, and other economic factors. However, Lukongo (2018) argued that it is reasonable to assume that individual leaders' decisions can impede the economic growth and development in weakly institutionalized countries. Many studies have explained how institutions shape individual behaviors and the way society evolves and affects economic performance (Lukongo, 2018; North, 1990; North and Weingast, 2004; Boetteke, Coyne, and Sautet, 2005; Boettke and Fink, 2011). It is very important to note that the lack of commitment to or enforcement of the constitutional arrangement and ease of changing or revising the constitutions have significant impact on the performance of a country compared to places where one is tied by the constitution to commit to or abode by the constitutional arrangement (Perkins, Radelet, and Lindauer, 1996; Lukongo, 2018; North and Weingast, 2004).

Many researchers examined trends in individual countries, but it was difficult to draw general conclusions from these case studies. A few revolutionary efforts, such as a book by Adelman and Morris (1967) titled *Society, Politics, and Economic Development. A Quantitative Approach cited* in Perkins, Radelet, and Lindauer (1996, p.75), paved the way for today's cross-country empirical growth research. In recent years, this type of research has grown very rapidly, in line with the emergence of many new and large datasets on income, education levels, health characteristics, quality of governance, politics, and a host of related items (Barro, 1991; Jeffrey and Warner, 1995; Mankiw, Romer, and Weil, 1992 cited in Perkins, Radelet, and Lindauer, 1996, p.75).

Meanwhile, Jones and Olken (2005) cited in Lukongo (2018) concluded that individual leaders played crucial roles in shaping the growth of nations. Lukongo (2018), illustratively stated that during the era between 1965 and 1997, Mobutu's presidency in the Congo is observed to be a good emblematic case. Very interestingly, Lukongo (2018) echoes the discussions in a book by

Friedman (2011, pp. 1–2) entitled *The Next Decade: Where We've Been...and Where We're Going*. The author emphatically explains that "human beings don't live in the long run. However, we live in the much shorter span in which our lives are shaped not so much by vast historical trends by the specific decisions of specific individuals . . . But rather in the shorter time frame of a decade, where individual decisions made by individual peoples, particularly those with political power, can matter enormously" (see Lukongo, 2018 for more details).

In a study conducted by Lukongo (2018) titled "Kleptocracy and Its Relation to Economic Performance, the Case of Congo" provides evidence of the existing literature in terms of institutional constraints and corrupt governments. Acemoglu, Robinson, and Verdier (2004) as cited in Lukongo (2018) provides an emblematic example of governments with corrupt leaders (kleptocracy) around the world to include the governances or rulings of DRC under SeseSeko Mobutu, the Dominican Republic under Rafael Truijillo, Haiti under the Duvaliers, Nicaragua under the Somozas, Uganda under Idi Amin, Liberia under Charles Taylor, and Philippines under Ferdinand Marcos. For the purpose of this publication, the Congolese and the Liberian cases become perfect cases or examples of institutional constraints to economic growth and development in the case of Africa.

## THE SOLOW GROWTH MODEL

The Solow Growth Model is a standard neoclassical model of explaining economic growth. This particular growth model was developed by Robert Solow in 1970 in a book titled *Growth Theory: An Exposition*. The theory has three basic sources or contributing factors to GDP or economic growth such as labor (L), capital (K) and knowledge (A). According to Solow (1970) "knowledge" is a sort of catch-all category used to augment labor (AL), called "effective labor" (Solow, 1970; Mankiw, 2012; Well, 2005). The Solow model is so straightforward; it is worth pointing out what it does not include. Government, multiple goods, changes in employment, natural resources, geography, and social institutions are main features the model ignores (Mankiw, 2012). It is, however, this simplification that allows researchers to better understand the role of capital, labor, and knowledge in the study of economic growth and development.

The Solow Growth Model has been used widely by many economists to explain the rise and fall of capital, income differences, and relative income growth rates (Well, 2005, pp. 57–69). The Solow Growth Model predicts conditional convergence (Solow, 1970; Mankiw, 2012; Well, 2005). This means that countries with similar characteristics converge to the same steady state (situation in which $k$ stays the same). Similar characteristics in this model imply that the savings rate of both countries is the same (Solow, 1970; Mankiw, 2012; Well, 2005). Applying this model to spatial spillover of war and life expectancy will categorize countries into coldspot and hotspot regions. For the case of spatial coldspot regions to occur at the steady state, such a country must have a low LEB, and must be surrounded by countries with similar characteristics of low LEB. Also for spatial hotspot regions to occur at the steady state, such a country must have high LEB and must be surrounded by countries with similar characteristics of high LEB. This particular spatial coldspot and hotspot analysis at the steady state has been extensively explained in chapters 3 and 4 of the monograph.

## LIFE EXPECTANCY IN AFRICA: RELEVANT LITERATURE REVIEW

In 1970, as the Africans' social indicators were slowly but progressively improved in all the years in many of African countries, the statistics of LEB among the Africa countries still, by today, shows a large disappointment (Roser, 2015). In fact, the top ten countries with lowest life expectancy happened to originate from the African continent, and those countries are Swaziland, Sierra Leone, Zimbabwe, Zambia, Namibia, and Botswana. There, on average, none of the male or female lives beyond 45 years. This is a far cry compared to some countries like Japan with 85 years of age as the life expectancy (Roser, 2015).

The stagnancy and fluctuations in life expectancy among Africa countries as compared to the other continents have been observed during several decades, centuries, and cycles; yet, little has been done to examine the dynamics in life expectancy among African countries. Also as shown in figure 1.1, the African countries among the countries in other continents have also shown a downward spiral of the relationship between life expectancy and income per persons (or GDP per capita) as at 2015.

Meanwhile, Lawrence Chia-Wei has revealed, in his 2009 publication, some possible factors that are likely to account for low life expectancy including famine, war, poor government spending, corruption, low level of education, availability of clean water, and spread of HIV/AIDs. Furthermore, according to WHO (2000) the key factors that are likely to contribute to low life expectancy are the big infectious disease killers such as HIV/AIDS, malaria, and tuberculosis as well as big child killers, including pneumonia and diarrhea. It was further argued that the health life expectancy in such countries as Botswana, Namibia, and Zimbabwe has been reduced by 14 years because of the impact of widespread AIDS (World Health Organization, 2000).

## AFRICAN POLITICAL CYCLES AND DIVISIONS: RELEVANT LITERATURE REVIEW OF COLONIAL PRESENCE

The map below shows the areas of Africa under the sovereignty or influence of the colonial powers in 1913, along with modern borders (Simon, 1995; Lucien, 2001). In the late nineteenth century, the European imperial powers engaged in a major territorial scramble and occupied most of the continent, creating many colonial territories, and leaving only two fully independent states: Ethiopia (known to Europeans as "Abyssinia") and Liberia. Egypt and Sudan were never formally incorporated into any European colonial empire; however, after the British occupation of 1882, Egypt was effectively under British administration until 1922 (Simon, 1995; Lucien, 2001).

## INDEPENDENCE STRUGGLES

The imperial rule by Europeans continues until after the conclusion of World War II, when almost all remaining colonial territories gradually obtained formal independence (Simon, 1995; Lucien, 2001). Independence movements in Africa gained momentum following World War II, which left the major European powers to weakened (Simon, 1995; Lucien, 2001; Aryeetey, Harrigan, and Nissanke, 2000). In 1951, Libya, a former Italian colony, gained independence. In 1956, Tunisia and Morocco won their independence from France (Simon, 1995; Lucien, 2001). Apparently, Ghana followed suit the next year (March 1957) becoming the first of the sub-Saharan colonies to be granted independence. Most of the rest of the continent became independent over the next decade (Simon, 1995; Lucien, 2001; Aryeetey, Harrigan, and Nissanke, 2000).

Therefore, Portugal's overseas presence in sub-Saharan Africa (most notably in Angola, Cape Verde, Mozambique, Guinea-Bissau and São Tomé, and Príncipe) lasted from the sixteenth century to 1975, after the Estado Novo regime was overthrown in a military coup in Lisbon (Simon, 1995; Lucien, 2001; Aryeetey, Harrigan, and Nissanke, 2000). Rhodesia unilaterally declared independence from the United Kingdom in 1965, under the white minority government of Ian Smith, but was not internationally recognized as an independent state (as Zimbabwe) until 1980, when black nationalists gained power after a bitter guerilla war (Simon, 1995; Lucien, 2001; Aryeetey, Harrigan, and Nissanke, 2000). Although South Africa was one of the first African countries to gain independence, the state remained under the control of the country's white minority through a system of racial segregation known as apartheid until 1994 (Simon, 1995; Lucien, 2001; Aryeetey, Harrigan, and Nissanke, 2000).

## POST-COLONIAL AFRICA

Today, Africa contains fifty-four sovereign countries, most of which have borders that were drawn during the era of European colonialism. Since colonialism, African states have frequently been hampered by instability (Gupta, 1967; Mbaku, 1988; Kieh, 2008), corruption (Transparency International, 2015; Lucien, 2001; Aryeetey, Harrigan, and Nissanke, 2000), violence, and authoritarianism (Simon, 1995; Lucien, 2001; Aryeetey, Harrigan, and Nissanke, 2000). The vast majority of African nations are republics that operate under some form of the presidential system of rule. However, few of them have been able to sustain democratic governments on a permanent basis, and many have instead cycled through a series of coups, producing military dictatorships (Simon, 1995; Lucien, 2001; Aryeetey, Harrigan, and Nissanke, 2000).

Great instability was mainly the result of marginalization of ethnic groups and graft under these leaders. For political gain, many leaders fanned ethnic conflicts, some of which had been exacerbated, or even created, by colonial rule. In many countries, the military was perceived as being the only group that could effectively maintain order, and it ruled many nations in Africa during the 1970s and early 1980s (Simon, 1995; Lucien, 2001; Aryeetey, Harrigan, and Nissanke, 2000). During the period from the early 1960s to the late 1980s, Africa had more than seventy coups and thirteen presidential assassinations (Simon, 1995; Lucien, 2001; Aryeetey, Harrigan, and Nissanke, 2000). Border and territorial disputes were also common, with the European-imposed borders of many nations being widely contested through armed conflicts (Simon, 1995; Lucien, 2001; Aryeetey, Harrigan, and Nissanke, 2000).

Cold War between the United States and the Soviet Union, as well as the policies of the IMF (Aryeetey, Harrigan, and Nissanke, 2000), also played a role in instability (Aryeetey, Harrigan, and Nissanke, 2000). When a country became independent for the first time, it was often expected to align with one of the two superpowers (Simon, 1995; Lucien, 2001; Aryeetey, Harrigan, and Nissanke, 2000). Many countries in Northern Africa received Soviet military aid, while others in Central and Southern Africa were supported by the United States, France, or both (Simon, 1995; Lucien, 2001; Aryeetey, Harrigan, and Nissanke, 2000). The 1970s saw an escalation of Cold War intrigues, as newly independent Angola and Mozambique aligned themselves with the Soviet Union, and the West and South Africa sought to contain Soviet influence by supporting friendly regimes or insurgency movements (Aryeetey, Harrigan, and Nissanke, 2000).

In the former Rhodesia (now Republic of Zimbabwe), Soviet and Chinese-backed leftist guerrillas of the Zimbabwe Patriotic Front waged a brutal guerrilla war against the country's white government (Simon, 1995; Lucien,

2001; Aryeetey, Harrigan, and Nissanke, 2000). There was a major famine in Ethiopia, when hundreds of thousands of people starved. Some claimed that Marxist economic policies made the situation worse (Simon, 1995; Aryeetey, Harrigan, and Nissanke, 2000; Patman, 1990). The most devastating military conflict in modern independent Africa has been the Second Congo War; this conflict and its aftermath have killed an estimated 5.5 million people (Varnis, 1990; Aryeetey, Harrigan, and Nissanke, 2000; Patman, 1990). Since 2003 there has been an ongoing conflict in Darfur, which has become a humanitarian disaster. Another notable tragic event is the 1994 Rwandan Genocide in which an estimated 800,000 people were murdered. AIDS in post-colonial Africa has also been a prevalent issue (Varnis, 1990; Patman, 1990).

In the twenty-first century, however, the number of armed conflicts in Africa has steadily declined. For instance, the civil war in Angola ended in 2002 after nearly 30 years (Varnis, 1990; Patman, 1990). This has coincided with many countries abandoning communist-style command economies and opening up for market reforms (Varnis, 1990; Patman, 1990). The improved stability and economic reforms have led to a great increase in foreign investment into many African nations, mainly from China (Varnis, 1990; Aryeetey, Harrigan, and Nissanke, 2000; Patman, 1990), which has spurred quick economic growth in many countries, seemingly ending decades of stagnation and decline. Several African economies are among the world's fastest growing as of 2016 (Varnis, 1990; Politze, 2008; Aryeetey, Harrigan, and Nissanke, 2000; Patman, 1990). A significant part of this growth, which is sometimes referred to as Africa Rising, can also be attributed to the facilitated diffusion of information technologies and specifically the mobile telephone (Alasdair and Blake, 1985; Varnis, 1990; Politze, 2008; Aryeetey, Harrigan, and Nissanke, 2000; Patman, 1990).

## LIFE EXPECTANCY AND ITS EMPIRICAL RELATIONSHIP WITH OTHER VARIABLES

Delavari et al. (2016) conducted a study on life expectancy and its socioeconomic determinants in Iran. These authors claimed that LEB is closely associated with the degree of economic and social development in developed and developing countries. The purpose of the study was to examine the socioeconomic factors affecting LEB in Iran from 1985 to 2013. Time series analysis was used to examine the effects of key explanatory factors (GDP per capita, number of doctors per 10,000 population, degree of urbanization, food availability, $CO_2$ emission, total fertility rate, inflation rate, and literacy rate) on LEB in Iran from 1985 to 2013. The data were retrieved from the Central Bank of Iran (CBI), Iranian Statistical Center (ISC), and World Bank.

Augmented Dickey Fuller (ADF) and Banergy, Dolado, and Master (BDM) tests, Engle Granger approach, and an ordinary least-square (OLS) model were used to achieve the aim of the study. The data analysis was performed by Stata, version 12 software. As part of the findings, the study revealed that GDP per capita ($p$ = 0.003), number of doctors per 10,000 population ($p$ = 0.036), literacy rate ($p$ = 0.0001), and food availability ($p$ = 0.0001) were statistically significant at the conventional levels. At the same time, all the variables exhibited a positive effect on LEB. They concluded that GDP per capita, number of doctors per 10,000 population, food availability, literacy rate, and total fertility were identified as the main factors affecting life expectancy in Iran. The study, however, suggests that life expectancy in Iran could be improved if attention is given to factors that reside outside of the health sector.

Chan and Devi (2012) did an investigation on factors affecting life expectancy. The authors examine the impact of demographic changes, socioeconomic inequality, and the availability of health care resources on life expectancy in Singapore, Malaysia, and Thailand. The authors did a cross-country study by collecting annual data from three Southeast Asian countries from 1980 to 2008. They theorized that life expectancy is the dependent variable with demographics, socioeconomic status, and health care resources as the three main determinants. A structural equation model was used, and results showed that the availability of more health care resources and higher levels of socioeconomic advantages are more likely to increase life expectancy. In contrast, demographic changes are more likely to increase life expectancy by way of health care resources. The authors suggest that more effort should be taken to expand and improve the coverage of health care programs to alleviate regional differences in health care use and improve the overall health status of people in these three Southeast Asian countries.

Kabir (2008) did a study titled, "Determinants of Life Expectancy in Developing Countries" and examined the socioeconomic determinants of life expectancy for ninety-one developing countries using the multiple linear regression and probit frameworks. The disaggregated probit regression was applied for three groups of countries with low, medium, and high life expectancy. As part of the findings, most of explanatory variables turned out to be statistically insignificant, which imply that relevant socioeconomic factors like per capita income, education, health expenditure, access to safe water, and urbanization cannot always be considered to be influential in determining life expectancy in developing countries. Based on the analyses it has been suggested that the countries should formulate and implement appropriate social sector policies and programs to increase physicians' availability and reduce adult illiteracy and undernourishment so as to improve their life expectancies.

Another study was conducted by Gilligan and Skrepnek (2015) titled, "Determinants of Life Expectancy in the Eastern Mediterranean Region." The researchers conducted this particular study based on the premise that the Eastern Mediterranean Region (EMR) health care sector has been expanding rapidly; however, many differences exist across socioeconomic status, clinical practice standards, and health care systems.

The objective of the study by Gilligan and Skrepnek was to predict the production functions of health by measuring socioeconomic and expenditure factors that impact life expectancy in the EMR. Data were sourced from the WHO, Global Health Observatory and the World Bank. A time-series study spanning twenty-one nations in the EMR from 1995 to 2010 was investigated. The primary outcome was LEB. The covariates of interest, which were employed in the study, included sociodemographic and health indicators. To both establish and validate appropriate categorization of countries, a cluster analysis was undertaken to group cases by taking selected characteristics into account. A variance-component, multilevel mixed-effects linear model was employed that incorporated a finite, Almon, distributed lag of 5 years and bootstrapping with 5,000 simulations to model the production function of life expectancy.

As part of Gilligan's and Skrepnek's findings, the cluster analysis found four groupings. That is, Clusters 1 and 2, composed of six total countries, generally represented as non-industrialized/least developed countries. Clusters 3 and 4, totaling fifteen nations, captured more industrialized nations. Overall, GDP ($p = 0.011$), vaccination averages ($p = 0.026$), and urbanization ($p = 0.026$) were significant positive predictors of life expectancy. No significant predictors existed for Cluster 1 countries. Among Cluster 2 nations, physician density ($p = 0.014$), and vaccination averages ($p = 0.044$) were significant positive predictors. GDP ($p = 0.037$) and literacy ($p = 0.014$) were positive significant predictors among Cluster 3 nations. GDP ($p = 0.002$), health expenditures ($p = 0.002$), and vaccination averages ($p = 0.014$) were significant positive predictors in Cluster 4 countries. The study concluded that predictors of life expectancy differed between non-industrialized and industrialized nations, with the exception of vaccination averages. Non-industrialized/least developed nations were associated with adjusted life expectancies of greater than 14% lower than their industrialized peers. The study suggested that continued work or research to address differences in the quality of and access to care in the EMR is required.

A study titled, "Determinants of Life Expectancy: A Panel Data Approach" was, for example, conducted by Monsef and Mehrjardi (2015). The authors examined the link between health status and economic, social, and environmental factors for 136 countries between 2002 and 2010. The LEB was considered as the proxy of health status. As part of the variables used in the study by the authors, the inflation rate, unemployment rate, gross capital formation, and gross national income were the main economic factors that previous existing literatures have used in examining LEB. However, these authors introduced two additional economic variables such as inflation and unemployment rate, and urbanization and $CO_2$ emission as the social and environmental factors that are likely to affect life expectancy. The panel data were processed using STATA software. The findings of the study showed that inflation rate and the unemployment rate have a significant negative impact on life expectancy in 136 selected countries, while the unemployment rate is more effective. The urban population factor, as a proxy for urbanization, as well as gross capital formation has a significant impact on life expectancy as well. For further in-depth analysis, the authors examined the degree of economic development impact on life expectancy across countries, by dividing the countries into two groups: (1) the countries that have the gross national income more than global average income and (2) the countries that have the gross national income less than global average income. The results indicated that the countries with more income than the global average income have a higher LEB than less income countries by 6.377 years.

Hassan et al. (2017) conducted a study on social and environment determinants of life expectancy in developing countries by using a panel data analysis. These authors observed that despite the remarkable improvements in health over the past 50 years, there still remain a great number of health challenges around the world. Therefore, their study examined the relationship between life expectancy rate (as a proxy for health status) with health expenditure, gross domestic product, education index, improved water coverage, and improved sanitation facilities in 108 selected developing countries using annual panel data within the period of 2006–2010. The empirical results from using the panel data approach showed a positive relationship between life expectancy rate and all of those explanatory variables. The relationship between life expectancy with education index and gross domestic product were significant at 1% and 5% significance levels, respectively. Furthermore, the causality finding showed that there is no short-run causality between life expectancy and its determinants. There was unidirectional causality running from the independent variables of health expenditure, education index, improved water, and improved sanitation to LEB. On the other hand, bidirectional causality exists between life expectancy and income in the long-run by employing Vector Error Correction Model (VECM) test. According to the authors of this article, these independent variables can be considered as important determinants for investment in health status in the long-run. They concluded that this study could be used as a guideline and may be significant for future researchers and policy makers who aim to improve the life expectancy in developing countries.

## CHAPTER SUMMARY AND GAP IDENTIFICATION

Perhaps, due to a thorough investigation of available development literature, health indicator model, and several of the articles in reputable journals, it was observed that life expectancy in many parts of the world has been increasing steadily over the past few decades, due to increases in technology, medicine, economic growth, food security, and international aid. Yet, enormous discrepancies still exist between first world nations and developing countries.

Chapter 2, indeed, underscored that several social, economic, environment, and health factors are likely to determine a country's LEB. Taking for example, socioeconomic factors, now the two relevant questions to be posed are the following: If societal health can be measured as LEB, then what are the various socioeconomic factors that are likely to increase or decrease it? Can the marginal effects of these factors be disentangled? If so, which of these factors produce the largest health benefits (or costs) to society? These questions are as important now as when first posed by Auster, Leveson, and Sarachek in 1969. Since Auster, Leveson, and Sarachek, and several economic studies have attempted to answer these questions using data from the United States or multiple countries, none of those attempts tried to use spatiotemporal analysis to examine the pattern of life expectancy in Africa.

Many of the authors, whose works have been reviewed to aid this chapter, have used aggregate data from the member countries of the OECD to explain cross-country life expectancies. While the empirical results are mixed, the derived general consensus is that a population's life expectancy, at birth, is a function of environmental measures (i.e., wealth, education, safety, regulation, infrastructure), lifestyle measures (i.e., tobacco or alcohol consumption), and health care consumption measures (i.e., medical expenditures). However, the appropriate econometric and spatial methodology for disentangling these effects and its meaning for relative importance (statistical or econometric) of the estimated effects is more contentious.

Furthermore, it was observed in the chapter that many of the Africa countries have engage in political disruptions or violence, civil war, and conflicts over the decades. Several of the articles have also proven that countries with close border are likely to have violence spillover to their neighboring countries. Perhaps, theories have suggested institutions, and safety among the measuring indicators of longevity (or LEB); yet, no attempt has been made to look into the spatial spillover of violence or conflicts and its impact on LEB (longevity) across countries in Africa.

Again, conflicts across borders and spillover of major armed wars in Africa have been covered in many of the available war literatures; political science studies, historical studies, and in popular press at the international fronts but uncommon in economics literature. Adding to that scholars like Easterly and

Levine (1997) and Murdoch and Sander (2002) have observed a systematic contamination of growth performance, negative spillovers in the short run stemming from neighbors' civil wars, and in the long run from neighbors' per capita income across the borders of Africa, Asia, and Latin America.

More recent studies have unearthed evidence of spillover of violence from conflict in the following: (1) Rwanda into the Eastern DRC in 1994, (2) Liberia into Sierra Leone in West Africa in 1991, (3) Bosnia into Kosovo, and (4) Burundi into Rwanda (Raleigh and Hegre, 2009; Gershoni, 1997; Schutte and Weidmann, 2011). Therefore, this publication contributes to existing literature on LEB, economic growth, and political disruption or wars in Africa in several ways, that is by testing for spatial dependence in LEB, identifying spatial clustering of low and high LEB regions, and finally, measuring the spatial spillover of violence in one country on its neighbors.

# *Chapter 3*

# Methodology and Models Specification of Spatiotemporal and Spatial Regression Analyses

By following the methodology discussed in this chapter, readers of the book are to have a full grasp of the models specification of spatiotemporal and spatial regression analysis. This chapter also includes the justification for each selected method to be utilized for the book. As chapter 3 of the book, it is divided into eight thematic sections, which bring home to readers the research design, background to the book's research area (i.e., Africa), the population that is scrutinized or studied, data sources, types and sample size, study hypotheses, model specifications, reliability as well as validity, and data analysis.

## OVERALL DESIGN AND METHODOLOGY

In this book, I have used spatiotemporal and spatial regression analyses to analyze the changes in life expectancy and its determinants across selected continental regions and time so that they will ultimately explain the public health policy in the African nations that have been studied. In the foregoing context, the research for the book has utilized an exploratory spatial data analysis as a form of quantitative design and, also, as the variables that the author of the book relied upon for both the spatiotemporal and spatial regression (or econometric) analyses, all of which are to be quantitative in nature, coupled with both interval and ratio level of measurement.

Overall, the exploratory spatial data analysis is based on decades of political and historical trends. However, the data being used in the research for the book stem from a secondary source of the World Bank, Barro and Lee, and the WHO. The analysis is based on a spatial unit (i.e., each country or region with close borders in Africa). Two strategies are adopted for the analysis of the research for the monograph, which include (1) spatiotemporal analysis (i.e., by creating different maps for life expectancy based on decades, Cold War and post-Cold War, Africa Renaissance, and divisions of Africa's political cycles) and (2) spatial regression (or econometric analysis) analysis.

## BACKGROUND TO THE BOOK'S RESEARCH AREA (AFRICA)

Africa, as the temporal and spatial unit of analysis, is the world's second largest and second most-populous continent (the first being Asia in both categories). At about 30.3 million $km^2$ (11.7 million square miles) including adjacent islands, it covers 6% of the global total surface area and 20% of its total land area (International Monetary Fund, 2017). With approximately a total of 1.2 billion people as of 2016 (United Nations Department of Economic and Social Affairs, 2017), it accounts for about 16% of the world's human population. The continent is surrounded by the Mediterranean Sea to the north, the Isthmus of Suez and the Red Sea to the northeast, the Indian Ocean to the southeast and the Atlantic Ocean to the west.

In totality, the African continent includes Madagascar and various archipelagos. Also, it contains fifty-four fully recognized sovereign states (or countries), nine territories and two de facto independent states with limited or no recognition (Sayre, 1999). The majority of the continent and its countries are in the Northern Hemisphere, with a substantial portion and number of countries in the Southern Hemisphere.

Africa's average population is the youngest among all of the continents (Swanson, 2015; Harry, 2013); the median age in 2012 was 19.7, when the worldwide median age was 30.4 (Abdoulie, 2012). Algeria is Africa's largest country by area, and Nigeria is its largest by population. Africa straddles the equator and encompasses numerous climate areas; it is the only continent to stretch from the northern temperate to southern temperate zones (Georges, 2015). Africa hosts a large diversity of ethnicities, cultures, and languages. In the late nineteenth century, European countries colonized almost all of Africa; most present states in Africa originated from a process of decolonization in the twentieth century. African nations cooperate through the establishment of the AU, which is headquartered in Addis Ababa (Georges, 2015; Lewis and Short, 1879).

Africa has abundant natural resources; yet, the continent remains the world's poorest and most underdeveloped continent, the result of a variety of causes that may include corrupt governments that have often committed serious human rights violations, failed central planning, high levels of illiteracy, lack of access to foreign capital, and frequent tribal and military conflict (ranging from guerrilla warfare to genocide) (Sandbrook, 1985). According to the United Nations' Human Development Report in 2003, the bottom twenty-four ranked nations (151st–175th) were all African (United Nations' Human Development Report, 2016).

Africans profess a wide variety of religious beliefs, and statistics on religious affiliation are difficult to come by since they are often a sensitive a topic for governments with mixed religious populations (Onishi, 2001). According to the World Book Encyclopedia, Islam is the largest religion in Africa, followed by Christianity. According to Encyclopedia Britannica, 45% of the populations are Christians, 40% are Muslims, and 10% follow traditional religions. A small number of Africans are Hindu, Buddhist, Confucianist, Baha'i, or Jewish. There is also a minority of people in Africa who are irreligious.

## POPULATION

The population researched for the book comprises the forty-seven regions or countries in Africa, starting from Algeria to Zimbabwe, specifically with regions of close borders. The population of the entire continent or region (or all of the fifty-four countries) is 1,225,080,510 (United Nations Department of Economic and Social Affairs, 2017), with a population density of 36.4/km$^2$ or 94/sq mi (United Nations Department of Economic and Social Affairs, 2017). Africa's population has rapidly increased over the last 40 years, and consequently, it is relatively young. In some African states, more than half the population is under 25 years of age (United Nations Department of Economic and Social Affairs, 2017). The total number of people in Africa increased from 229 million in 1950 to 630 million in 1990 (United Nations Department of Economic and Social Affairs, 2017). Africa's total population surpassing other continents is fairly recent; African population surpassed Europe in the 1990s, while the Americans were overtaken sometime around the year 2000 (United Nations Department of Economic and Social Affairs, 2017).

### Data Sources, Type, and Sample Size

The research for the book uses an existing dataset to estimate the spatio-temporal analysis of LEB as well as the spatial regression (or econometric) model. It also uses secondary sources of data between the years of 1960 and 2015 from the WHO, World Bank, IMF, and Barro and Lee (2010) data on world education attainment (1950–2010). The data type is quantitative in nature, but the longitudinal datasets are spanning from the period of 1960–2014 across the aforementioned agencies. The sampling units (or variables) of the datasets were measured in both interval and ratio levels. The total sample size considered for the purpose of the analysis span for fifty-four countries. A sample size of forty-seven out of the fifty-four regions or countries in Africa is selected, based on the consistency in data on availability of the selected variables for the analysis. Furthermore, the data were organized based on Cold War and post-Cold War, over decades starting from 1960s to 2000s, divisions of African political cycles, contemporary independence era (phases 1 and 2), and African Renaissance period for all variables.

## Study Hypotheses

The research for the monograph has three main hypotheses. Based on the first and the second hypotheses, the researcher employs the spatiotemporal analysis to examine the spatial pattern and randomness of LEB model across all regions in Africa. The third hypothesis uses spatial error model to examine the spatial spillover of major armed war (or conflicts) on LEB across all regions in Africa. The hypotheses are as follows:

1. $H_0$: There is no detectable spatial pattern, or concentration, from the LEB across all regions in Africa.
   $H_1$: There is a detectable spatial pattern, or concentration, from the LEB across all regions in Africa.
2. $H_0$: There is spatial randomness in the LEB across all regions in Africa.
   $H_1$: There is spatial autocorrelation in the LEB across all regions in Africa.
3. $H_0$: There is no effect of spatial spillover of major armed war (or conflict) on LEB across all regions in Africa.
   $H_1$: There is a negative effect of spatial spillover of major armed war (or conflict) on LEB across all regions in Africa.

## Models Specification of Spatiotemporal and Spatial Regression Analyses

Two empirical strategies are adopted for the analysis of the research for the monograph, namely (1) spatial regression (econometric) analysis and (2) spatiotemporal analysis. As it relates to spatial analysis, three steps are important to carry out the empirical analysis (or strategies). First, the researcher tests for spatial dependence in LEB across regions and identifies spatial clustering of high and low LEB regions. Second, the researcher estimates the spatial generating process for LEB in Africa. Third, the research for the book measures the spillover of violence (conflict, civil war, major and minor wars) in one country on its neighbors. The research for the monograph takes advantage of developments in applied spatial econometrics and geographic information systems and uses case studies of historical conflicts, divisions of Africa's political cycles, contemporary independence eras I and II, and African Renaissance to measure LEB in the county involved in conflict and surrounding countries.

## SPATIAL DEPENDENCE, LEB, AND CONFLICT/CIVIL WAR

In perusing numerous conflicts, and spatial analysis research, it was observed that spatial spillovers or diffusion of conflicts in Africa have been covered in war literature, political science studies, historical studies, and economics of war publications. In fact, such examination is relatively rare in the economics literature. In one study, Easterly and Levine (1997) finds a systematic contagion of growth performance and underperformance across borders in Africa. Similarly, using data from Africa, Asia, and Latin America, Murdoch and Sander (2002) find negative spillovers in the short run stemming from neighbors' civil wars and in the long run from neighbors' per capita income. More recently, Raleigh and Hegre (2009) find evidence of spillover of violence from conflict in Rwanda into the Eastern DRC in 1994. Similarly, the war in Liberia spilled over to Sierra Leone in West Africa in 1991 (Gershoni, 1997). In studying violence in civil wars, Schutte and Weidmann (2011) find abundant evidence for spatial autocorrelation and diffusion of conflict in the literature. The authors find evidence of diffusion of war between Bosnia and Kosovo and also Burundi and Rwanda. According to the authors, changes in the political dynamics in zones of control likely escalate violence to new or nearby locations. This type of diffusion has been referred to as escalation (Cohen and Tita, 1999; Lukongo and Rezek, 2016) or expansion (Gould, 1988; Lukongo and Rezek, 2016).

In applied spatial econometrics literature, a spatial weight matrix, W, represents the connectivity relationship between neighboring units. It plays a critical role in defining the neighborhood structure, identifying the spatial dependence between geographic units or regions, and specifying the extent of spatial spillovers across a group of countries. The design of the spatial weight matrix and the adoption of a suitable spatial regression model are extremely important in conducting the type of analysis described in this monograph. In applied spatial research on Africa, including publications of economic growth and per capita income, other weighting schemes, such as the length of common borders (Murdoch and Sander, 2002; Lukongo and Rezek, 2016), or the weighted growth of surrounding countries (Easterly and Levine, 1997; Lukongo and Rezek, 2016), have been used rather than the widely used spatial weight matrices. Easterly and Levine (1997) and Lukongo and Rezek (2016) recognize that their chosen weighting scheme magnifies the direct effects of shock and acknowledge that their approach violates the proper spatial arrangement in which, by construction, a country cannot be its own neighbor. Anselin (2002) writes that there is no clear guidance in the choice of spatial weight matrix, but it adds that the applied researcher should maintain the exogeneity of the spatial weight matrix.

The research for the monograph focuses the analysis on LEB over the period from 1960 to 2015 for forty-seven neighboring African countries. In the research for the book, the effects of the spatial diffusion of political disruption and other factors are explicitly considered, as the performance of one country may be related to the geographic proximity and economic relationships it has with other countries (Morrill, Gaile, and Thrall, 1988; Easterly and Levine, 1997; Lukongo and Rezek, 2016). In performing this analysis, the researcher tests for the proper spatial weight matrix and model. The advantage of this approach is the inclusion of the spatial impacts in the modeling strategy, which allows for the quantification of the spillover and the direct, indirect, and total impacts.

After the spatial weight matrix is specified, exploratory spatial data analysis is conducted to verify whether or not spatial clustering patterns exist in the data. Using a global Moran's I statistic, the researcher first tests for the existence of spatial autocorrelation. Then, using a local Moran or Local Indicators of Spatial Autocorrelation (LISA) statistic, as developed by Anselin (1995), the researcher identifies the location of spatial clusters, such as hotspots (high LEB clusters), cold spots (low LEB clusters), and spatial outliers.

Meanwhile, the generating processes of the spatial patterns are investigated next, and the most appropriate spatial econometric model is selected. The two models that have been widely used in the literature are (1) the spatial autoregressive model and (2) the spatial error model. A suitable model is chosen based on the goodness of fit, including the log likelihood, Akaike Information Criterion (AIC), and Schwarz criterion or Bayesian Information Criterion (BIC), as well as the significance of coefficients associated with the models. Also, the researcher has taken steps to evaluated the models and, in the process, concluded that the spatial error model is preferred for calculating the extent of spatial spillover across Africa. Furthermore, the researcher has calculated the impacts associated with the model to determine the extent of spatial spillovers using the spatial econometrics package GeoDa.

## SPATIAL MODELING: SPATIAL DEPENDENCE AND CLUSTERING

In this research for the monograph, identifying and classifying spatial patterns in the data enhance the understanding of the factors and processes contributing to changes in LEB over time and space. Changes in LEB may result from several factors; however, the analysis conducted here seeks to capture the spatial extent of a shock caused by war or similar political disruption on the existing patterns and processes of LEB. The relationship among countries is identified through a spatial weight matrix. This matrix, W, has been used in the literature to organize spatial relationships and specify the spatial extent of spillovers among units (Anselin, 2002; Lee and Wong, 2001; LeSage and Pace, 2009). The elements, $w_{ij}$, of the spatial weight matrix W are positive for all neighbors $i \neq j$, and by construction, $w_{ij}$ equal zero for $i = j$ because a country I cannot be its own neighbor. There are several ways of representing this matrix depending on the research objective and spatial information product. The researcher tests four types of spatial weight matrices: queen contiguity, rook contiguity, general distance, and k-nearest neighbors. The spatial dependence, p, between observations at locations i and j is given by:

$$y_i = p\sum_j w_{ij}y_j, \text{ with } i \neq j \tag{1}$$

Where $w_{ij}$ are the elements of the spatial weight matrix showing the structure of connectivity among countries, i, j = 1, 2, 3 . . . 47 represent neighboring African countries, y represents the LEB, and p is a measure of the strength of spatial autocorrelation in the sample of observations. Using the row standardization technique, the total of each row is normalized to one. The spatial lag term, $\Sigma_j w_{ij} y_j$, for country i represents the spatially weighted average LEB of neighboring countries.

Once a spatial weight matrix is specified, spatial patterns are typically identified and quantified through global and local statistics as well as a map analysis. Therefore, both Moran's I statistic and the Moran scatterplot (Anselin, 1995, 2003) are used here to measure and test the hypothesis of spatial randomness in life expectancy in Africa from 1960 to 2015. These two Moran statistics complement each other. Moran's I allows the detection of the spatial autocorrelation in the life expectancy across the study area, but it offers little insight into the specific location of clusters of high or low LEB. The researcher uses Moran's I with the spatial weights matrix row normalized to one given below:

$$\text{Moran's I} = y^{1}Wy/y^{1}y \tag{2a}$$

Where, "y" represents the LEB, "W" is the spatial weight matrix, "Wy" represents the spatial lag or weighted average of the LEB in neighboring counties or regions in Africa (or the study area). Moran's I here measures the degree of linear association between the LEB (y) and the spatially weighted average of life expectancy of the neighboring countries according to Anselin (1995). This measure provides a global view of the presence or absence of spatial autocorrelation and its strength. The researcher also utilize Moran's I statistic (Equation 2b) to test for spatial autocorrelation in an ordinary least squares (OLS) residuals (e), spatial lag model residuals, and spatial error model residuals.

$$\text{Moran's I} = e^{1}We/e^{1}e \qquad (2b)$$

Where "e" represents ordinary least squares (OLS) residuals, "W" is the spatial weight matrix, and "We" represents the spatial lag or weighted average of the OLS residuals of LEB in neighboring counties or regions in Africa.

Following Lukongo and Rezek (2016), the Moran scatterplot, on the contrary, supplements Moran's I in providing additional insight into high LEB areas, low LEB areas, and areas of mixed LEB in four types of local spatial association.

- The first type of cluster is composed of high LEB countries (high-high). The countries that appear here post high average LEB from 1960 to 2015 and are surrounded by high LEB countries (HH in the Moran scatterplot); these represent a hotspot.
- The second type of cluster indicates that low LEB countries are surrounded by high LEB countries (LH) and there is a local negative spatial autocorrelation.
- The third type of cluster is composed of high LEB country surrounded by low LEB countries (HL) and there is also local negative spatial autocorrelation.
- The fourth type of cluster occurs when low LEB country has other low LEB countries as neighbors (LL); these represent the cold spot. There is a positive spatial autocorrelation.

It is very important to note that the identification of the spatial autocorrelation by the Moran scatterplot and Moran's I makes it feasible for the application of the spatial econometrics. The use of the spatial econometrics aids in the quantification of the following: (1) spatial dependency, (2) uncovering the data-generating process, and (3) the spatial spillover. Adding to that whenever a researcher decides to test for spatial autocorrelation at both global and local level, the specification of spatial weight matrix is very significant because it captures the spatial relationship among geographic units.

Evaluation of the spatial dependence during the process uses both the Moran's I statistic and their associated $p$ values at the traditional type I error levels of 1% (0.01), 5% (0.05), and 10% (0.10). However, the Moran's I statistical values range between −1 and 1. For interpretation or decision purposes, when the Moran's I statistic is greater than 0, it implies that countries with similar LEB are clustered, and whenever Moran's I statistical values are less than 0, it implies the level of dispersion, that is, a group of countries that exhibit dissimilar LEB, such as high and/or low LEB are found together (Mitchell, 2005, p. 124). Finally, the Moran's I statistical values of zero imply a random pattern.

## SPATIAL AUTOREGRESSIVE MODEL, SPATIAL LAG MODEL, AND SPATIAL ERROR MODEL

The research for the monograph follows the procedures of Anselin (1988) and Lukongo and Rezek (2016) as well as the standard practice of the generalized spatial model discussed in the spatial econometrics literature, publications, and journals for examining spatial dependence. The researcher starts the analytical processes with the generalized spatial model and its reduced form used by the Anselin (1988) and Lukongo and Rezek (2016). According to Anselin and Berra (1988) and Lukongo and Rezek (2016), the application of model procedure takes into account three competing models that differ by their respective restrictions. The three competing models are (1) the traditional linear regression model, (2) the linear spatial lag model, and (3) the spatial error model. Therefore, the generalized model is stated in equation 3as follows:

$$y = pWy + X\beta + u, \quad u = \lambda Wu + \varepsilon, \tag{3}$$

In relation to the model (or equation 3) "y" represents LEB; "X" is a matrix of commonly used LEB predictors or indicator variables such as socioeconomic variables (education, growth in health, and political unrest variables such as civil war or conflicts, minor and major wars); β is a vector of parameter coefficient associated with the explanatory or predictive variables; u is the innovation or a shock to be introduced; ε represents the error term or white noise or otiose that follows the normal distribution; and λ is the measure of the strength of spatial dependence in the disturbances (or error term) of the model. The model (equation 3) is estimated by using the maximum likelihood estimation procedure (Anselin, 1988; Lukongo and Rezek, 2016).

## VARIABLES USED IN THE SPATIOTEMPORAL ANALYSIS

The research for the book used LEB as the dependent or criterion variable. According to World Health Organization (2000) "LEB" is defined as the mean number of years still to be lived by a person at birth. The researcher used LEB because Mathers et al. (2003) strongly argued that even though this measure of health outcome is not perfect, it is probably the best available indicator to reflect the health status of the population in a given country.

However, the explanatory variables or regressors or independent variables used in the research for the manuscript were obtained from several kinds of literature of eminent authorities and agencies such World Bank, WHO, Barro and Lee, and IMF datasets and published articles. The explanatory variables include growth in health (i.e., changes in LEB), education, war, and conflict in Africa.

There is a wide consensus in the literature on educational attainment as an input in the health production function. Empirical evidence on both developed and developing countries shows that education is significantly positively correlated with health outcomes and is likely to be a causal factor in the production of health (Aka and Dumont, 2008; Becker, 2007; Cutler and Leras-Muney, 2006; Grossman, 2000; Adu-Frimpong, 2016; Guisan and Exposito, 2007). According to Barro and Lee (2010, 2012), Grossman (2000), and World Health Organization (2000), education is expected to improve quality of life (or life expectancy). These and other publications have suggested that better educated people generally have healthier behaviors. For example, they are more likely to eat a healthier diet, exercise, seek preventive care, and better understand and comply with medical treatments.

Nonetheless, according to Health Systems Performance Assessment (2003), income is correlated with health outcomes (i.e., life expectancy). It has been argued that higher income by itself does not make people healthier (Grossman, 2000; World Bank, 2016; Lauritsen, 2016; Wangwe, 1998; World Health Organization, 2000). It does, however, affect health by facilitating access to the goods and services that contribute to improving health and longevity, such as better nutrition and housing (Health Systems Performance Assessment, 2003, p. 686). It also enables the society to develop better health technologies (Health Systems Performance Assessment, 2003, p. 686). In addition, the level of income per capita may also reflect general working conditions in the country, as wealthier economies tend to have a higher share of service industries and occupations, which are considered to be less health damaging than manufacturing or construction (Grossman, 2000; World Bank, 2016; Lauritsen, 2016; Wangwe, 1998; World Health Organization, 2000).

Taking also into account such political and civil unrest variables as civil war, political instability, general warfare, and conflict are all expected to have a negative association with life expectancy (or health outcome). These instability components of an economy are likely to lead to misallocation of health care resources by channeling them to defense or military sector instead of health care to ensure quality of life among citizens (Lauritsen, 2016; Ali and Matthews, 1999; World Health Organization, 2000; Elbadawi and Sambanis, 2000; Annan, 2014; Jeffrey, 2010). World Health Organization 2000 report revealed that war (or conflict) is also a major source of low life expectancy and economic growth in Africa. In 2000, the WHO reported that children growing up in Sierra Leone (or any of the war-torn zones) can expect to live healthily for fewer years than in any other country in the world.

## RELIABILITY AND VALIDITY

According to Babbie and Schutt (2012), reliability and validity are related or intertwined, while Neuman (2012) has argued that they are not related. Both theoretical and empirical reviews from renowned scholars revealed that data must be both valid and reliable before it can be used in inferential analysis. With that in mind, reliability is also understood as the duplicable nature of findings (Babbie and Schutt, 2012). The research for the monograph used an existing concept and definition of reliability suggested by Nachmias and Nachmias (2008, p. 155). Nachmias and Nachmias (2008) defined reliability as the ratio of the true score to observe score variance (Nachmias and Nachmias, 2008, p. 155), expressed as:

Reliability = $\sigma_t^2/\sigma_x^2 = (\sigma_x^2 - \sigma_e^2)/\sigma_x^2$ where, $\sigma_t^2$ = variance of true score, $\sigma_e^2$ = variance of errors, and $\sigma_x^2$ = variance of observed scores. Therefore, according to Nachmias and Nachmias (2008, p. 155) the reliability measure varies on a scale from 0 to 1, having the value zero (0) when the measurements display nothing but error, and reaching the value 1 when the measurements display no variable error at all. Practically, the researcher adopted the test-retest method for the data sets across two separate independent authorities, to compute for the correlation between the two sets of observations (scores). The researcher obtains a reliability estimate of 0.98, which is close to 1. Therefore, there is a strong evidence of reliability on the instruments, techniques, as well as the data sets utilized.

Conversely, validity is also understood as the capacity of an instrument or procedure to measure accurately. According to Cronbach (1984, p. 121) and Nachmias and Nachmias (2008, p. 150) empirical validity is concerned with the relationship between a measuring instrument and the measuring outcome.

These scholars as well as scientists assume that if a measuring instrument is valid, the results produced by applying the instrument and the relationships existing among the variables measured in the real world should be quite similar. This particular assumption of empirical validity is consistent with the book's findings such that spatial spillover of civil war value is a strong predictor of LEB. This is practically true because outbreaks of war affect the quality of healthy life due to issues in food security and outbreaks of diseases and deteriorate the standard of living of a given nation. For the purpose of predictive validity, the researcher estimated the predictive validity by assessing the results that this book expects to obtain against some other external measure or criterion and by comparing them to estimate the correlation coefficient. Here, the researcher finds a high degree of correlation value of 0.89 between the two observations. Finally, regarding the construct validity, the researcher establishes construct validity by relating the measuring instrument (spatiotemporal packages such as GIS, ArcGIS, GeoDa, LISA, Moran's I statistics, etc.) to the general theoretical framework (spatial analytics) to determine their logical and empirical ties to concepts and theoretical assumptions. This current research for the monograph satisfies the reliability and validity conditions at all levels.

## BOOK'S DATA ANALYSIS

The research for the book employs two empirical strategies for data analysis. The first strategy is the use of the spatiotemporal analysis to create different maps in LEB across all regions in Africa based on the following divisions: (1) over decades starting 1960s–2000s, (2) Cold War and post-Cold War, (3) divisions of African political cycles, and (4) contemporary independence era (phases 1 and 2) and African Renaissance period.

Furthermore, the research for the monograph adopts Moran's I statistics and Moran scatterplot to test for spatial autocorrelation and measures whether the spatial pattern of the variables are clustered, dispersed, or random. Finally, for the book, spatial specification search is utilized to identify the best fit spatial regression model by examining the following: (1) spatial autoregressive model, (2) spatial lag model, and (3) spatial error model.

*Chapter 4*

# Spatiotemporal Analysis of Life Expectancy and Conflict-*cum*-War in Africa

This part of the book—also known as chapter 4—presents the main findings of my research for the publication in an exhaustive discussion. That is made up of the descriptive statistics and the spatial regression analyses. Changes in LEB, which happens to be across the African countries, are presented by using five decades, which start from the 1960s to 2000s. It should, however, be noted that percent changes have been obtained in order to show the progress made, if only to prolong lives through the provision of sound public policy, which enhances among other factors of sustainable development, the public health across the continent. Very briefly, as stated earlier in chapter 1, the purpose of the research in this book is to understand the changes in life expectancy across regions and time in Africa, mostly in order to inform public policy.

## ADDRESSING THE BOOK'S RESEARCH QUESTIONS AND HYPOTHESIS

In fact, three research questions were outlined for the purposes of completing the final research for the book. The first two questions are subject to in-depth spatial temporal and regression analyses of LEB data sets. The third research question is perhaps being used to observe the extent to which geospatial and econometric models may inform public health policy in Africa.

## DYNAMICS AND TRENDS MAPS OF LEB OVER THE PAST FIVE DECADES, 1960–2015

This segment of the analysis for the book has two parts. The first describes changes in LEB across the African countries as shown in figures 4.1–4.5. The second part reveals the percent change (increase or decrease) of the LEB across the study area by using the difference in the average LEB over the past five decades. In order to address the fundamental research questions guiding the study, forty-seven African countries were used.

It is very important to note that the 1960s—as described by researchers, including historians and political scientists—happened to be a decade of the Gregorian calendar that began on January 1, 1960, and ended on December 31, 1969 (Zeitz, 2010), a nine-year period. The term "1960s" also refers to an era more often called the sixties, denoting the complex of inter-related cultural and political trends around the globe (Barth, 1984; Janet, 2007; Zeitz, 2010). In Africa, the 1960s was a period of radical political change as thirty-two countries gained independence from their European colonial rulers (see Barth, 1984; Janet, 2007; Zeitz, 2010 for more details). The transformation of Africa from colonialism to independence, which was termed as the era of decolonization of Africa, dramatically accelerated during the decade (i.e., 1960s), with thirty-two countries gaining independence between 1960

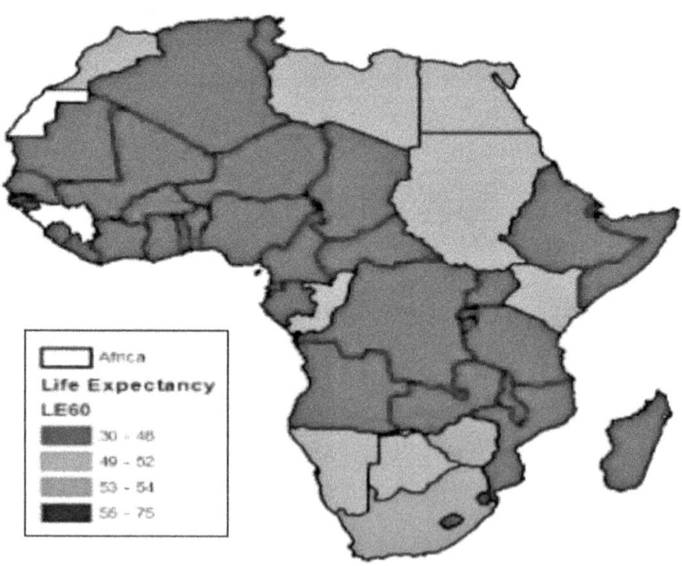


**Figure 4.1 Life Expectancy at Birth from 1960 to 1969 (1960s).** Data source: World Bank, 2016.

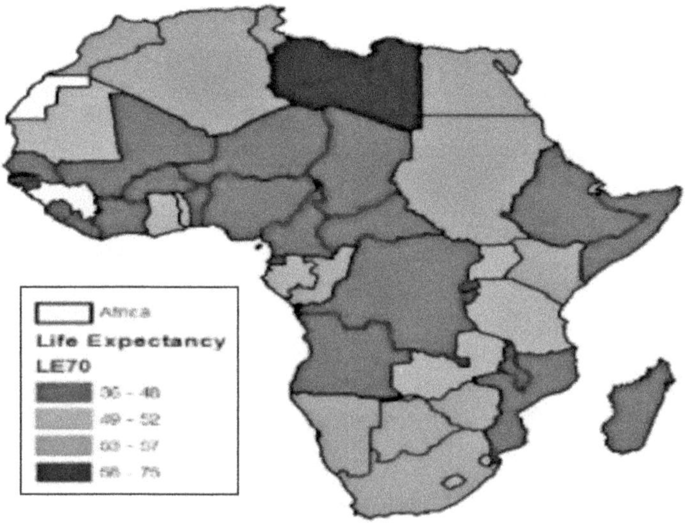


**Figure 4.2 Life Expectancy at Birth from 1970 to 1979 (1970s).**

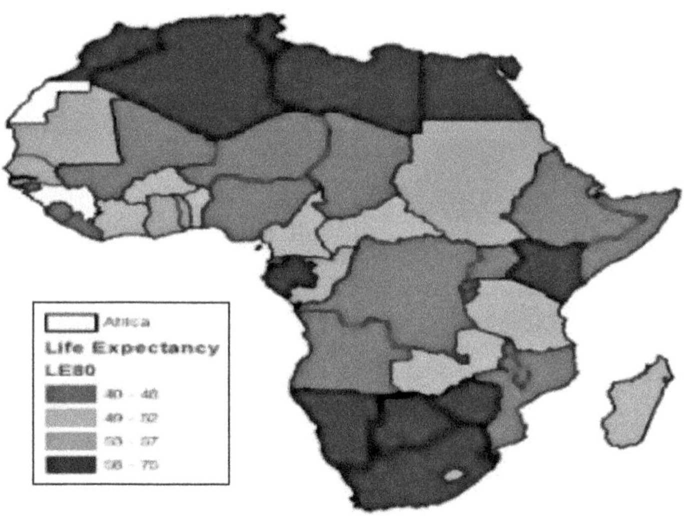


**Figure 4.3 Life Expectancy at Birth from 1980 to 1989 (1980s).**

and 1968, marking the end of the European empires that once dominated the African continent (Barth, 1984; Janet, 2007; Zeitz, 2010).

However, the ambitious political aspirations of these new nations quickly faded or diminished for various reasons (Barth, 1984; Janet, 2007; Marwick, 1998; Zeitz, 2010), and in the end, many of the nations descended

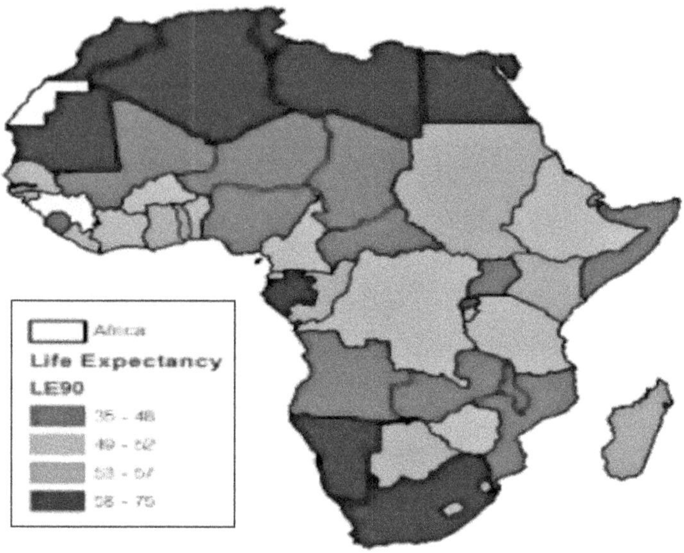


**Figure 4.4 Life Expectancy at Birth from 1990 to 1999 (1990s).**

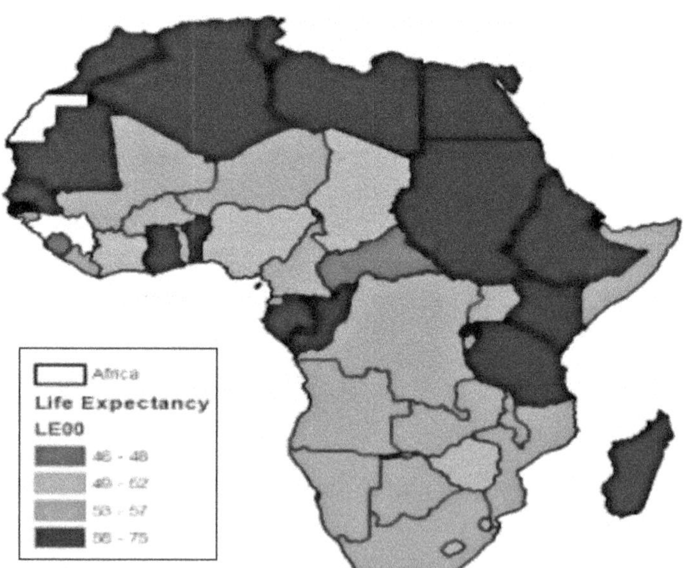


**Figure 4.5 Life Expectancy at Birth from 2000 to 2015 (2000s).**

into anarchy (United Nations, 2013), as well as kleptocracy, dictatorships, and/or civil war (Barth, 1984; Janet, 2007; Marwick, 1998; United Nations, 2013; Zeitz, 2010). Unfortunately, the road to prosperity has been difficult; during the 1960s, by many measures including LEB. To be specific, Africa continues to possess the poorest population in the world as well as the lowest LEB (Barth, 1984; Janet, 2007; Marwick, 1998; Zeitz, 2010). The foregoing evidence is from the World Bank data source of LEB in the first decade (1960–1969).

For the sake of consistency across decades, four quartiles have been applied to the life expectancy data throughout this study. The first quartile ranges from 30 to 49 (i.e., lowest LEB or 25 percentile), while the second quartile ranges from 49 to 52 (i.e., middle LEB or 50 percentile). It should be noted that the third quartile goes from 53 to 54 (i.e., high LEB or 75 percentile), and the last one ranges from 55 to 75 (i.e. very high LEB or 100 percentile). In fact, in relation to the data analysis, the majority of the African countries were not doing well in terms of the number of years, an average African is likely to live between 56 years (minimum) and 75 years (maximum). That is, about 84% of the African countries (i.e., forty-five countries) were located or centered at the lowest level or 25 percentile of the LEB distribution. As shown in figure 4.1, during the 1960s, the majority of African countries (i.e., 84%) had a minimum LEB of 30 years and a maximum of 48 years. It is important to stress that the 84% of the countries include countries in the western region of Africa and Central Africa (except Republic of Congo), in the Indian Ocean Island (i.e. Madagascar), eastern part of Africa, and some parts of southern Africa (i.e., Angola, Zambia, Malawi, Mozambique, and Tanzania), and the northern part of Africa (i.e., Algeria and Tunisia).

Meanwhile, only 15% of the African countries were located at the 50 percentile of the LEB distribution, with a minimum number of years a person can live in those countries pegged at 49 years. But, none can exceed a maximum of 52 years. These median life expectancy countries include Republic of Congo, Morocco, Libya, Egypt, Sudan, Kenya, Namibia, and Botswana. However, there were two countries in southern Africa (i.e., South Africa and Zimbabwe), which are in the 75 percentile of the LEB, with a minimum number of years a person can live in these two countries being 53 years and a maximum of 54 years. Based on the data, none of the African countries was located within the 100 percentile. This implies that the average number of years an average African is likely to live in the 1960s was less than 56 years, and this can be attributed to the political upheavals or instability, independence struggles, poverty, and minor as well as major wars experienced by many of the African countries.

Taking for example between 1951 and 1962, the following countries experienced bitter war for independence: Libya (in 1951), Morocco (in 1956),

Tunisia (in 1956), Sudan (in 1956), Ghana (in 1957), and Algeria (in 1962). Therefore, within the subsequent decades of 1960s (or between 1961 and 1967) the following African countries also went through independence struggles and finally attained their freedom from their colonial powers: Congo DRC (in 1960), Nigeria (in 1960), Somalia (in 1960), Tanzania (in 1961), Uganda (in 1962), Sierra Leone (in 1961), Rwanda (in 1962), Burundi (in 1962), Kenya (in 1963), Malawi (1964), Zambia (in 1964), Gambia (in 1965), Zimbabwe (in 1965), Lesotho (in 1966), Botswana (in 1966), and Swaziland (in 1968). Additionally, many of the African countries, in the 1960s, encountered a series of wars (minor or major) and conflicts. Some examples of the series of major and minor wars encountered by some of the African countries include the 1960s civil war in South Sudan as well as the civil war in Congo, formerly Belgian Congo (between 1960 and 1965) and the Nigeria-Biafra civil war in Nigeria (1967).

It is important to point out the fact that the political upheavals or instability, struggles for independence, poverty, geopolitics, and minor as well as major civil wars or conflicts in Africa were the possible major causes of the downward spiral of LEB in Africa during the first decades (1960s). To be very specific, relating to wars or conflicts in the 1960s, about fourteen African countries engaged in minor wars, nine African countries engaged in civil wars, fifteen African countries engaged in conflicts, and five African countries engaged in major wars (Angola, DRC, Egypt, Nigeria, and Sudan).

Among crucial events which took place in the 1960s were the Organization of Africa Unity (OAU), which was formed in Ethiopia in 1963 by African leaders, and the discovery of oil in some parts of Africa. Some of the oil-discovered African countries between the 1960s and 1970s include the following: Tanzania, Kenya, Uganda, Ethiopia, Somalia, Somaliland, and Eritrea, commencing with the 1950s, Nigeria (in 1950s), Libya (in 1960s), Sierra Leone (in 1960s), Liberia (in 1960s), and Ethiopia (in 1960s). Also, in the subsequent decade of 1970s (between 1970 and 1979), Africans experienced an improvement in LEB. An example is what happened in the northern part of Africa as shown in figure 4.2, whereby almost all the countries have an average minimum LEB of 55 years in the 1970s and a maximum of 57 years. Notice that a decade ago; the majority of Africans were not able to live beyond 50 years. However, Libya was an exceptional African country in the 1970s to be placed in the 100 percentile, with a minimum of 58 years of LEB and a maximum of 75 years of LEB. Additionally, 41% of the African countries were located between 50 and 75 percentile of the LEB distribution with a minimum number of years a person can live in those countries being put at 49 years and a maximum of 57 years.

Unlike the 1960s, whereby about 84% of the Africa countries (i.e., forty-five countries) were located or placed at the lowest level or 25 percentile of the LEB distribution with a minimum years of 36 years and a maximum years of 48, in 1970s about 57% of the African countries (i.e., thirty-one countries) were located or centered at the lowest level or 25 percentile of the LEB distribution. Subsequently, the reduction in the 25 percentile of the LEB distribution implies an improvement in 27% of African countries with the expectation that people were living a bit longer than before. Meanwhile, the improvement in LEB in the 1970s could be attributed to several factors, including the political freedoms (or independence) many of the African countries (i.e., thirty-one countries) have obtained prior to the 1970s as well as the discovery of natural resources (especially oil in the northern part of Africa), improvement in per capita income from $997 (in 1960s) to $ 1,385 (in 1970s), and the formation of the OAU in 1963, which championed Africa's growth in the various economies and expanded the quality of life for the citizenry.

In the 1980s (thus, between 1980 and 1989), Africa experienced a significant improvement in the people's LEB. Looking at figure 4.3 for example, in all of Northern Africa, with an exception of Sudan, the average minimum LEB was 58 years in the 1980s, with a maximum of 75 years as compared to the 1960s where none of the African countries were living above 55 years. See figures 4.1 and 4.3, respectively, for a detailed account. Additionally, countries like Namibia, South Africa, Botswana, Zimbabwe, and Swaziland in the southern region of Africa, Kenya in East Africa, and Gabon in Central Africa, with 100 percentile, saw a minimum of 58 years of LEB and a maximum of 75 years of LEB. Furthermore, about 24% of the African countries (i.e., thirteen countries) were placed between 50 and 75 percentile of the life expectancy cycle at birth distribution with a minimum number of years a person can live in those countries being 49 years, but with a maximum of 57 years.

Unlike the 1960s, whereby about 84% of the African countries (i.e., forty-five countries) experienced the lowest level (or 25 percentile) of the LEB, with a minimum of 36 years and a maximum of 48 years, in 1980s about 33% of the African countries (i.e. eighteen countries) also experienced the lowest level (or 25 percentile) of the LEB distribution. Overall, the reduction in the 25 percentile of the LEB distribution implies an improvement in LEB in Africa generally, but with the expectation that people were living a bit longer than before.

Indeed, the improvement in LEB in the 1980s could as well be attributed to the attainment of political freedom (or independence) by many of the African countries prior to the 1970s, coupled with the discovery of natural resources (including oil several places in the Northern Africa), improvement in per capita income, private sector development (i.e., in the case of Botswana) and the formation of the OAU in 1963, which championed improvement in the lifestyles and growth in the economies of various Africans nations.

Figure 4.4 describes the 1990s' LEB across Africa. In fact, the 1990s was also termed as Africa's Renaissance period (see Schraeder, 2014, p. 6; Vale and Maseko, 1998 for more details). The Africa's Renaissance period (or 1990s) marks the rebirth of economic, social, and political freedom that had been extinguished during the colonial era and subsequently denied to African peoples by dictatorial elites during the initial decades of the contemporary independence era (see Schraeder, 2014, p. 6; Vale and Maseko, 1998 for more details). With reference to the World Bank's data sources between 1990 and 1999, Africa experienced a high improvement in LEB. Taking for example, in the Northern Africa, about 99% of the countries in the region had an average minimum LEB of 58 years in the 1990s, and a maximum of 75 years, with an exception of Sudan, which has an average minimum LEB of 53 years in the 1990s and a maximum of 57 years.

Unfortunately, countries like Swaziland and Botswana, which were within the 100 percentile in the 1980s, did fall back to the 75 percentile in the 1990s. However, the decline in LEB is attributed to the status of the *HIV/AIDS* epidemic in some of the sub-Saharan African countries. These include South Africa, Lesotho, *Swaziland*, *Botswana*, Namibia, Zambia, and Zimbabwe (USAID, 2001; Caldwell and Caldwell, 1996). Madagascar moved from the 50 percentile in the 1980s to 75 percentile in the 1990s. Meanwhile, Zimbabwe also fell back from 100 percentile in the 1980s to 50 percentile in the 1990s, while Kenya also fell back from 100 percentile in the 1980s to 75 percentile in the 1990s.

Additionally, countries like Namibia and South Africa in the southern part of Africa, Mauritania in Western Africa, and Gabon in the Central Africa were also placed within the 100 percentile with a minimum of 58 years of LEB, and also a maximum of 75 years of LEB. This improvement in LEB could be attributed to improvement in quality health care in those countries. That is, the Healthcare Access and Quality (HAQ) Index in Gabon and some part of the region provided a summary measure of health care access and quality for a given location. This measure was based on risk-standardized mortality rates or mortality-to-incidence ratios from causes that, in the presence of quality health care should not result in death—also known as amenable mortality (Healthcare Access and Quality Index, 2016).

Unlike the 1980s, whereby 33% of the African countries (i.e., eighteen countries) were located or placed at the lowest level (or 25 percentile) of the LEB distribution, with a minimum of 36 years but a maximum of 48 years, the 1990s saw about 24% of the African countries (i.e., thirteen countries) within the lowest level (or 25 percentile) of the LEB distribution. Although a slight increment (or improvement) is observed in the LEB across all of the African countries, but the increment could be termed as increase in LEB with a decreasing rate (this typically confirms the setback observed between the 1980s and the 1990s).

Figure 4.5 illustrates life expectancy rates at birth for Africans in the 2000s (or the last decade) within the study area. The 2000s' diagram (or map) reveals substantial gains in LEB across the African continent as reported in figure 4.5. For instance, in the 1980s, almost all of the southern part of Africa were within 100 percentile with a minimum of 58 years of LEB but a maximum of 75 years of LEB, a high rate which started fading in the 1990s, and finally settled at 75 percentile with a minimum of 53 years of LEB and a maximum of 57 years of LEB.

The first part of the 2000s (2000–2010) was marked by a great improvement in the LEB across the study area, as compared to the past four decades. This is because, in the 2000s, about 15% of the African countries (i.e., a total of eight countries) were within 100 and 75 percentile with a minimum of 46 years of age in the LEB and a maximum of 52 years of LEB. While 85% of the citizens of several African countries were likely to live up to 75 years (maximum), countries like Sierra Leone in West Africa and Central African Republic did not show any improvement, in the LEB over the past five decades. Also, countries like Lesotho, Swaziland, Ivory Coast, Nigeria, Chad, and Zimbabwe showed downward spiral, with respect to life expectancy, over the past four decades with a slight increase from 25 percentile (bottom) to the middle 50 percentile. In a nutshell, the majority of the countries across Africa are facing ups-and-downs spiral in LEB for the past five decades. However, the ups-and-downs spiral in the LEB, for the past five decades, could be attributed to the political upheavals or instability the continent was facing, coupled with the cost of their independence struggles, societal poverty, lack of economic growth, as well as devastating civil wars experienced by many of the African countries from the 1960s to the present.

## EMPIRICAL TEST OF CHANGES IN LEB OVER THE PAST FIVE DECADES

Table 4.1 reveals the average number of years the African continent gained or obtained within its life expectancy rates over the past five decades. In fact, after the ending of the independence struggles of the 1960s in many of the African countries, Africa continent gained or saw an increase in the average age of about 5 years (or 4.615 years) between 1960s and 1970s (thus, during the era of the struggle for independence).

This is evidenced by a significant difference between 1960s and 1970s (4.615) with an associated $p$ value of 0.000 less than 5% significance level.

**Table 4.1 Changes in Life Expectancy at Birth between Decades and over Africans Political Divisions or Cycles**

| | *Paired Differences* | | | | | | | |
|---|---|---|---|---|---|---|---|---|
| | | | | *95% Confidence Interval of the Difference* | | | | |
| *Changes in Life Expectancy at Birth over the Five Decades* | *Mean* | *Std. Deviation* | *Std. Error Mean* | *Lower* | *Upper* | *t* | *Df* | *Sig. (2-tailed)* |
| Between 1960s and 1970s (Struggle for Independence) | 4.615 | 1.859 | 0.258 | 4.098 | 5.133 | 17.900 | 51 | 0.000 |
| Between 1970s and 1980s (Start of Political Competitions, 1970–1989) | 4.308 | 2.414 | 0.335 | 3.636 | 4.980 | 12.871 | 51 | 0.000 |
| Between 1980s and 1990s (End of Cold War, 1947–1991) | 1.189 | 3.883 | 0.533 | 0.118 | 2.259 | 2.229 | 52 | 0.030 |
| Between 1990s and 2000s (African Renaissance Period from 1990 to present) | 4.208 | 4.829 | 0.663 | 2.876 | 5.539 | 6.343 | 52 | 0.000 |

*Note:* Ho: $\mu_{1960s} = \mu_{1970s}$; Ha: $\mu_{1960s} \neq \mu_{1970s}$; $t = \left(\bar{X}_{1970s} - \bar{X}_{1960s}\right) - \left(\mu_{1970s} - \mu_{1960s}\right) / se\left(\bar{X}_{1970s} - \bar{X}_{1960s}\right)$. For decision rule of the paired differences are significant if the calculated t-values are greater than two or the associated $p$ values are less than 0.01 (or 1%), 0.05 (or 5%), and 0.10 (or 10%).

Also, between the 1970s and 1980s (which is also termed as the "start of political competition, 1970–1989"), the African continent gained an average age rate of about 4 years (or 4.308 years), which was less than the improvement in the mean age gained between the 1960s and the 1970s (i.e., 4.615). This is confirmed by a significant difference between the 970s and the1980s (4.308), with an associated $p$ value of 0.000 less than 5% significance level. However, between the 1980s and the 1990s, there was a sharp drop in the average age gain from barely 5 years to 1 year. This implies that the continent lost an average age of 4 years in its life expectancy rate between the 1960s and the 1990s. Particularly, this section of the analysis confirms the ups and downs in the LEB across the study area and the changes in the patterns of the various decades map. Nonetheless, this could be attributed to the numerous political upheavals, including coups d'état that occurred during the period. In many of the African countries, between the 1960s and the 1990s, the military was perceived as being the only group that could effectively maintain law and order; as a result, it ruled many nations in Africa during the 1970s and early 1980s (Simon, 1995; Lucien, 2001; Aryeetey, Harrigan, and Nissanke, 2000). During the period between the early 1960s and the late 1980s, Africa experienced more than seventy coups and thirteen presidential assassinations (Simon, 1995; Lucien, 2001; Aryeetey, Harrigan, and Nissanke, 2000).

Finally, there was a rebound in LEB across the African continent between the 1990s and 2000s, thus in the contemporary independent era (phase II, 1990s–present) or the beginning of the African Renaissance period in 1990. It also showed that between the 1990s and the 2000s, the African continent gained an average age of 4.208 years, which is as well less than the average age gained between the 1960s and 1970s. This analysis is, therefore, consistent with the assertion by Roser (2015) about LEB across Africa. The author argued that in 1970, as the social indicators of Africans were slowly but progressively improved in all the years in many of the African countries, the statistics of LEB among these countries still, by today's standard, showed a large disappointment (Roser, 2015).

Meanwhile, World Health Organization, WHO (2000) and Chia-Wei (2009) have revealed some possible factors, which were likely to account for the low life expectancy across Africa. They included famine, war, poor government spending, corruption, low level of education, availability of clean water, and the wide-spread of several devastating diseases, including HIV/AIDs and the Ebola disease. However, due to improvement in the provision of medical care and the living standards of the citizenry in many African countries, life expectancy has seen a steady growth.

## ADDRESSING RESEARCH QUESTION 1: TO WHAT EXTENT CAN SPATIOTEMPORAL ANALYSES BE USED TO COMPREHEND BETTER LIFE EXPECTANCY IN AFRICA?

Two main analyses were used to address the research question one: (1) analysis of testing for spatial dependence and (2) identification of spatial clusters.

### Testing for Spatial Dependence

In the process of answering the research question one, the study begins by first testing for the hypothesis of spatial randomness in LEB across Africa against the alternative hypothesis of spatial autocorrelation or dependence. These tests were conducted using twelve alternative specifications of spatial weight matrix: queen of Order 1–4, k-nearest neighbors of 1–4, and general distance threshold with 734-mile, 800-mile, 850-mile, and 900-mile radius between two countries for all decades between 1960 and 2015. The test results are presented in table 4.2. The first panel in table 4.2 represents the spatial weight matrix; the second panel describes the global Moran's I output for 1960s and 1990s, respectively. The third panel represents the results of the LISA for 1960s and 1990s, respectively, and the fourth panel describes the Moran's I output for 1970s and 2000s, respectively. The fifth panel represents the results of the LISA for 1970s and 2000s respectively and the sixth panel illustrates the global Moran's I output for 1980s and the seventh panel represents the results of the LISA for 1980s.

As for the 1960s and 1980s (or contemporary independence phase I), the results of the spatial dependence or autocorrelation are presented in table 4.2 from columns 1 to 15. Columns 1, 6, and 11 of table 4.2 present the global Moran's I output, while columns 2–5 in 1960s, columns 7–10 in 1970s, and columns 12–15 in 1980s of table 4.2 present the LISA results. Meanwhile, columns 2, 7, and 12 of table 4.2 represent the HH LEB African countries. This means that high life expectancy countries are surrounded by high life countries.

Columns 3, 8, and 13 of table 4.2 represent high-low (HL) LEB African countries, which indicate that high life expectancy countries are neighbors to low life expectancy countries. Columns 4, 9, and 14 of table 4.2 represent low-high (LH) LEB African countries, which suggest that low life expectancy countries are neighbors to high life expectancy countries. Columns 5, 10, and 15 of table 4.2 represent low-low (LL) LEB African countries, that is, low life expectancy countries are neighbors to low life expectancy countries. For the purposes of statistical significance of the global Moran's I statistics as shown in table 4.2, the researcher compares the calculated $p$ values associated

**Table 4.2 Detecting Spatial Autocorrelation Using the Life Expectancy at Birth and Its Spatially Weighted Average, 1960–1989 (or Contemporary Independence Phase I) and 1990–2015 (or Contemporary Independence Phase II)**

| *Decades* | *1960s* | | | | | *1970s* | | | | | *1980s* | | | | | *1990s* | | | | | *2000s* | | | | |
|---|---|---|---|---|---|---|---|---|---|---|---|---|---|---|---|---|---|---|---|---|---|---|---|---|---|
| | | *LISA* | | | | | *LISA* | | | | | *LISA* | | | | | *LISA* | | | | | *LISA* | | | |
| *Spatial Weight Matrix* | *Moran's I* | *HH* | *HL* | *LH* | *LL* | *Moran's I* | *HH* | *HL* | *LH* | *LL* | *Moran's I* | *HH* | *HL* | *LH* | *LL* | *Moran's I* | *HH* | *HL* | *LH* | *LL* | *Moran's I* | *HH* | *HL* | *LH* | *LL* |
| Queen | [1] | [2] | [3] | [4] | [5] | [6] | [7] | [8] | [9] | [10] | [11] | [12] | [13] | [14] | [15] | [16] | [17] | [18] | [19] | [20] | [21] | [22] | [23] | [24] | [25] |
| Queen of Order 1 | 0.1439** | 5 | 0 | 2 | 4 | 0.1058* | 5 | 2 | 1 | 4 | 0.0402 | 3 | 2 | 1 | 2 | 0.0441 | 2 | 1 | 1 | 2 | 0.0190 | 2 | 1 | 1 | 0 |
| | (0.0490) | | | | | (0.0770) | | | | | (0.2050) | | | | | (0.2260) | | | | | (0.4590) | | | | |
| Queen of Order 2 | 0.1024** | 9 | 2 | 3 | 6 | 0.0451* | 4 | 2 | 4 | 6 | 0.0281 | 1 | 2 | 1 | 1 | 0.0534 | 0 | 1 | 1 | 0 | 0.0843* | 2 | 1 | 2 | 0 |
| | (0.0180) | | | | | (0.0740) | | | | | (0.4930) | | | | | (0.2510) | | | | | (0.0620) | | | | |
| Queen of Order 3 | 0.1196*** | 14 | 4 | 3 | 8 | 0.0684** | 9 | 3 | 7 | 5 | 0.0044 | 2 | 1 | 4 | 2 | 0.0495 | 0 | 2 | 0 | 0 | 0.0332 | 0 | 1 | 2 | 1 |
| | (0.0020) | | | | | (0.0120) | | | | | (0.1510) | | | | | (0.1760) | | | | | (0.3930) | | | | |
| Queen of Order 4 | 0.0780*** | 16 | 7 | 5 | 13 | 0.0414** | 11 | 4 | 7 | 5 | 0.0009 | 4 | 3 | 7 | 2 | 0.0415 | 1 | 1 | 2 | 1 | † | † | † | † | † |
| | (0.0020) | | | | | (0.0110) | | | | | (0.1300) | | | | | (0.1590) | | | | | | | | | |
| K-nearest neighbors | | | | | | | | | | | | | | | | | | | | | | | | | |
| 1-nearest neighbor | 0.2195* | 2 | 1 | 0 | 0 | 0.1885* | 1 | 1 | 0 | 0 | 0.2188** | 4 | 1 | 0 | 1 | 0.3434** | 2 | 1 | 0 | 0 | 0.2609** | 4 | 2 | 0 | 1 |
| | (0.0650) | | | | | (0.0610) | | | | | (0.0450) | | | | | (0.0150) | | | | | (0.0380) | | | | |
| 2-nearest neighbor | 0.1132* | 3 | 2 | 0 | 1 | 0.0988 | 7 | 1 | 0 | 1 | 0.1069 | 5 | 0 | 0 | 1 | 0.1481* | 3 | 0 | 0 | 0 | 0.0522 | 3 | 0 | 1 | 1 |
| | (0.0950) | | | | | (0.1240) | | | | | (0.1260) | | | | | (0.0900) | | | | | (0.1890) | | | | |
| 3-nearest neighbor | 0.1385* | 4 | 1 | 1 | 5 | 0.1166* | 4 | 1 | 1 | 5 | 0.0884* | 4 | 1 | 0 | 2 | 0.0799 | 3 | 0 | 1 | 2 | 0.0099 | 3 | 1 | 1 | 1 |
| | (0.0650) | | | | | (0.0730) | | | | | (0.0980) | | | | | (0.1420) | | | | | (0.3210) | | | | |
| 4-nearest neighbor | 0.1514** | 3 | 1 | 1 | 5 | 0.1043* | 2 | 2 | 0 | 5 | 0.0519 | 3 | 2 | 0 | 3 | 0.0383 | 1 | 2 | 0 | 1 | 0.0028 | 3 | 3 | 1 | 0 |
| | (0.0450) | | | | | (0.0850) | | | | | (0.1570) | | | | | (0.1990) | | | | | (0.3470) | | | | |
| Distance Threshold | | | | | | | | | | | | | | | | | | | | | | | | | |
| 734 miles | 0.1137* | 3 | 2 | 0 | 6 | 0.1006* | 6 | 2 | 0 | 5 | 0.0628 | 7 | 2 | 0 | 2 | 0.0666 | 4 | 2 | 1 | 0 | 0.0258 | 3 | 2 | 1 | 0 |
| | (0.0640) | | | | | (0.0750) | | | | | (0.1480) | | | | | (0.1600) | | | | | (0.2330) | | | | |
| 800 miles | 0.1470** | 2 | 1 | 1 | 6 | 0.1246** | 5 | 3 | 1 | 5 | 0.0843* | 5 | 3 | 0 | 3 | 0.0795 | 3 | 3 | 0 | 1 | 0.0394 | 3 | 4 | 0 | 1 |
| | (0.0390) | | | | | (0.0370) | | | | | (0.0890) | | | | | (0.1150) | | | | | (0.1870) | | | | |
| 850 miles | 0.1395** | 5 | 3 | 2 | 6 | 0.1121** | 4 | 3 | 1 | 4 | 0.0640 | 2 | 3 | 0 | 4 | 0.0597 | 4 | 3 | 0 | 0 | 0.0220 | 3 | 4 | 0 | 0 |
| | (0.0360) | | | | | (0.0420) | | | | | (0.1100) | | | | | (0.1150) | | | | | (0.2280) | | | | |
| 900 miles | 0.1383** | 5 | 2 | 2 | 7 | 0.0978* | 5 | 2 | 1 | 4 | 0.0448 | 2 | 4 | 1 | 3 | 0.0396 | 2 | 4 | 0 | 0 | † | † | † | † | † |
| | (0.0220) | | | | | (0.0510) | | | | | (0.1520) | | | | | (0.1660) | | | | | | | | | |

*Note:* $p$ values are reported in parentheses underneath the Moran's I statistic, $p$ value $< 0.01$; $0.01 < p$ value $< 0.05$; $0.05 < p$ value $< 0.10$; $p$ value $> 0.10$. Figures in columns 16 and 21 represent the estimated value of the Moran's I. Moran's I $> 0$ indicates a clustered pattern where similar values are together. Moran's I $= 0$ indicates that there is no obvious pattern or a random arrangement of data, and Moran's I $< 0$ shows a dispersed pattern where high and low values are interspersed. *, **, *** statistically significant at 10%, 5%, and 1% respectively. † indicates that the results are not attainable based on the neighborhood structure showed with queen of Order 4, fourth nearest neighbor, and the threshold distance of 900 mile-radius between two African countries.

with the global Moran's I statistics against the convention critical values of 0.01, 0.05, and 0.10 as the basis for evaluation. The manuscript establishes strong evidence of significant spatial clustering of LEB across countries and time, specifically in the 1960s. That is, the LEB is similar in neighboring countries in the 1960s. Regarding the spatial dependency test for the1960s, column 1 of table 4.2 shows evidence of spatial clustering with queen contiguity of Order 1, 2, 3, and 4. The Moran's I ranges from 0.0780 to 0.1439 and are significant for positive spatial autocorrelation at the 1%, 5%, and 10% levels as shown in column 1 of table 4.2. Furthermore, in the 1960s, the author tests for spatial dependence using the k-nearest-neighbor specification of the weighted matrix, with k ranging from 1 (minimum neighbor) to 4 (maximum neighbors).

The results, also shown in column 1 of table 4.2, indicate strong spatial dependence in LEB when considering 1 to 4 nearest neighbors in specification. The Moran's I statistics range from 0.1132 to 0.2195 and are significant at the 5% and 10% significance levels. Again, in the 1960s, the general distance threshold approach yields similar results. As shown in column 1 of table 4.2, using the arc distance weight matrix with maximum distances of about 734, 800, 850, and 900 miles between capital cities, the researcher also detects the presence of clustering in LEB. The Moran's I ranges from 0.1137 to 0.1470 and are significant at the 5% and 10% levels. These results in the 1960s corroborate the view that a positive and significant spatial clustering exists between African countries with similar health outcomes (or LEB). That is, neighboring African countries tend to have similar LEB (or health outcomes). Furthermore, based on these results, the queen Order 4 spatial weight matrix and, 900-mile distance weight matrix appear to be the best choice to be carried forward in the regression analysis for 1960s. This is because the queen Order 4 spatial weight matrix reveals a very similar high LEB in sixteen countries that constitute the hotspot of life expectancy in Africa and, thirteen countries are the coldspots, that is, low LEB countries surrounded by low LEB countries. In addition, similar results were obtained when using the 900-mile distance weight matrix. It should be noted that five high LEB countries surrounded by high LEB countries, which represent the hotspot and seven low LEB countries surrounded by low LEB countries, which form the coldspot.

For the case of the spatial dependence test for the1970s, column 6 of table 4.2 shows evidence of spatial clustering with queen contiguity of Order 1, 2, 3 and 4. The Moran's I ranges from 0.0414 to 0.1058 and are significant for positive spatial autocorrelation at the 5%, and 10% levels as shown in column 6 of table 4.2. Again, in the 1970s, the manuscript tests for spatial dependence using the k-nearest-neighbor specification of the weighted matrix, with k ranging from 1 (minimum neighbors) to 4 (maximum neighbors). The results, also shown in column 6 of table 4.2, indicate some degree of spatial dependence in LEB when considering 1 to 4 nearest neighbors in specification. The Moran's I statistics range from 0.1043 to 0.1885 and are significant at the 10% significance level. Moreover, in the 1970s, the general distance threshold approach is shown in column 6 of table 4.2, using the arc distance weight matrix with maximum distances of about 734, 800, 850, and 900 miles between capitals cities. The general distance threshold approach detects the presence of clustering or strong spatial dependence in LEB in the 1970s. The Moran's I ranges from 0.0978 to 0.1246 and are significant at the 5% and 10% levels. These results in the 1970s reveal strong positive and significant spatial clustering among African countries with similar health outcomes (or LEB). That is, neighboring African countries tend to have similar LEB (or health outcomes). Toward this end, the results of the queen Order 4 spatial weight matrix and, 734-mile distance weight matrix appear to be the best choice to be carried forward in the regression analysis for 1970s.

Furthermore, in relation to the spatial dependence test for the1980s, column 11 of table 4.2 shows no evidence of spatial clustering with queen contiguity of Order 1, 2, 3, and 4. Again, in the 1980s, the study tests for spatial dependence using the k-nearest-neighbor specification of the weighted matrix, with k ranging from 1 neighbor to 4 neighbors. The results, also shown in column 11 of table 4.2, indicate strong evidence of spatial dependence in LEB when considering 1 and 3 nearest neighbors in specification. The Moran's I statistics range from 0.0884 to 0.2188 and are significant at the 5% and 10% significance levels. Moreover, in the 1980s, the general distance threshold approach is shown in column 11 of table 4.2, using the arc distance weight matrix with maximum distances of about 734, 800, 850, and 900 miles between capitals cities.

Indeed, the general distance threshold approach detects the presence of clustering or strong spatial dependence in LEB in the 1980s for only 800 miles, with a Moran's I value of 0.0843 at 10% significance level. These results in the 1980s reveal weak positive and significant spatial clustering among African countries with similar health outcomes (or LEB). That is, neighboring African countries tend to have similar LEB (or health outcomes). Toward this end, the results of the first nearest neighbor spatial weight matrix and 800-mile distance weight matrix appear to be the best choice to be carried forward in the regression analysis for 1980s.

Regarding the 1990s and 2000s, also known as the contemporary independence phase II, the results of the spatial dependence or autocorrelation are presented in table 4.2 from columns 16 to 23. Columns 16–21 of table 4.2 present the global Moran's I output, while columns 17–20 and 22–25 of table 4.2 present the LISA results for the 1990s and the 2000s, respectively. Note that the 2000s covers years 2000–2015.

Columns 17 and 22 of table 4.2 represent HH LEB African countries, and columns 18 and 23 of table 4.2 represent HL LEB African countries. Columns 19 and 24 of table 4.2 represent LH LEB African countries, and columns 20 and 25 of table 4.2 represent LL LEB African countries. Here, the researcher also compares the calculated *p* values associated with the global Moran's I statistics in columns 16 and 21 against the convention critical values of 0.01, 0.05, and 0.10 to evaluate their significance level.

For the case of the spatial dependence test for the1990s, column 16 of table 4.2 shows no evidence of spatial clustering with queen contiguity of Order 1, 2, 3, and 4. In addition, the general distance threshold approach (about 734, 800, 850, and 900 miles between capitals cities) yields similar results. The general distance threshold approach discovers no evidence of the presence of clustering in LEB. This is because given the available data, the LEB is not statistically correlated with the neighboring countries' "weighted average LEB" within the 1990s.This could be related to the economic, social, and political transformations that many of the African countries were going through in the 1990s termed as the African Renaissance (see Schraeder, 2004, p. 6 for more details).

Above all, the researcher tests for spatial dependence using the k-nearest-neighbor specification of the weighted matrix, with k ranging from 1 to 4. The results, also shown in column 16 of table 4.2, indicate some degree of spatial dependence in the LEB when considering 1–2 nearest neighbors in specification. The Moran's I statistics range from 0.1481 to 0.3434 and are significant at the 5% and 10% significance levels. These results in the 1990s reveal weak positive and significant spatial clustering among African countries with similar health outcomes (or LEB). That is, African countries with a minimum of one neighbor and a maximum of two neighbors in the 1990s tend to have similar LEB (or health outcomes).

Subsequently, regarding the spatial dependence test for the 2000s, column 21 of table 4.2 shows no evidence of spatial clustering using queen contiguity of Order 1, 2, 3, and 4. Furthermore, the general distance threshold approach yields similar results. As shown in column 21 of table 4.2, the general distance threshold approach also discovers no evidence of spatial clustering in LEB in the 2000s using the arc distance weight matrix with maximum distances of about 734, 800, 850, and 900 miles between capital cities. This is because given the available data, the LEB is not statistically correlated with the neighboring countries "weighted average LEB" during the last decade (2000s). This could be related to the economic, social, and political transformations many of the African countries were going through in the 1990s that were extended to the 2000s (see Schraeder, 2004, pp. 6–7 for more details).

Finally, the author tests for spatial dependence using the k-nearest-neighbor specification of the weighted matrix, with k ranging from 1 to 4. The results, also shown in column 21 of table 4.2, indicate some degree of spatial dependence in the LEB when considering 1 nearest neighbor in specification. The Moran's I statistic for the 1 nearest neighbor is 0.2609 and is statistically significant at the 5% significance level. Therefore, the results of the first nearest neighbor spatial weight matrix appear to be the best choice to be carried forward in the regression analysis for 2000s.

## IDENTIFICATION OF SPATIAL CLUSTERS OF LEB IN AFRICA, 1960–2015

As the Moran's I statistic is a global measure of the spatial dependence, it does not indicate where high or low LEB countries are located. The author used Moran scatterplot and LISA to gain insights into clustering at the local level for all decades. The results are shown in figure 4.6A for 1960s and figure 4.6B for 2000s, as shown sequentially below starting from 1960s to 2000s (see Appendix I for more details). The four quadrants of the figure 4.6 display four types of spatial clusters: HH, LL, HL, and LH. These figures

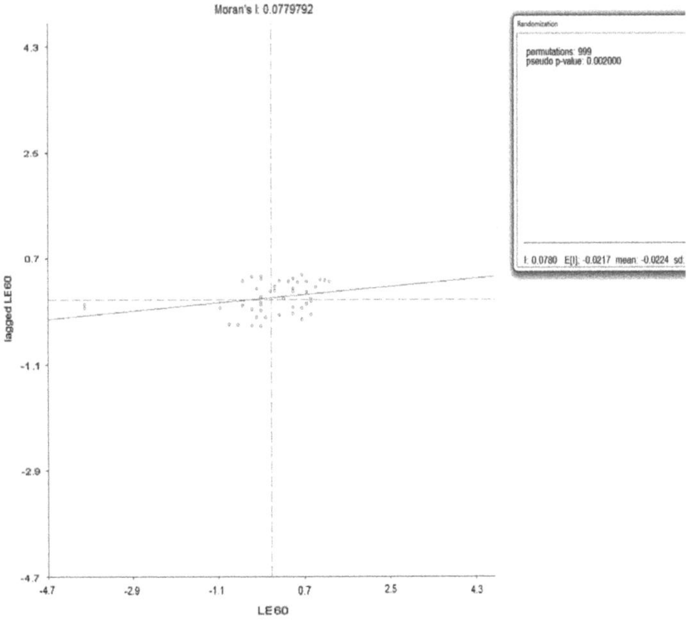


**Figure 4.6A Moran Scatterplot of Life Expectancy at Birth in Africa, 1960s.** *Note:* Scatterplot with a Moran's I = 0.0780*** using queen of Order 4 spatial weight matrix. The queen of Order 4 spatial weight matrix is because it reveals the highest hotspot and coldspot with a statistical significance at 10%, 5%, and 1%.

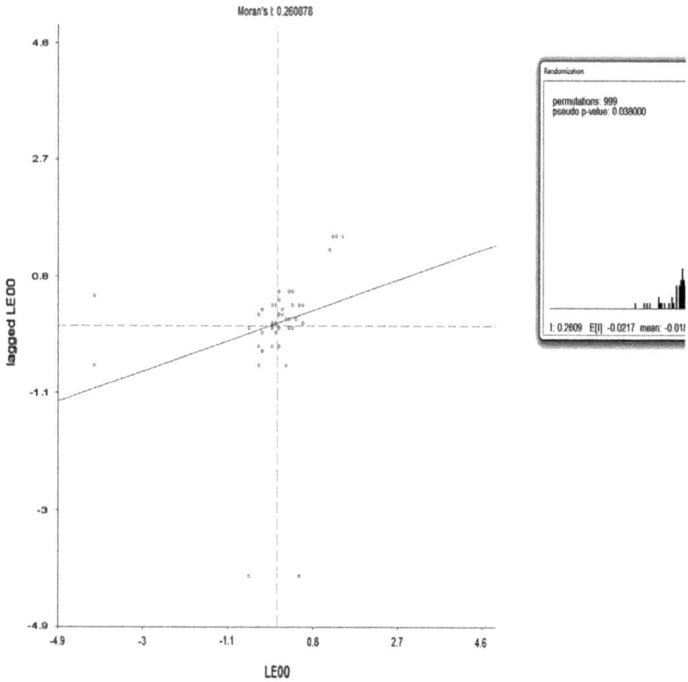


**Figure 4.6B Moran Scatterplot of Life Expectancy at Birth in Africa, 2000s.** *Note:* Scatterplot with a Moran's I = 0.2609** using k-nearest neighbor of Order 1 spatial weight matrix. The 1-nearest neighbor of spatial weight matrix is used in the analysis because it reveals the highest hotspot and coldspot with a statistical significance at 10% and 5%.

have standardized deviation from the mean of LEB on the x-axis and spatially lagged LEB on the y-axis, which is the standardized deviation from the mean of LEB multiplied by the spatial weight matrix. Therefore, HH implies that high LEB take place in countries, which are neighbors to other high LEB countries that are located in the northeast quadrant (HH). Furthermore, the high LEB countries surrounded by low LEB countries located in the southeast quadrant (HL). Low LEB countries surrounded by high LEB countries were also found in northwest quadrant (LH). Finally, low LEB countries that neighbor other low LEB countries were also found in the southwest quadrant (LL).

For the case of the 1960s, figure 4.6A reveals high LEB countries that neighbor other high LEB countries located in the northeast quadrant (HH) to include Kenya, Uganda, Djibouti, Burundi, Rwanda, DRC, Gabon, Congo, Zambia, Zimbabwe, Botswana, Namibia, South Africa, Lesotho, and Swaziland. Meanwhile, the High LEB countries which were surrounded by low LEB countries located in the southeast quadrant (HL) include Ghana, Togo,

Libya, Tunisia, Algeria, Morocco, and Mauritania. However, the low LEB countries which were surrounded by high LEB countries were found in northwest quadrant (LH) and include Angola, Malawi, Mozambique, Ethiopia, and Somalia. Finally, the low LEB countries that neighbor other low LEB countries were found in the southwest quadrant (LL) and include Chad, Niger, Nigeria, Benin, Burkina Faso, Mali, Senegal, Gambia, Guinea Bissau, Guinea, Sierra Leone, Liberia, and Ivory Coast (or Côte d'Ivoire).

In relation to the 1970s, LEB dataset, the result demonstrates high LEB countries that neighbor other high LEB countries located in the northeast quadrant (HH) to include Kenya, Gabon, Congo, Zambia, Zimbabwe, Tanzania, Botswana, Namibia, South Africa, Lesotho, and Swaziland. Between the 1960s and 1970s, the following countries drop from the northeast quadrant (HH)—Djibouti, Uganda, DRC, Burundi, and Rwanda. Meanwhile, the high LEB countries which were surrounded by low LEB countries located in the southeast quadrant (HL) in the 1970s include Ghana, Tunisia, Algeria, and Mauritania. Also, between the1960s and 1970s, the following countries drop from the southeast quadrant (HL)—Togo, Libya, and Morocco. However, the Low LEB countries which were surrounded by high LEB countries were found in northwest quadrant (LH) and include Equatorial Guinea, Angola, Malawi, Rwanda, Burundi, Mozambique, and Somalia. Finally, the low LEB countries that neighbor other low LEB countries were found in the southwest quadrant (LL) and include Niger, Gambia, Guinea Bissau, Sierra Leone, and Liberia. In a nutshell, between the 1960s and 1970s the following countries drop from the southwest quadrant (LL)—Nigeria, Chad, Benin, Burkina Faso, Mali, Senegal, Guinea, and Ivory Coast (or Côte d'Ivoire). Additionally, Ethiopia also drops from the northwest quadrant (LH) between the 1960s and 1970s.

Furthermore, in relation to the 1980s, the analysis of the LEB dataset demonstrates high LEB countries that neighbor other high LEB countries located in the northeast quadrant (HH) to include Algeria, Tunisia, Libya, Egypt, and Lesotho. Between the 1960s and 1980s, the following countries drop from the northeast quadrant (HH)—Kenya, Gabon, Congo, Zambia, Zimbabwe, Tanzania, Botswana, Namibia, South Africa, Djibouti, Uganda, DRC, Burundi, and Rwanda. Meanwhile, the high LEB countries which were surrounded by low LEB countries located in the southeast quadrant (HL) in the 1980s include Ghana, Senegal, and Mauritania. Also, between the1960s and 1980s, the following countries drop from the southeast quadrant (HL)—Tunisia, Algeria, Togo, Libya, and Morocco. However, there were no low LEB countries which were surrounded by high LEB in 1980s. Finally, the low LEB countries that neighbor other low LEB countries were found in the southwest quadrant (LL) and include Gambia, Guinea Bissau, and Sierra Leone. In a nutshell, between the 1960s and 1980s the following countries drop from the southwest quadrant (LL)—Nigeria, Liberia, Niger, Chad, Benin, Burkina Faso, Mali, Senegal, Guinea, and Ivory Coast (or Côte d'Ivoire). Additionally, Equatorial Guinea, Angola, Malawi, Rwanda, Burundi, Mozambique, and Somalia Ethiopia also drop from the northwest quadrant (LH) between the 1960s and 1980s.

Regarding the 1990s' LEB dataset, the result demonstrates high LEB countries, which are neighbors of other high LEB countries, are located in the northeast quadrant (HH) to include Algeria, Tunisia, and Egypt. Between the 1960s and 1990s, the following countries drop from the northeast quadrant (HH)—Libya, Kenya, Gabon, Congo, Zambia, Zimbabwe, Tanzania, Botswana, Namibia, Lesotho, South Africa, Djibouti, Uganda, DRC, Burundi, and Rwanda. In addition, there were no high LEB countries which were surrounded by low LEB countries located in the southeast quadrant (HL) in the 1990s. Additionally, there were no low LEB countries which were surrounded by high LEB in 1990s. Finally, there were no low LEB countries which were surrounded by low LEB in 1990s.

In relation to the 2000s LEB dataset, figure 4.6B illustrates the Moran Scatterplot of LEB from 2000 to 2015. The result demonstrates high LEB countries that neighbor other high LEB countries located in the northeast quadrant (HH) to include Egypt and Sudan. Between the 1960s and 2000s, the following countries drop from the northeast quadrant (HH)—Morocco, Algeria, Tunisia, Libya, Kenya, Gabon, Congo, Zambia, Zimbabwe, Tanzania, Botswana, Namibia, Lesotho, South Africa, Djibouti, Uganda, DRC, Burundi, and Rwanda. Meanwhile, per the data, Senegal was the only high LEB country surrounded by low LEB countries located in the southeast quadrant (HL) in the 2000s. Additionally, Chad was the only low LEB country which was surrounded by high LEB in 2000s. Finally, there were no low LEB countries which were surrounded by low LEB in the 2000s.

## SPATIAL CLUSTERS AND IDENTIFICATION OF HOTSPOTS AND COLDSPOTS IN LEB IN AFRICA, 1960–2015

Hotspots and coldspots are composed of significant clusters of HH and LL LEB countries. According to Anselin (1995) the permutation approach is used to calculate for the local Moran's I in order to identify the significant clusters of HH and LL LEB countries.

In the 1960s, fifteen countries passed the test of significance at 10%, 5%, and 1% levels for the formation of the hotspots: Kenya, Uganda, Djibouti, Burundi, Rwanda, DRC, Gabon, Congo, Zambia, Zimbabwe, Botswana, Namibia, South Africa, Lesotho, and Swaziland (see figure 4.7A for more

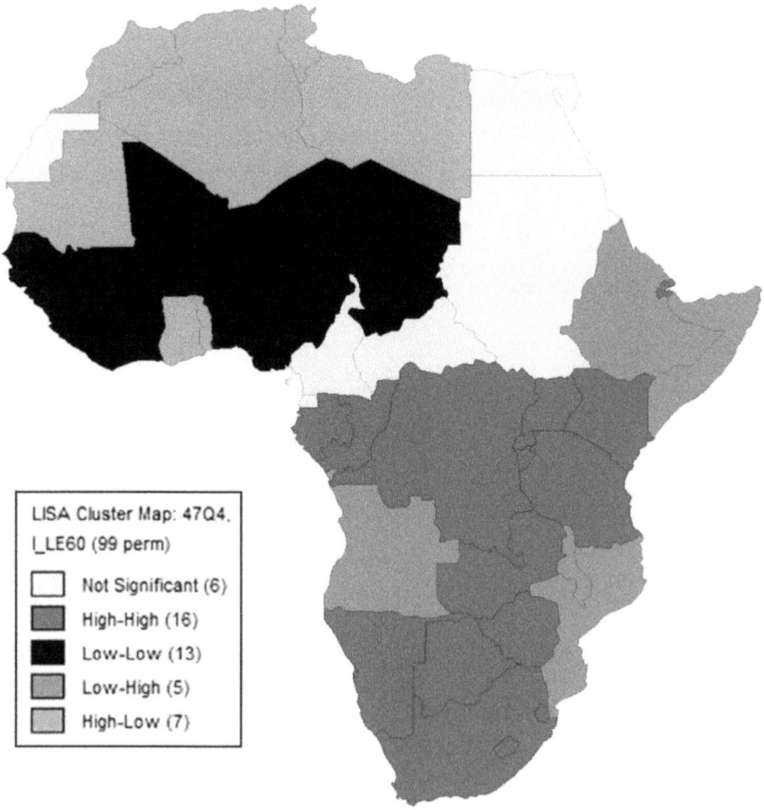


**Figure 4.7A Spatial Clusters and Identification of Hotspots and Coldspots in Life Expectancy at Birth in Africa, 1960s.** *Source*: The spatial weight matrix queen of Order 4 was employed on LISA cluster map.

details). However, the coldspots were located by using similar analysis. The following African countries form the coldspot by passing the significant test at the 10%, 5%, and 1% levels of significance: Chad, Niger, Nigeria, Benin, Burkina Faso, Mali, Senegal, Gambia, Guinea Bissau, Guinea, Sierra Leone, Liberia, and Ivory Coast (see figure 4.7A for more details). These results shown in figure 4.7A are consistent with previously reported World Bank (2016) data on LEB in the 1960s.

In the 1970s, eleven countries pass the test of significance at 10%, 5%, and 1% levels for the formation of the hotspots: Kenya, Gabon, Congo, Zambia, Zimbabwe, Tanzania, Botswana, Namibia, South Africa, Lesotho, and Swaziland (see figure 4.7B more details). However, the coldspots were located by using similar analysis. Five African countries form the coldspot by passing the significant test at the 10%, 5%, and 1% levels of significance—Niger,

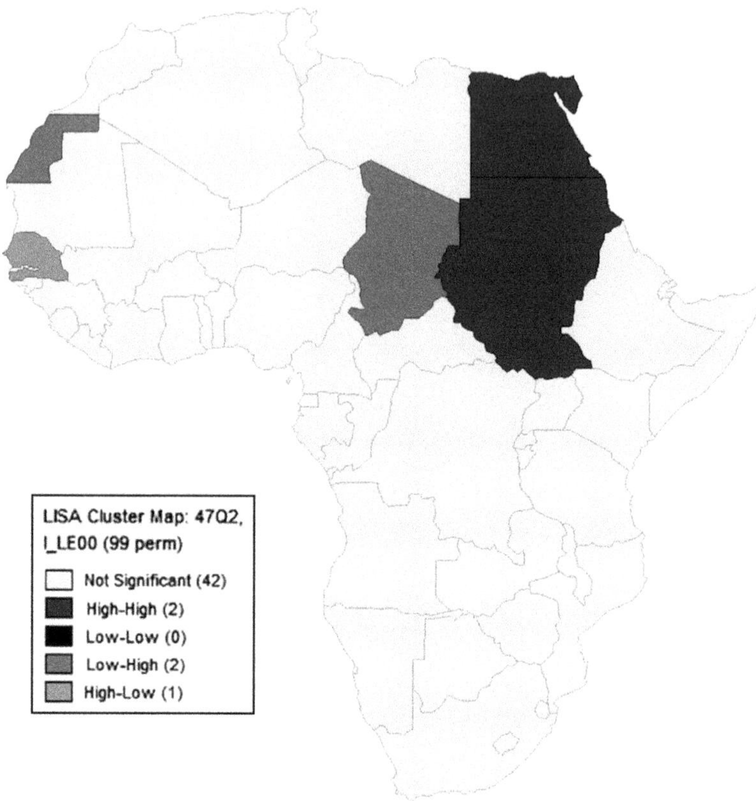


**Figure 4.7B Spatial Clusters and Identification of Hotspots and Coldspots in Life Expectancy at Birth in Africa, 2000s.** *Source*: The spatial weight matrix queen of Order 2 was employed on LISA cluster map.

Gambia, Guinea Bissau, Sierra Leone, and Liberia (see table 4.2 for more details).

In the 1980s, five African countries pass the test of significance at 10% and 5% levels for the formation of the hotspots: Algeria, Tunisia, Libya, Egypt, and Lesotho (see table 4.2 for more details). However, the coldspots were located by using similar analysis. Perhaps, three African countries form the coldspot by passing the significant test at the 10% and 5% levels of significance: Gambia, Guinea Bissau, and Sierra Leone.

In the 1990s, three African countries pass the test of significance at 10% and 5% levels for the formation of the hotspots: Algeria, Tunisia, and Egypt (see table 4.2 for more details). However, given the available information (or data) there was no statistically significant coldspots formation in the 1990s.

In the 2000s, two African countries pass the test of significance at 10%, and 5% levels for the formation of the hotspots: Egypt and Sudan (see figure 4.7B for more details). However, given the available information (or data) there was no statistically significant coldspots formation in the 2000s (see figure 4.7B for more details). Nonetheless, the ups-and-downs spiral of the spatial dependence and clustering tests during the Cold War era (1947–1989) and/or contemporary independence phase I (1960s–1989), could be attributed to the numerous political upheavals, including coups d' etat that occurred during the period. In many of the African countries, between the 1960s and the 1990s, the military was perceived as being the only group that could effectively maintain law and order; as a result it ruled many nations in Africa during the 1970s and early 1980s (Simon, 1995; Lucien, 2001; Aryeetey, Harrigan, and Nissanke, 2000). During the period between the early 1960s and the late 1980s, Africa experienced more than seventy coups and thirteen presidential assassinations (Simon, 1995; Lucien, 2001; Aryeetey, Harrigan, and Nissanke, 2000). Furthermore, during the African Renaissance period (1990–present) or the post-Cold War era (1990–present), the African countries transformation process in terms of social, economic, political, and health have slowed down over the last two decades. This is empirically observed in the statistical significant of the hotspot and the coldspot clustering location of LEB in the 1990s and 2000s (see Schraeder, 2004, pp.6–8 for more details).

## ADDRESSING THE BOOK'S RESEARCH QUESTION 2: WHAT IS THE BEST SPATIAL ECONOMETRIC MODEL THAT IS SUITABLE FOR EXPLAINING LIFE EXPECTANCY IN AFRICA?

The main purpose of the spatial econometric models is to investigate the spatial consequence or dependence of the education and political unrest factors (conflicts, civil war, minor and major wars, etc.) on the health outcome, LEB, across the study area. In order to answer the research question two, the researcher searched for a best spatial model portraying spatial dependence.

## SEARCH FOR A BEST SPATIAL MODEL PORTRAYING SPATIAL DEPENDENCE

The results of the previous section suggest spatial dependence in the data. The researcher of the monograph estimates three competing equations to determine how to best model this spatial dependence: (1) a standard regression model, (2) a spatial lag model, and (3) a spatial error model. The researcher evaluates these three models based on the significance of their coefficients and applies the standard procedures for assessing their goodness of fit and detecting spatial autocorrelation in the models' residuals. For the comparison purposes, the researcher uses the same explanatory variables in the standard model, the spatial lag model, and the spatial error model. Similarly, the research for the monograph uses the same spatial weight matrices in estimating the spatial lag model and the spatial error model and in investigating spatial autocorrelation among the residual of the standard model. The explanatory and control variables include education, previous state of LEB, and war or conflict dummy variable.

A second layer of search for the spatial model consists of testing spatial autocorrelation in the residuals of the standard regression model, the spatial lag model, and the spatial error model. Empirical research for the monograph suggests that the best spatial model should be free of spatial autocorrelation in its residuals. According to Anselin (1995, 1988), Anselin and Berra (1998), and Lukongo and Rezek (2016), among others, the presence of significant residual spatial clustering undermines the potential of model to be the best candidate for portraying the generating process in the data. The standard practice in data-driven spatial empirical studies is to report the best model based on the optimal spatial weight matrix. As mentioned previously, the matrix is the queen Order 4. However, distance-based weight matrix fails to identify the spatial effects. To conserve space, these results are not shown here but are available upon request.

## LEB EQUATION

The results of the standard regression model are shown in columns 1–4 of table 4.3. I find that war reduces LEB by 1.31%. I also find that growth in health care (or historical trend of LEB) increases the present LEB by 1.084 % per year. An additional year of average education increases LEB by 0.863% per year.

The Moran's I statistic for the residuals of the standard regression model, as shown on the bottom panel of table 4.3, indicates the presence of spatial autocorrelation (1.853* in column 2, 1.939* in column 3, and 4.107*** in column 4 in table 4.3). Given these results, the standard practice in applied spatial research is to conduct a specification search, using alternative models (spatial lag model or spatial error model) with the same spatial weight matrix, and validate the preferred model based on diagnostics for spatial dependence and measures of fits.

Based on the higher Moran's I statistic, the researcher use the queen contiguity spatial weight matrix of Order 4 in the LEB-war regression analysis to estimate both the spatial lag model and the spatial error model. The results are presented in columns 5–12 of table 4.3.

**Table 4.3 Life Expectancy at Birth and War: Standard Regression Model, Spatial Lag, and Spatial Error Model**

| *Variables* | *Standard Model (OLS)* | | | | *Spatial Lag Model (MLE)* | | | | *Spatial Error Model (MLE)* | | | |
|---|---|---|---|---|---|---|---|---|---|---|---|---|
| *Dependent Variable: LFB, 1970–1979* | *(1)* | *(2)* | *(3)* | *(4)* | *(5)* | *(6)* | *(7)* | *(8)* | *(9)* | *(10)* | *(11)* | *(12)* |
| | *Q1* | *Q2* | *Q3* | *Q4* | *Q1* | *Q2* | *Q3* | *Q4* | *Q1* | *Q2* | *Q3* | *Q4* |
| Explanatory Variables | | | | | | | | | | | | |
| Major War | −1.307** | −1.307** | −1.307** | −1.307** | † | −1.0193* | † | −0.3078** | † | −1.3665** | † | −1.256** |
| | (0.0282) | (0.0282) | (0.0282) | (0.0282) | | (0.0533) | | (0.0015) | | (0.00969) | | (0.0173) |
| LFB60 | 1.084*** | 1.084*** | 1.084*** | 1.084*** | † | 1.0934*** | † | 1.1023*** | † | 1.1029*** | † | 1.1043*** |
| | (0.000) | (0.000) | (0.000) | (0.000) | | (0.0000) | | (0.0000) | | (0.0000) | | (0.0000) |
| Control Variable | | | | | | | | | | | | |
| Education | 0.863 | 0.863 | 0.863 | 0.863 | † | 0.8297 | † | 0.7859 | † | 0.8304 | † | 0.7665 |
| | (0.132) | (0.132) | (0.132) | (0.132) | | (0.1307) | | (0.1502) | | (0.1331) | | (0.1641) |
| Constant | 1.528 | 1.528 | 1.528 | 1.528 | † | 7.7935** | † | 14.9202*** | † | 0.7581 | † | 0.5838 |
| | (0.181) | (0.181) | (0.181) | (0.181) | | (0.0020) | | (0.0006) | | (0.5087) | | (0.6391) |
| Specification Search | | | | | | | | | | | | |
| Spatial lag effects (Rho) | - | - | - | - | † | −0.1484 * * | † | −0.3078 * * | † | - | † | - |
| | | | | | | (0.0067)[a] | | (0.0015)[a] | | | | |
| Spatial Error Effects (Lambda) | - | - | - | - | † | - | † | - | † | 0.4132* | † | 0.6223 * * |
| | | | | | | | | | | (0.0976)[a] | | (0.0116)[a] |
| Measure of Fit Log Likelihood | −94.963 | −94.963 | −94.963 | −94.963 | † | −91.651 | † | −93.860 | † | −94.180 | † | −90.4423 |
| AIC | 195.926 | 195.926 | 195.926 | 195.926 | † | 191.302 | † | 193.719 | † | 194.361 | † | 188.885 |
| BIC | 201.476 | 201.476 | 201.476 | 201.476 | † | 198.703 | † | 199.270 | † | 199.911 | † | 196.285 |
| Spatial Dependence | | | | | | | | | | | | |
| LM (Lag) | 0.763 | 5.135** | 1.341 | 6.225** | | | | | | | | |
| | (0.382)[b] | (0.024)[b] | (0.247)[b] | (0.013)[b] | | | | | | | | |
| Robust LM (Lag) | 0.932 | 6.130** | 2.988* | 7.798** | | | | | | | | |
| | (0.335)[b] | (0.013)[b] | (0.084)[b] | (0.005)[b] | | | | | | | | |

(Continued)

**Table 4.3 Life Expectancy at Birth and War: Standard Regression Model, Spatial Lag, and Spatial Error Model** *(Continued)*

| *Variables* | *Standard Model (OLS)* | | | | *Spatial Lag Model (MLE)* | | | | *Spatial Error Model (MLE)* | | | |
|---|---|---|---|---|---|---|---|---|---|---|---|---|
| *Dependent Variable: LFB, 1970–1979* | *(1)* *Q1* | *(2)* *Q2* | *(3)* *Q3* | *(4)* *Q4* | *(5)* *Q1* | *(6)* *Q2* | *(7)* *Q3* | *(8)* *Q4* | *(9)* *Q1* | *(10)* *Q2* | *(11)* *Q3* | *(12)* *Q4* |
| LM (Error) | 0.247 | 1.300 | 0.697 | 2.3739 | | | | | | | | |
| | (0.619)[b] | (0.254)[b] | (0.404)[b] | (0.123)[b] | | | | | | | | |
| Robust LM (Error) | 0.415 | 2.296 | 2.344 | 3.947** | | | | | | | | |
| | (0.519)[b] | (0.130)[b] | (0.126)[b] | (0.047)[b] | | | | | | | | |
| LM (SARMA) | 1.1789 | 7.431** | 3.685 | 10.172** | | | | | | | | |
| | (0.555)[b] | (0.024)[b] | (0.158)[b] | (0.006)[b] | | | | | | | | |
| Moran's I for residuals | 0.774 | 1.853* | 1.939* | 4.107*** | | 6.6238** | | 9.0412** | | 1.5649 | | 2.2066 |
| | (0.439)[b] | (0.064)[b] | (0.052)[b] | (0.000)[b] | | (0.0101) | | (0.0026) | | (0.2110) | | (0.1374) |
| Spatial Weight Matrix | Queen of Order 1 | Queen of Order 2 | Queen of Order 3 | Queen of Order 4 | | Queen of Order 2 | | Queen of Order 4 | | Queen of Order 2 | | Queen of Order 4 |

*Note:* LFB = life expectancy at birth; OLS = ordinary least square; MLE = maximum likelihood estimation; AIC = Akaike information criterion; BIC = Bayesian information criterion; LM = Lagrange multiplier test for spatial dependence; SARMA = spatial autoregressive moving average. $p$ values are reported in parentheses underneath the three regression estimation values, $p$ value $< 0.01$; $0.01 < p$ value $< 0.05$; $0.05 < p$ value $< 0.10$; $p$ value $> 0.10$. † indicates that the results are not attainable based on the neighborhood structure showed with queen of Order 1 and 3 between two African countries for both spatial lag and error models. [a]$p$ values of spatial lag and error models are in parentheses. I use forty-seven contiguous countries in Africa. [b]$p$ values are reported in brackets to evaluate spatial dependence in columns 1–4. *, **, *** statistically significant at 10%, 5%, and 1%.

The specification search suggests that the coefficient associated with the spatial error effects (lambda, 0.6223**) is statistically significant at 5% and 10% conventional levels. The standard errors for lambda and rho are listed in parentheses next to these coefficients as shown in columns 5–12 of table 4.3. Given the results in columns 5–12 of table 4.3, the spatial error model is the preferred model. In the specification search process, applied researchers also utilize other measures of fit, such as log likelihood, Akaike information criterion (AIC), and Schwarz criterion or Bayesian information criterion (BIC), to guide their decisions. The research for the monograph follows the standard rule for computing spatial error and spatial lag models: the higher the log likelihood the better fit and the lower the AIC and Schwarz criterion or BIC, the better the fit. Here, the log likelihood, AIC and Schwarz criterion or BIC (−90.4423, 188.885, and 196.285) in the spatial error model are preferred to the same statistics (−93.860, 193.719, and 199.270) in the spatial lag model for queen of Order 4. The diagnostics for spatial autocorrelation and the evaluation of the model based on the measures of fit and specification search statistics suggest that the spatial error model is the model that depicts the spatial process best in cross-country LEB in Africa. The results of a final spatial autocorrelation test on the spatial error model residuals using the Moran's I are shown at the bottom of table 4.3. The researcher fail to find evidence of spatial dependence among the residuals of this model (Moran's I = 2.2066, not statistically significant) and, therefore, the research for the monograph concluded that the spatial error model is the proper specification for LEB equation relative to spatial lag model and standard model. It is very crucial to underscore that the importance of the spatial modeling strategy is not necessary more precisely estimated coefficients, but the uncovering of spatial spillovers. This particular assumption helps the researcher to answer the book's research question three.

## ADDRESSING THE BOOK'S RESEARCH QUESTION 3: TO WHAT EXTENT CAN I APPLY GEOSPATIAL AND ECONOMETRIC MODELS TO INFORM PUBLIC HEALTH POLICY IN AFRICA?

In this particular section of the monograph, whereby the researcher tends to answer the research question, to what extent can I apply geospatial and econometric models to inform public health policy in Africa, the research for the book used the spatial error model to determine the extent of spatial spillovers to inform public policy in Africa.

## DETERMINING THE EXTENT OF SPATIAL SPILLOVERS

The spatial error model appears to be the proper specification for the spatial spillover analysis. As a data-generating process, the spatial error model introduces a random shock to the three vignettes of contemporary Africa (DRC, Burundi, and Liberia), and captures both their direct impact and the propagation of that shock throughout Africa. The model also allows us to calculate the overall impact of a major armed conflict by summing the direct impacts and its diffusion across the continent. Based on the results from the column 12 of table 4.4, a major armed conflict results in a LEB shock of −1.256 %. Meanwhile, the researcher has introduced this shock into the LEB equation to model the direct impact of war. The intuition here is that a war may reduce longevity or quality of life or probability of a person being alive in a given country, but its real effects are larger because it also affects its neighbors. The indirect consequences of major armed conflicts are less visible but equally serious. To show the destructive impact of war on LEB, a spatial spillover model is used. It is written as:

$$\hat{y}^{(i)} = (I_n - \hat{\lambda}W)^{-1}\tilde{\mu}^{(j)}, \tag{4}$$

Where $\hat{y}^{(i)}$ represents the spatial spillovers or the predicted LEB, i is a given country, $I_n$ is the identity matrix, $\hat{\lambda}$ is the maximum likelihood estimated value of spatial error model coefficient (0.6223), $\tilde{\mu}^{(j)}$ is the vector that imbeds the LEB shock (−1.256%) in a specific country (j), and W represents the row-standardized spatial weight matrix-queen of Order 4.

The spatial error model allows the researcher to introduce a random shock to a specific country and capture the spatial spillovers through the entire study area. This application, including aspects of spatial (physical distance, mountains, jungles, etc.) and relational (insurgency, ethnicity, fractionalization, wealth inequality, cross-border sanctuaries, etc.) proximity often overlooked in previous studies, is not possible when using the standard regression model. The spatial spillovers are better explained by the recent civil wars in the DRC, Rwanda, Burundi, Sierra Leone, Liberia, Sudan, and Angola, where the major rebel movements have military bases in their homelands or nearby countries. The spillovers of violence are well documented in the war literature (Raleigh and Hegre, 2009). The results of the research for the monograph improves the researcher understanding of the destructive effects of civil wars on the LEB introduced in this particular study as a random shock in several ways. Studying a sample of Central African countries, Raleigh and Hegre (2009) pointed that civil conflicts are more prevalent in locations with valuable natural resources, locations distant from the capital city, or close to the borders.

**Table 4.4 Loss in Life Expectancy at Birth (LEB) in Africa due to War**

| | *Reduction in Life Expectancy at Birth* | | |
|---|---|---|---|
| *Affected African Countries (1)* | *War in Democratic Republic of Congo (2)* | *War in Burundi (3)* | *War in Liberia (4)* |
| Algeria | −0.3407 | −0.0370 | −0.0500 |
| Angola | −0.2389 | −0.2226 | −0.2603 |
| Benin | −0.3215 | −0.2956 | −0.2666 |
| Botswana | −0.5128 | −0.3724 | −0.3728 |
| Burkina Faso | −0.1484 | −0.1666 | −0.1650 |
| Burundi | −0.0835 | −0.8054 | −0.0995 |
| Cameroon | −0.5949 | −0.3741 | −0.2755 |
| Central African Republic | −0.3617 | −0.2281 | −0.4818 |
| Chad | −0.4908 | −0.3037 | −0.2306 |
| Congo, Dem. Rep. | −1.4076 | −0.2883 | −0.4002 |
| Congo, Rep. | −0.2786 | −0.2967 | −0.4134 |
| Cote d'Ivoire | −0.1331 | −0.1323 | −0.2604 |
| Djibouti | −0.3910 | −0.0210 | −0.0965 |
| Egypt, Arab Rep. | −0.2831 | −0.2553 | −0.2784 |
| Equatorial Guinea | −0.3020 | −0.2622 | −0.3014 |
| Ethiopia | −0.4511 | −0.3363 | −0.2650 |
| Gabon | −0.1992 | −0.2684 | −0.2590 |
| Gambia, The | −0.2712 | −0.1835 | −0.1170 |
| Ghana | −0.1331 | −0.1323 | −0.2604 |
| Guinea | −0.1331 | −0.1323 | −0.2604 |
| Guinea-Bissau | −0.1331 | −0.1323 | −0.2604 |
| Kenya | −0.2655 | −0.0613 | −0.1905 |
| Lesotho | −0.7065 | −0.1630 | −0.0787 |
| Liberia | −0.1818 | −0.1275 | −0.9704 |
| Libya | −0.1687 | −0.1282 | −0.1754 |
| Malawi | −0.2980 | −0.3313 | −0.2685 |
| Mali | −0.1484 | −0.1666 | −0.1650 |
| Mauritania | −0.3061 | −0.2613 | −0.3620 |
| Morocco | −0.3061 | −0.2613 | −0.3620 |
| Mozambique | −0.3367 | −0.2001 | −0.1011 |
| Namibia | −0.3573 | −0.1810 | −0.2120 |
| Niger | −0.3557 | −0.3448 | −0.3404 |
| Nigeria | −0.3557 | −0.3448 | −0.3404 |
| Rwanda | −0.1875 | −0.0314 | −0.0693 |
| Senegal | −0.1331 | −0.1323 | −0.2604 |
| Sierra Leone | −0.0057 | −0.0448 | −0.0756 |
| Somalia | 0.4052 | −0.4990 | −0.4191 |
| South Africa | −0.5241 | −0.2798 | −0.2399 |
| Sudan | −0.4591 | −0.4492 | −0.7083 |
| Swaziland | −0.6629 | −0.3673 | −0.4247 |
| Tanzania | −0.1599 | −0.0718 | −0.0002 |
| Togo | −0.2185 | −0.1850 | −0.1131 |
| Tunisia | −0.4745 | −0.0786 | −0.2372 |
| Uganda | −0.0055 | −0.0012 | −0.1603 |
| Zambia | −0.1895 | −0.2334 | −0.1617 |
| Zimbabwe | −0.5128 | −0.3724 | −0.3728 |

*Note*: Total loss in terms of life expectancy at birth or development as a result of major war from Democratic Republic of Congo, Liberia, and Burundi are presented in the above table. Numbers of columns are in parentheses from 1 to 4. The shock of −1.256 to life expectancy at birth across Africa was introduced into the three vignettes.

War can depress the productivity, human capital, food security, infrastructures, economic growth, literacy rate, cultural capital, tourism, social capital, and trade networks. It also damages the overall sectors (primary, secondary, and tertiary) productivity through the destruction of infrastructure (roads, bridges, etc.) and uncertainty, which increase the transaction costs and the input prices, production costs and discourages food production and investments. The spread of diseases is prevalent among internally displaced persons, families, and community due to lack of adequate shelter (malaria), and the lack of safe clean drinking water and poor sanitation (diarrhea, cholera, etc.) both on their homeland and inside the refugee camps. War depresses LEB, longevity, and the probability of a person living a healthy good life or being alive in a given country due to spread of diseases, insecurity, fear of death, systematic rapes increase spread of HIV/AIDs, and psychological trauma triggered by frequent violence. The spillovers of violence or wars have forced many citizens to flee for their lives into other areas in the same country, to refugee camps, deep into the forest, or neighboring countries they depend on humanitarian assistance or they have access to marginal land and resources just to survive.

Furthermore, war does hold backs commerce, destroys or disrupts trade networks, and distorts investments incentives or opportunities. The diversion of public resources from growth-enhancing projects (research and extension, and so on, public infrastructure) to military goods (weapons, ammunitions, etc.) and refugee care in wartime has negative impacts on life expectancy or longevity or the probability of a person in a given country to live longer. The duration of war depress productivity, brings about starvation, disease outbreak, and which in effect reduces the survival rate or the number of years a person born in a given country live longer (or reduces LEB). It is very important at this stage to theorize that the longer a war lasts, the more devastating it is on longevity or LEB. This is because almost all the atrocities and human suffering such as disease outbreak, spread of HIV/AIDs, starvation, and constants gun shots occurs in all nook and cranny in a given country whenever there is a war outbreak.

To demonstrate how the model works and to calculate the impacts of historical conflicts, the author of the manuscript infuses a LEB or longevity shock totaling −1.256% in the three vignettes in the contemporary Africa society which were part of the deadly post-World War countries: DRC, Burundi, and Liberia. The longevity or life expectancy shock is introduced in one country at a time, while the remainder of the elements of the random shock is set to zero. Rey and Montouri (1999) use the same approach to stimulate the propagation of economic growth across the United States. Lukongo and Rezek (2016) also use the same approach to stimulate the propagation of total food production growth across Africa. Therefore, at this juncture, the researcher calculates the predicted LEB for each country in the sample using equation (4). The results are reported in table 4.4.

## THE THREE VIGNETTES IN CONTEMPORARY AFRICA: THREE CASE STUDIES

### Democratic Republic of Congo

Figure 4.8A and column 2 of table 4.4 show the results of the stimulated LEB shock in the DRC caused by a major armed conflict. Plugging a shock of −1.256 into equation 4, which represents the estimated LEB shock associated with war, yields a decline in the LEB by about 1.4076 % per year. This represents a direct impact of a major armed conflict on the DRC's LEB. Estimates suggest that a LEB shock in the DRC has a particularly strong effect on Lesotho (−0.7065%), Swaziland (−0.6629%), Cameroon (−0.5949%), South Africa (−0.5241%), Botswana (−0.5128%), Zimbabwe (−0.5128 %), Chad (−0.4908%), Tunisia (−0.4745%), Sudan (−0.4591%), Ethiopia (−0.4511%), Somalia (0.4052%), and much lower than 0.4000% in the rest of the study area. These losses represent a significant reduction to LEB in Africa.

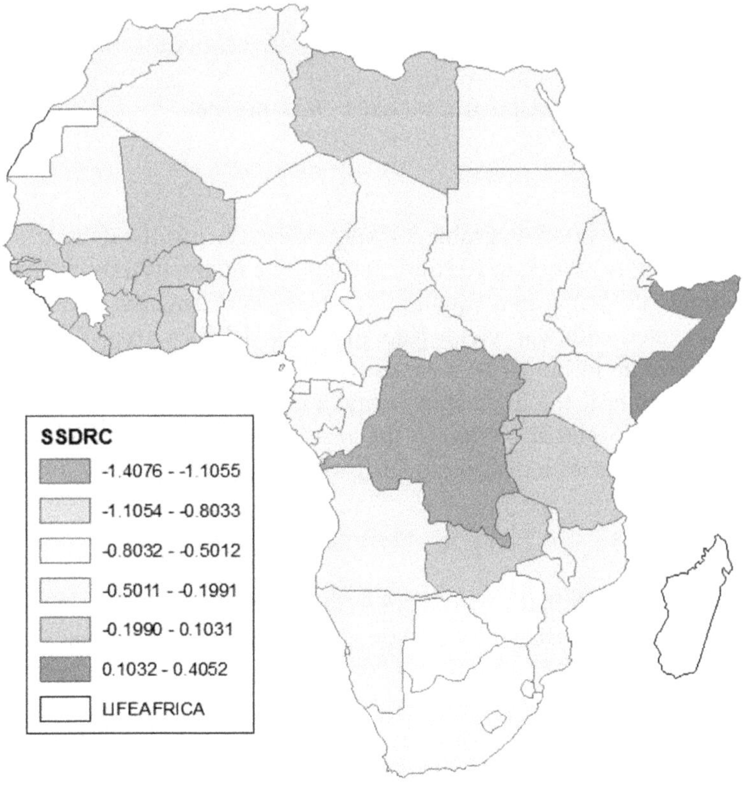


**Figure 4.8A Spillover of Major Armed Conflict from Democratic Republic of Congo.**

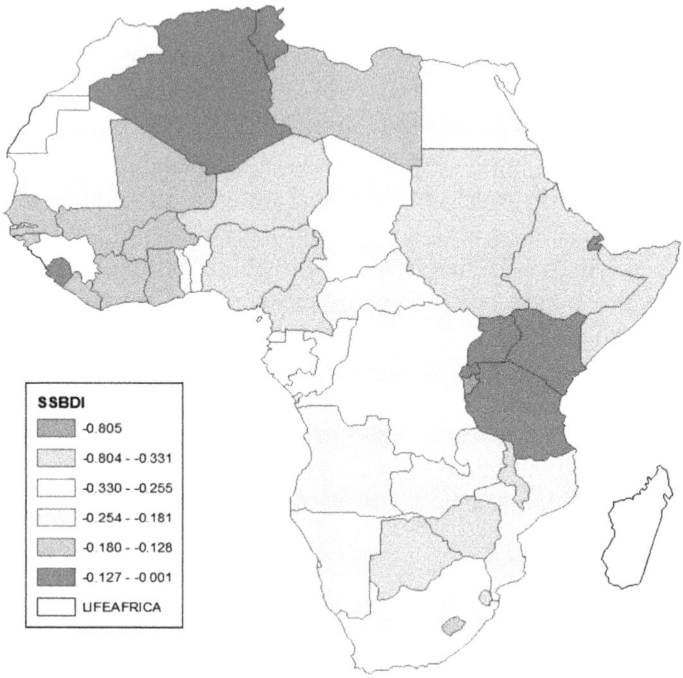


**Figure 4.8B Spillover of Major Armed Conflict from Burundi.**

## Burundi

Figure 4.8B and column 3 of table 4.4 summarize the results of the stimulated LEB (or longevity) shock in Burundi caused by a major armed conflict. Plugging a shock of −1.256 into equation 4, which represents the estimated LEB shock associated with war, yields a decline in the LEB by about 0.8054 % per year. The decline in the LEB, as a result of a war-sized growth shock introduced in Burundi, is the highest in Somalia (−0.4990%), Sudan (−0.4492%), and much lower than 0.4000% in the rest of the study area. These losses represent a significant reduction to LEB in Africa.

## Liberia

Figure 4.8C and column 4 of table 4.4 show the results of the stirred LEB shock in the Liberia caused by a major armed conflict. Plugging a shock of −1.256 into equation 4, which represents the estimated LEB shock associated with war, yields a decline in the LEB by about 0.9704 % per year. This represents a direct impact of a major armed conflict on the Liberia's LEB. Estimates suggest that a LEB shock in the Liberia has a particularly strong effect on Sudan (−0.7083%), Central African Republic 0.4818%), Swaziland

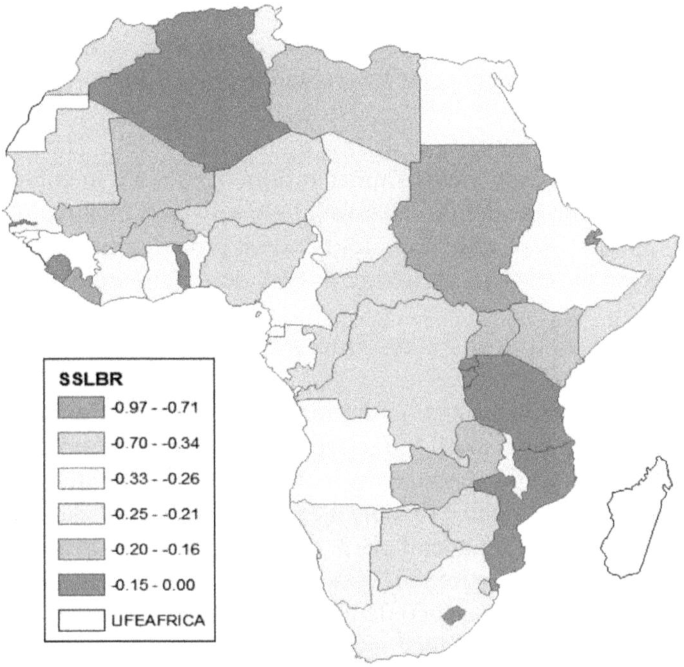


**Figure 4.8C Spillover of Major Armed Conflict from Liberia.**

(−0.4247%), Somalia (−0.4191%), Republic of Congo (−0.4134 %), DRC (−0.4002 %), and much lower than 0.4000% in the rest of the study area. These losses represent a significant reduction to LEB in Africa.

## DISCUSSION OF HYPOTHESES FOR THE BOOK'S RESEARCH

Hypothesis 1: There is No Visible Spatial Pattern, or Concentration, from the LEB across the Study Area.

For the exact purpose of investigating the first hypothesis, Moran's I statistics was used. In fact, there is evidence to reject the null hypothesis which states that "there is no visible spatial pattern, or concentration, from the LEB across the study area." This is because, as part of the findings, the study discovers a strong evidence of a significant spatial clustering of life expectancy across the study area. Taking for example, the global Moran's I statistics for the 1960s and 1970s shown in columns 1 and 6 of table 4.2. The researcher compares the calculated *p* values associated with the global Moran's I statistics against the convention critical values of 0.01, 0.05, and 0.10 to evaluate their significance. The researcher establishes a strong evidence of significant spatial clustering of LEB across countries and time. That is, the LEB is correlated with neighboring countries' "weighted average LEB." Again, columns 1 and 6 of table 4.2 show evidence of spatial clustering with queen contiguity of Order 1, 2, 3, 4 at both 5% and 10% significance levels. The general distance threshold approach yields similar results. As shown in columns 1 and 6 of table 4.2, using the arc distance weight matrix with maximum distances of about, 734, 800, 850, and 900 miles between capitals cities, the researcher also detects the presence of clustering in LEB across the study area.

Hypothesis 2: There Is Spatial Randomness in the LEB across the Study Area.

For the purpose of investigating the second hypothesis, Moran scatter plot and LISA statistics were used. In fact, there is enough evidence to reject the claim that "there is spatial randomness in the LEB across the study area." This is because as columns 1 and 6 of table 4.2 show evidence of spatial clustering with queen contiguity of Order 1, 2, 3, 4 and the general distance threshold of 734, 800, 850, 900-mile for the1960s and the 1970s. The Moran's I values for the 1960s which range from 0.0780 to 0.1439, and the 1970s which range from 0.0414 to 0.1058, exhibited significant positive spatial autocorrelation at the 1%, 5%, and 10% levels as shown in columns 1 and 6 of table 4.2. Furthermore, the study tests for spatial dependence using the general distance thresholds specification of the weighted matrix, with 734, 800, 850, and 900 miles for the 1960s and the 1970s. The results, also shown in columns 1 and 6 of table 4.2, indicate a strong spatial dependence in LEB when considering the distance between 734 and 900 miles in specification. The Moran's I statistics range from 0.1137 to 0.1470 for 1960s and from 0.0978 to 0.1246 for 1970s and are significant at the 5% and 10% significance levels. Therefore, there is enough evidence to conclude that LEB across countries are not random, rather they exhibited elements of spatial dependence or autocorrelation.

Hypothesis 3: There Is No Effect of Spatial Spillover of Major Armed War (or Violence) on LEB across the Study Area.

There is enough evidence to reject the claim that there is no effect of spatial spillover of major armed war on LEB across the study area, and fail to reject the alternate hypothesis based on the available data and analyses. This is because the researcher tested this particular hypothesis by using the identified spatial error model for the specification of the spatial spillover analysis using queen of Order 4. As a data-generating process, the spatial error model introduces a random shock to a specific country and captures both its direct impact and the propagation of that shock (major armed war) throughout Africa.

Based on the results from the column 3 of table 4.4, a major armed conflict results in a LEB shock was −0.3829%. The researcher tested the impacts of historical conflicts (major armed conflicts), by infusing a LEB or longevity shock totaling −1.256 % in the three vignettes in the contemporary Africa society which were part of the deadly post-World War countries, DRC, Burundi, and Liberia. The estimates suggest that a LEB shock in the DRC has a particularly strong effect on Lesotho (−0.7065%), Swaziland (−0.6629%), Cameroon (−0.5949%), South Africa (−0.5241%), Botswana (−0.5128%), Zimbabwe (−0.5128 %), Chad (−0.4908%), Tunisia (−0.4745%), Sudan (−0.4591%), Ethiopia (−0.4511%), Somalia (0.4052%), and much lower than 0.4000% in the rest of the African countries. These losses represent a significant reduction to LEB in Africa due to the spatial spillover of major armed war or conflict that emanated from DRC.

Again, the decline in the LEB, as a result of a war-sized growth shock introduced in Burundi, is highest in Somalia (−0.4990 %), Sudan (−0.4492 %), and much lower than 0.4000% in the rest of the African countries. These losses represent a significant reduction to LEB in Africa as a result of spatial spillover of major armed war or conflict that came from Burundi. Finally, regarding the case of Liberia, the estimates suggest that a LEB shock in Liberia has a particularly strong effect on Sudan (−0.7083%), Central African Republic 0.4818 %), Swaziland (−0.4247%), Somalia (−0.4191%), Republic of Congo (−0.4134 %), DRC (−0.4002 %), and much lower than 0.4000% in the rest of the African countries. These losses represent a significant reduction to LEB in Africa resulting from spatial spillover of major armed war or conflict that arose from Liberia.

## CONCLUSION

The contents of the conclusion for this part of the book extend the discussion of the LEB analysis into the spatial dimension by applying exploratory and confirmatory spatial data analysis. It capitalizes on successful implementation of spatial techniques and analytical tools proven in other fields or subfields of geospatial science. The exploratory spatial data analysis provides evidence of spatial autocorrelation in African LEB over the period of 1960–2015. That is, neighboring (or contiguous) African countries tend to have similar LEB, whether high or low. The research for the monograph takes a step further by conducting a hot and coldspots analysis on LEB in Africa. The research for the book finds that in the 1960s, fifteen countries pass the test of significance at 10%, 5%, and 1% levels for the formation of the hotspots: Kenya, Uganda, Djibouti, Burundi, Rwanda, DRC, Gabon, Congo, Zambia, Zimbabwe, Botswana, Namibia, South Africa, Lesotho, and Swaziland (see figure 4.7A for more details). However, the following African countries form the coldspot by passing the significant test at the 10%, 5%, and 1% levels of significance—Chad, Niger, Nigeria, Benin, Burkina Faso, Mali, Senegal, Gambia, Guinea Bissau, Guinea, Sierra Leone, Liberia, and Ivory Coast (see figure 4.7A for more details). These results shown in figure 4.7A are consistent with previously reported World Bank (2016) data on LEB in the 1960s.

In the 1970s, the hotspots countries reduce to a total of eleven, and they include Kenya, Gabon, Congo (DRC), Zambia, Zimbabwe, Tanzania, Botswana, Namibia, South Africa, Lesotho, and Swaziland (see table 4.2 for more details). Five African countries form the coldspot, and they are Niger, Gambia, Guinea Bissau, Sierra Leone, and Liberia (see table 4.2 for more details). Additionally, there was a significant decline in both the hotspots and coldspots in the 1980s. That is, in the 1980s, five African countries constitute the formation of the hotspots: Algeria, Tunisia, Libya, Egypt, and Lesotho (see table 4.2 for more details). Perhaps, three African countries form the coldspots—Gambia, Guinea Bissau, and Sierra Leone (see table 4.2 for more details). In the 1990s, three African countries constitute the formation of the hotspots: Algeria, Tunisia, and Egypt (see table 4.2 for more details).

However, given the available information (or data) there was no statistically significant coldspots formation in the 1990s. In the 2000s, two African countries form the hotspots: Egypt and Sudan (see figure 4.7B for more details). However, given the available information (or data) there was no statistically significant coldspots formation in the 2000s (see figure 4.7B for more details). Nonetheless, the ups-and-downs spiral of the spatial dependence and clustering tests during the Cold War era (1947–1989) and/or contemporary independence phase I (1960s–1989), could be attributed to the numerous political upheavals, including coups d'etat that occurred during the period. Between the 1960s and the 1990s, the ruling by military was perceived among many of the African countries as being the only group that could effectively maintain law and order; as a result it ruled many nations in Africa during the 1970s and early 1980s (Simon, 1995; Lucien, 2001; Aryeetey, Harrigan, and Nissanke, 2000). During the period between the early 1960s and the late 1980s, Africa experienced more than seventy coups and thirteen presidential assassinations (Simon, 1995; Lucien, 2001; Aryeetey, Harrigan, and Nissanke, 2000). Furthermore, during the African Renaissance period (1990–present) or the post-Cold war era (1990–present), the African countries transformation process in terms of social, economic, political, and health have slowed down over the last two decades. This is empirically observed in the statistical significant of the hotspot and the coldspot clustering location of LEB in the 1990s and 2000s (see Schraeder, 2004, pp.6–8 for more details).

The spatial econometrics approach suggests that the spatial error model provides the best fit for the data after the evaluation of the alternative specifications, including the standard regression model and the spatial lag model. The determination of the spatial error model as the optimal model allows for the possibility of introducing a random shock in the system of countries under analysis, as they are connected through the spatial weight matrix. The quantification of the spatial spillover of a random shock helps develop the understanding of the underlying processes of the decline in the LEB in Africa. Although still rudimentary, my book provides useful information as well as suggestions with vistas to help with future research of this important topic.

The provided facts in the book make a case for the fact that a war or major conflict may reduce LEB (or longevity) in a given country, but its real effects, which are overlooked by alternative modeling strategies, are larger. During wartime, citizens (individuals or families or communities) are forced to flee for their lives and others are killed. The displaced persons and families (or citizens of a given country) flee deep into the bush or to other countries, which exposed them to poor living lifestyles, malnutrition, famine (or starvation), and outbreak of diseases such as malaria, cholera, diarrhea, and HIV/AIDs. All these factors contribute to bad health outcome such as high mortality rate, high morbidity rate, and low LEB. This disruption (or major armed wars or conflicts) introduced in this particular research for the book as a random shock to the changes in life expectancy of a given country can affect LEB not only in the affected country but also in surrounding countries that are affected by the spillover of violence (or major armed war) and refugees.

The research for the book used applied spatial econometrics to uncover the spatial effects in the life expectancy analysis of the African countries over the period of 1960–2015. Estimates reveal that the growth shock (or war spillover) not only shifts a country away from attaining or experiencing improvement in LEB (or recording low LEB), but also affects the LEB of other countries. According to the findings, the Africa continent suffers substantial losses in the LEB when certain countries experience major armed conflict. A major armed conflict in the DRC caused its LEB to a decline by about 1.41% per year on average. A major armed conflict war in Burundi caused its LEB to decline by about 0.81% per year on average. Additionally, a major armed conflict war in Liberia caused its LEB to decline by about 0.97% per year on average. The results provided under the spillover analysis of the three vignettes of contemporary Africa represents first attempt in the literature to identify the life expectancy impacts of war in Africa including spatial spillovers in the analysis. That is, taking for example, column 2 of table 4.5 shows that the reduction in LEB to the eleven nearest neighbor ranges from 0.4052% in Somalia to 0.7065% in Lesotho.

The chapter, as things stand, has discussed all the three research questions stated in chapter 1 in detail, coupled with the various hypotheses outlined in chapter 3. The chapter, as well, very exhaustively answered all the earmarked research questions for the book, and it also examined the various hypotheses using spatiotemporal and regression analyses, Moran's I statistics and Moran scatterplot. Toward the end, the chapter discussed the study findings in detail. The chapter concluded that spatial analysis has been observed by the researcher as an important analysis in explaining the changes in LEB and its determinants across the regions of Africa. Finally, the book's chapter has provided an in-depth spatial spillover analysis of the three vignettes of contemporary Africa. Also, the chapter, above all, established that the spatial spillover analysis of major armed war or conflict represents the first attempt in the literature to identify the life expectancy impacts of war in Africa.

# *Chapter 5*

# Epilogue

## *Book's Conclusion, Policy Recommendation, and Implications*

This part of the book (chapter 5), which serves as the conclusion as well, is being utilized to discuss the following three crucial issues: (a) the rationale for embarking on the research for the book, the purpose of the research, the relevant research questions examined, or discussion and summary of the data analysis, (b) significance and limitations of the overall research for the book and, above all, (c) the implications and suggestions for future research in the thematic area of the book.

### DISCUSSION AND SUMMARY OF THE DATA ANALYSIS

Very importantly, one of the key policy initiatives in development policy is improvement in quality of life through high-quality health care provision. Policymakers, in the developing world, harbor key development goals of improving peoples' (or citizens') economic well-being and health conditions. As a result, LEB is one of the outcome indicators of development. In 2000, the WHO reported that children, growing up in war-torn zones, can expect to live healthy lives for fewer years than in any other country in the world.

Despite the numerous factors that have been suggested in the literature about LEB, little or no attempt has been made to investigate factors that determine the spatial and temporal components of life expectancy among African countries, and the spatial spillover of major wars or conflicts frequently recorded in Africa. That is, indeed, part of the reason the research for the book conducted the spatiotemporal analyses for a better understanding of the dynamics in life expectancy in Africa in order to inform public policy with enlightenment.

Therefore, the exact purpose of the research for the book was, indeed, to provide an understanding of the changes of life expectancy across regions and time in Africa, mostly in order to inform public policy in Africa. The research for the book was driven by the following research questions, namely: (a) To what extent can spatiotemporal analyses be used to comprehend better LEB in Africa? (b) What is the best spatial econometric model that is suitable for explaining LEB in Africa? And (c) to what extent can I apply geospatial and econometric models to inform public health policy in Africa?

In the process of answering the three important research questions, the contents of the book extend the discussion of LEB analysis into the spatial dimension by applying exploratory and confirmatory spatial data analysis. It capitalizes on successful implementation of spatial techniques and analytical tools proven in other fields or subfields of geospatial science. The exploratory spatial data analysis provides evidence of spatial autocorrelation in African LEB over the period of 1960–2015. That is, neighboring (or contiguous) African countries tend to have similar LEB, whether high or low.

Also, the contents of the publication, indeed, take a step further by conducting a hot and coldspots analysis on LEB in Africa, from which the findings include the following: (a) in the 1960s, fifteen countries constituted the formation of the hot spots: Kenya, Uganda, Djibouti, Burundi, Rwanda, DRC, Gabon, Congo, Zambia, Zimbabwe, Botswana, Namibia, South Africa, Lesotho, and Swaziland; while the following African countries form the coldspots: Chad, Niger, Nigeria, Benin, Burkina Faso, Mali, Senegal, Gambia, Guinea Bissau, Guinea, Sierra Leone, Liberia, and Ivory Coast; (b) in the 1970s, the hotspot countries include Kenya, Gabon, Congo, Zambia, Zimbabwe, Tanzania, Botswana, Namibia, South Africa, Lesotho, and Swaziland (see figure 4.7B more details), while five African countries form the coldspot, and they are Niger, Gambia, Guinea Bissau, Sierra Leone, and Liberia. (c) In the 1980s, five African countries constitute the formation of the hotspots: Algeria, Tunisia, Libya, Egypt, and Lesotho, while three African countries form the coldspots: Gambia, Guinea Bissau, and Sierra Leone. (d) In the 1990s, three African countries were included in the formation of the hotspots: Algeria, Tunisia, and Egypt, while no country was part of the coldspots formation in the 1990s. (e) In the 2000s, the number of African countries forming the hotspots zones reduced to two: Egypt and Sudan.

The spatial econometrics approach suggests that the spatial error model provides the best fit for the data after the evaluation of the alternative specifications, including the standard regression model and the spatial lag model. The determination of the spatial error model as the optimal model allows for the possibility of introducing a random shock in the system of countries under analysis, as they are connected through the spatial weight matrix. The quantification of the spatial spillover of a random shock helps develop the understanding of the underlying processes of the decline in the LEB in Africa. Although still rudimentary, this exercise suggests an avenue that may be pursued in future research. The findings make a case for the fact that a war may reduce LEB (or longevity) in a given country, but its real effects, which are overlooked by alternative modeling strategies, are larger. As stated earlier in Chapter 4, during wartime, citizens (or members of a given country) are forced to flee for their lives, and others are killed. Therefore, the nature of disruption (or major armed wars or conflicts) introduced in this publication as a random shock to measure the changes in LEB of a given country is perceived to affect LEB not only in the affected country but also in surrounding countries that are affected by the spillover of violence (or major armed war).

The research for the book used applied spatial econometrics to uncover the spatial effects in the life expectancy analysis of the African countries over the period of 1960–2015. Estimates reveal that the growth shock (or war spillover) not only shifts a country away from attaining or experiencing improvement in LEB (or recording low LEB), but also affects the LEB of other countries.

According to the findings, the African continent suffers substantial losses in the LEB when certain countries experience major armed conflict. For example, a major armed conflict in the DRC caused its life expectancy, at birth, to a decline by about 1.41% per year on average. Additionally, a major armed conflict or war in Burundi caused its LEB to decline by about 0.81% per year on average. Furthermore, a major armed conflict or war in Liberia caused its LEB to decline by about 0.97% per year on average. The results provided under the spillover analysis of the three vignettes of contemporary Africa represents the first attempt in the literature to identify the LEB impacts of war in Africa including spatial spillovers in the analysis. That is, taking for example, a spillover effect of a major war in DRC reveals a reduction in LEB to eleven nearest neighbor ranges from 0.4052% in Somalia to 0.7065% in Lesotho.

## OVERALL CONCLUSION

Toward the foregoing analyzed end, it is very important to note that three relevant research questions and three tentative research hypotheses were designed to drive the research for the book, which a data-driven research for the monograph is meant to inform public policy. In a nutshell, it can be underscored promptly that the research for the monograph reveals that all types of wars (civil war, conflicts, minor or major wars) and growth in health care (or previous information of LEB) were statistically significant determinants of LEB across all regions in Africa. However, education was not very significant, but its expected goal or sign was achieved to be positively related to LEB across Africa. Very importantly, the findings go a long way to conclude that spatial spillovers of major wars in a given country are likely to cause substantial losses in LEB of the affected country as well as its neighboring countries. Above all, the researcher has utilized all the available resources, despite time and resource constraints, to explain and also help readers, academics, development students, and other scholars, as well as the local and international policymakers, to understand better the role and effects of spatial spillover of rampant major armed conflicts, and the differences in LEB (or longevity) in Africa over time.

## OVERALL RESEARCH FINDINGS OF THE BOOK: SIGNIFICANCE AND LIMITATIONS

The overall research for the book is very relevant because it has filled the gap in the literature, which lacks the spatiotemporal components in the life expectancy discourse in Africa. Again, depending on the political will of the various African countries, the study is expected to benefit the following specific stakeholders: the various researchers, policymakers, academia in general and its academics, and the delineated international bodies. Furthermore, the conclusions reached and disseminated through the book are expected to contribute tremendously to the prevailing economic development literature, applied geospatial analytics literature, and international development literature.

Furthermore, the findings are expected to feed the policymakers with relevant information of the underlining factors that determine LEB among the African countries in order to bring about growth and development to the continent. As disclosed in the chapter 1, it was observed that there was a positive association between low income countries and low LEB among many of the African countries, including Zambia, Zimbabwe, and Somalia.

Above all, the research and its conclusions comprehensively add to the existing literature by using spatial analytic capabilities to leverage the existing computing platform, or apparatus to inform better public policy design and implementation. Students, scholars, and academics in academia are, as well, likely to benefit and learn from the geospatial and spatiotemporal techniques of analyzing development data (such as life expectancy data).

However, the known minor limitation of my effort was the processing as well as the grouping of the data based on decades and periods of the war times (i.e., Cold War and post-Cold War era), which demanded unusual strenuous effort. Also, three periodic war zone countries were lacking some data consistency from 1960 to 2015 from the World Bank traditional source; hence, journal publications, articles, and newspaper reports were reluctantly substituted to fill part of the gaps of the data sets. Above all, the study also faced time and, to some extent, research funding resource constraints. Yet, I did my best to make sure that the available resources were prudently utilized to produce a reliable book, which will benefit all the previously named interest groups, including policy makers and researchers.

## POLICY IMPLICATIONS AND RECOMMENDATIONS

Based on the ultimate findings of the earmarked research, very strenuous efforts have been expended to provide varied crucial and very relevant policy recommendations. Indeed, with all other things being equal, coupled with the fact that there is an existence of goodwill among African leaders as well as an availability of funds for the provision of very strong institutional structures, the under-listed sets of policy recommendations are expected to yield both positive results and very certain outcomes; they include the following spotted factors:

- That the governments of the various African countries as well as policymakers, international peace-making/keeping advocates and such crucial organizations as the UN and the Ethiopia-based AU are to ensure effective constitutional arrangement of peaceful transfer of power among African countries. This will, in the long run, bring about political stability in order to minimize civil wars as well as minor and major ethnic and cross-border warfare on the continent of Africa. A typical case in point is the well-known peaceful constitutional transfer of power that has been observed in the Republic of Ghana since 1992 (i.e., with the promulgation of the country's Fourth Republican constitutional design of 1992).
- In relation to the numerous war or conflict theories, and economics of war, grievances about regime changes in the political cycles and hardship or poverty are to constitute key factors to trigger the scramble of either the citizenry or concerned patriots to rise-up to have access to resources. Consequently, the research for the monograph strongly advocates that governments of the various African countries, policymakers, and such institutions as the UN, the AU and the Economic Commission of West African States (ECOWAS) are expected to assist in the designing of policies that will introduce copyright laws to safeguard both the resources and the created entities. With viable copyright laws in place, Africans and their leaders can define explicit ownerships of resources and the created items in African countries in order to minimize the incidence warfare or conflicts over assets and resources on the continent. A case in point is what exists in Botswana, whereby access to resources has been explicitly defined between the private

sector and the ruling government, a transparent policy that will usher in place stable economy and political stability in order to ensure growth and development. Therefore, the foregoing in designed policies or programs are likely to have the following policy implication in various areas of the continent: (1) people will have a lot more time to become educated, (2) that there will be sustained peace to ensure growth, and (3) that people will also be in peace to live longer.

- That conflict resolution policies and programs can be introduced for the war-torn zones in Africa, coupled with the introduction of a comprehensive resource on how to manage and resolve conflict under the supervision of ECOWAS, international peace-making advocates, UN, and the AU. A case in point is what exists in Rwanda, whereby access to resources, resolution policies, and programs has helped the country to rebuild the infrastructures that were at the messy of the numerous civil wars.
- That there will be a provision for institutional strengthening in order to enforce the existing laws, regulations, and legislation, measures expected to improve upon accountability in order to ensure free and fair elections, efficient allocation of resources, and political stability. Cases in point are what exist in Ghana and Botswana, whereby institutions in these two countries have been strengthened to enforce the existing laws, regulations, and legislation, measures expected to improve upon accountability in order to ensure free and fair elections, efficient allocation of resources, and a transparent policy that have to usher in place stable economies and political stability.
- That there will be the understanding that contemporary violent situations are unacceptable, as each has been known to have its own origin that is often embedded in unique socio-economic, political, military, and cultural setting. Furthermore, I have demonstrated through the research for the book that the complex reality of contemporary conflict and its effect on LEB are to require a thorough and detailed analysis of the context in which rehabilitation programs are inserted. In essence, I will also recommend rehabilitation or recovery programs for the war-torn zones in Africa in order to salvage the countries from hardships, poverty, and food insecurity, situations that will bring about improvement in infrastructure building, economic growth, and longevity (or LEB). An example is to emanate from the fact that in 1947, the American Secretary of State George C. Marshall did propose the European Recovery Program (later known as the Marshall Plan), indeed after 5 years of war had obviously destroyed Europe's physical infrastructure, social, and economic systems. In Africa, there will be a need for a proposal of rehabilitation program for various war-torn zones as part of collective efforts from such stakeholders as ruling governments of the various African countries, policymakers, and such international peace-making advocates as the UN, AU, the World Bank, WHO, and IMF.

- That there is to be balance of ethnic dominance in governance for every political entity or regime to bridge the poverty gap between tribes or ethnic groups, as doing so will minimize political unrest and also control the spilling over of war across Africa; a case in point is the instance of Burundi, since the inception of the country's independence in 1962, as it has been engulfed by bloody civil wars, leaving its people to be counted among some of the poorest people in the world. The implementation of this particular policy will be a possible solution to the problem of disproportion of ethnic dominance in governance for every political entity or regime to bridge the poverty gap between tribes or ethnic groups of countries such as Nigeria, Burundi, DRC, and many others. This is because equality, they say is equity, that is, a nation cannot sow rivalry and expect peace to prevail on the land.
- That, in the process, the various African countries, policymakers, and international peace-making advocates as well as the UN, the AU and such other international bodies as the World Bank, WHO, and the IMF are to revamp the UN strategy that aims at addressing the root causes of major armed conflicts or wars, which include (1) the "conflict prevention agenda," (2) the "youth agenda," and (3) "development agenda." The hope is that the UN's reset 2018 action plans are to address the root causes of such complex crises in Africa as in such Sahel or semi-arid regions as Senegal, Mauritania, Mali, Burkina Faso, Niger, Chad, Sudan, Nigeria, and Eritrea; in the end, the UN's reset strategies are likely to bring about the following progressive measures: (1) improve physical infrastructure and (2) to improve social and economic structures, improvement in education, increase housings, increase food supplies, and stable currencies.
- Above all, it is hoped that there will be a diffusion of social pressures through corporate social responsibility, which is most likely to ease the burden of either the less privileged or the poor to also feel part of the ownership of the national resources. In the process, there can be the setting-up of more scholarship funds, health care funds, and many others in the poor communities to enhance their living standards. This is very important because the fair share of the national cake is likely to bring about peace and stability to the respective nations of the continent of Africa.

## CONCLUSION

Currently, there is no clearly defined or known specific international framework for analyzing and responding to the problems of Africa's youthful populace (or youngsters), including unemployment and utter violent conflicts. However, the UN has proposed three main policy streams (or reset strategies) to address such African crisis or issues as: (1) the "conflict prevention agenda," which places the youths within causes, conditions, and dynamics of conflicts; (2) the "youth agenda," which treats conflicts or post-conflict situations as simply one of the many environments that young people as a distinct group must navigate as they grow up; and above all (3) have a "development agenda," as defined by the Millennium Development Goals of the UN, which focus mainly on employment as a solution for perceived youth crisis as well as other obvious violent crisis.

Sadly, there exists a lack of knowledge and operational guidance on how to integrate Africa's adolescents, as part of the youthful age group, in cluster work in order to bring about growth and development as well as to ensure improvement in life expectancy from birth, coupled with efforts to minimize violence, conflicts, and spatial spillover of major armed conflicts across the borders of African countries. Therefore, it is part of the urgent proposal of the research for the monograph to ensure additional well-structured future research, with the above narrative directions in mind.

# Appendix I

## *Spatiotemporal Analysis Data Output*

### DESCRIPTIVE SECTION

[DataSet1] E:\SpatioTempAfricaLifeExpJune072018\LIFE.sav

*Statistics*

| | | *LE60* | *LE70* | *LE80* | *LE90* | *LE00* |
|---|---|---|---|---|---|---|
| N | Valid | 52 | 52 | 53 | 53 | 53 |
| | Missing | 1 | 1 | 0 | 0 | 0 |
| Mean | | 43.56 | 48.17 | 52.79 | 53.98 | 58.19 |
| Median | | 43.00 | 48.00 | 52.00 | 54.00 | 57.00 |
| Mode | | 39 | 51 | 46[a] | 47[a] | 55 |
| Std. Deviation | | 6.430 | 6.600 | 7.422 | 8.477 | 7.267 |
| Variance | | 41.350 | 43.558 | 55.091 | 71.865 | 52.810 |
| Range | | 32 | 28 | 29 | 36 | 28 |
| Minimum | | 30 | 36 | 40 | 35 | 46 |
| Maximum | | 62 | 64 | 69 | 71 | 74 |
| Percentiles | 25 | 39.00 | 43.00 | 47.00 | 48.00 | 54.00 |
| | 50 | 43.00 | 48.00 | 52.00 | 54.00 | 57.00 |
| | 75 | 48.75 | 53.75 | 59.00 | 58.50 | 61.00 |

a. Multiple modes exist. The smallest value is shown.

[DataSet1] E:\SpatioTempAfricaLifeExpJune072018\LIFE.sav

*Paired Samples Statistics*

| | | *Mean* | *N* | *Std. Deviation* | *Std. Error Mean* |
|---|---|---|---|---|---|
| Pair 1 | LE70 | 48.17 | 52 | 6.600 | .915 |
| | LE60 | 43.56 | 52 | 6.430 | .892 |
| Pair 2 | LE80 | 52.48 | 52 | 7.136 | .990 |
| | LE70 | 48.17 | 52 | 6.600 | .915 |

| | | | | | |
|---|---|---|---|---|---|
| Pair 3 | LE90 | 53.98 | [illegible] | 8.477 | 1.164 |
| | LE80 | 52.79 | 53 | 7.422 | 1.020 |
| Pair 4 | LE00 | 58.19 | 53 | 7.267 | .998 |
| | LE90 | 53.98 | 53 | 8.477 | 1.164 |

*Paired Samples Correlations*

| | | *N* | *Correlation* | *Sig.* |
|---|---|---|---|---|
| Pair 1 | LE70 & LE60 | 52 | .960 | .000 |
| Pair 2 | LE80 & LE70 | 52 | .941 | .000 |
| Pair 3 | LE90 & LE80 | 53 | .889 | .000 |
| Pair 4 | LE00 & LE90 | 53 | .823 | .000 |

*Paired Samples Test*

| | | *Paired Differences* | | | | | | | |
|---|---|---|---|---|---|---|---|---|---|
| | | | | | *95% Confidence Interval of the Difference* | | | | |
| | | *Mean* | *Std. Deviation* | *Std. Error Mean* | *Lower* | *Upper* | *t* | *df* | *Sig. (2-tailed)* |
| Pair 1 | LE70 - LE60 | 4.615 | 1.859 | .258 | 4.098 | 5.133 | 17.900 | 51 | .000 |
| Pair 2 | LE80 - LE70 | 4.308 | 2.414 | .335 | 3.636 | 4.980 | 12.871 | 51 | .000 |
| Pair 3 | LE90 - LE80 | 1.189 | 3.883 | .533 | .118 | 2.259 | 2.229 | 52 | .030 |
| Pair 4 | LE00 - LE90 | 4.208 | 4.829 | .663 | 2.876 | 5.539 | 6.343 | 52 | .000 |

## SPATIAL REGRESSION ESTIMATION SECTION

### SUMMARY OF OUTPUT: ORDINARY LEAST SQUARES ESTIMATION

Data set: AFRLIVE47
Dependent Variable: LE70
Mean dependent var: 45.7021
S.D. dependent var: 11.3323

Number of Observations: 47
Number of Variables: 3
Degrees of Freedom: 44

R-squared: 0.974067
Adjusted R-squared: 0.972888
Sum squared residual: 156.529
Sigma-square: 3.55749
S.E. of regression: 1.88613
Sigma-square ML: 3.33041
S.E of regression ML: 1.82494

F-statistic: 826.327
Prob(F-statistic):1.27321e-035
Log likelihood: -94.9629
Akaike info criterion: 195.926
Schwarz criterion: 201.476

| Variable | Coefficient | Std.Error | t-Statistic | Probability |
|---|---|---|---|---|
| CONSTANT | 1.52844 | 1.123437 | 1.360503 | 0.18060 |
| LE60 | 1.083992 | 0.0268948 | 40.30491 | 0.00000 |
| CONF70 | -1.307219 | 0.5759782 | -2.269563 | 0.02819 |

REGRESSION DIAGNOSTICS
MULTICOLLINEARITY CONDITION NUMBER 9.090302
TEST ON NORMALITY OF ERRORS

| TEST | DF | VALUE | PROB |
|---|---|---|---|
| Jarque-Bera | 2 | 5.5875 | 0.06119 |

DIAGNOSTICS FOR HETEROSKEDASTICITY
RANDOM COEFFICIENTS

| TEST | DF | VALUE | PROB |
|---|---|---|---|
| Breusch-Pagan test | 2 | 8.9551 | 0.01136 |
| Koenker-Bassett test | 2 | 6.4738 | 0.03929 |

DIAGNOSTICS FOR SPATIAL DEPENDENCE
FOR WEIGHT MATRIX : 47Q1.gal
(row-standardized weights)

| TEST | MI/DF | VALUE | PROB |
|---|---|---|---|
| Moran's I (error) | 0.0692 | 0.9169 | 0.35919 |
| Lagrange Multiplier (lag) | 1 | 0.9673 | 0.32535 |
| Robust LM (lag) | 1 | 1.2161 | 0.27012 |
| Lagrange Multiplier (error) | 1 | 0.4252 | 0.51434 |
| Robust LM (error) | 1 | 0.6741 | 0.41164 |
| Lagrange Multiplier (SARMA) | 2 | 1.6414 | 0.44013 |

==================== END OF REPORT ====================

SUMMARY OF OUTPUT: SPATIAL LAG MODEL - MAXIMUM LIKELIHOOD ESTIMATION

Data set: AFRLIVE47
Spatial Weight: 47Q1.gal
Dependent Variable: LE70 Number of Observations: 47
Mean dependent var: 45.7021 Number of Variables: 4
S.D. dependent var: 11.3323 Degrees of Freedom: 43
Lag coeff. (Rho): -0.0324818

R-squared: 0.974619
Sq. Correlation: -
Sigma-square: 3.25948
S.E of regression: 1.8054

Log likelihood: -94.4626
Akaike info criterion : 196.925
Schwarz criterion: 204.326

| *Variable* | *Coefficient* | *Std.Error* | *z-value* | *Probability* |
|---|---|---|---|---|
| W_LE70 | -0.03248177 | 0.03219459 | -1.00892 | 0.31301 |
| CONSTANT | 2.813281 | 1.669509 | 1.685094 | 0.09197 |
| LE60 | 1.088325 | 0.02608638 | 41.72003 | 0.00000 |
| CONF70 | -1.296252 | 0.5516934 | -2.349588 | 0.01879 |

REGRESSION DIAGNOSTICS
DIAGNOSTICS FOR HETEROSKEDASTICITY
RANDOM COEFFICIENTS

| *TEST* | *DF* | *VALUE* | *PROB* |
|---|---|---|---|
| Breusch-Pagan test | 2 | 9.5013 | 0.00865 |

DIAGNOSTICS FOR SPATIAL DEPENDENCE
SPATIAL LAG DEPENDENCE FOR WEIGHT MATRIX : 47Q1.gal

| *TEST* | *DF* | *VALUE* | *PROB* |
|---|---|---|---|
| Likelihood Ratio Test | 1 | 1.0006 | 0.31716 |

==================== END OF REPORT ====================

SUMMARY OF OUTPUT: SPATIAL ERROR MODEL - MAXIMUM LIKELIHOOD ESTIMATION

Data set: AFRLIVE47
Spatial Weight: 47Q1.gal
Dependent Variable: LE70
Mean dependent var: 45.702128
S.D. dependent var: 11.332339
Lag coeff. (Lambda) : 0.187443

Number of Observations: 47
Number of Variables: 3
Degrees of Freedom: 44

R-squared: 0.974629
Sq. Correlation: -
Sigma-square: 3.25823
S.E of regression: 1.80506

R-squared (BUSE): -
Log likelihood: -94.643793
Akaike info criterion : 195.288
Schwarz criterion: 200.838

| *Variable* | *Coefficient* | *Std.Error* | *z-value* | *Probability* |
|---|---|---|---|---|
| CONSTANT | 1.276546 | 1.111211 | 1.148789 | 0.25064 |
| LE60 | 1.088825 | 0.02607472 | 41.75789 | 0.00000 |
| CONF70 | -1.09278 | 0.5318857 | -2.054539 | 0.03992 |
| LAMBDA | 0.1874432 | 0.1866915 | 1.004027 | 0.31537 |

REGRESSION DIAGNOSTICS
DIAGNOSTICS FOR HETEROSKEDASTICITY
RANDOM COEFFICIENTS

| *TEST* | *DF* | *VALUE* | *PROB* |
|---|---|---|---|
| Breusch-Pagan test | 2 | 8.4653 | 0.01451 |

DIAGNOSTICS FOR SPATIAL DEPENDENCE
SPATIAL ERROR DEPENDENCE FOR WEIGHT MATRIX : 47Q1.gal

| *TEST* | *DF* | *VALUE* | *PROB* |
|---|---|---|---|
| Likelihood Ratio Test | 1 | 0.6382 | 0.42437 |

==================== END OF REPORT ====================

SUMMARY OF OUTPUT: ORDINARY LEAST SQUARES ESTIMATION

Data set: AFRLIVE47
Dependent Variable: LE70
Mean dependent var: 45.7021
S.D. dependent var: 11.3323

Number of Observations: 47
Number of Variables: 3
Degrees of Freedom: 44

R-squared: 0.974067
Adjusted R-squared: 0.972888
Sum squared residual: 156.529
Sigma-square: 3.55749
S.E. of regression: 1.88613
Sigma-square ML: 3.33041
S.E of regression ML: 1.82494

F-statistic: 826.327
Prob(F-statistic):1.27321e-035
Log likelihood: -94.9629
Akaike info criterion : 195.926
Schwarz criterion: 201.476

| *Variable* | *Coefficient* | *Std.Error* | *t-Statistic* | *Probability* |
|---|---|---|---|---|
| CONSTANT | 1.52844 | 1.123437 | 1.360503 | 0.18060 |
| LE60 | 1.083992 | 0.0268948 | 40.30491 | 0.00000 |
| CONF70 | -1.307219 | 0.5759782 | -2.269563 | 0.02819 |

REGRESSION DIAGNOSTICS
MULTICOLLINEARITY CONDITION NUMBER 9.090302
TEST ON NORMALITY OF ERRORS

| *TEST* | *DF* | *VALUE* | *PROB* |
|---|---|---|---|
| Jarque-Bera | 2 | 5.5875 | 0.06119 |

DIAGNOSTICS FOR HETEROSKEDASTICITY
RANDOM COEFFICIENTS

| *TEST* | *DF* | *VALUE* | *PROB* |
|---|---|---|---|
| Breusch-Pagan test | 2 | 8.9551 | 0.01136 |
| Koenker-Bassett test | 2 | 6.4738 | 0.03929 |

DIAGNOSTICS FOR SPATIAL DEPENDENCE
FOR WEIGHT MATRIX : 47Q2.gal
(row-standardized weights)

| *TEST* | *MI/DF* | *VALUE* | *PROB* |
|---|---|---|---|
| Moran's I (error) | 0.0701 | 1.8533 | 0.06384 |
| Lagrange Multiplier (lag) | 1 | 5.1346 | 0.02345 |
| Robust LM (lag) | 1 | 6.1302 | 0.01329 |
| Lagrange Multiplier (error) | 1 | 1.3003 | 0.25416 |
| Robust LM (error) | 1 | 2.2959 | 0.12972 |
| Lagrange Multiplier (SARMA) | 2 | 7.4305 | 0.02435 |

=================== END OF REPORT ===================

SUMMARY OF OUTPUT: SPATIAL LAG MODEL - MAXIMUM LIKELIHOOD ESTIMATION

Data set: AFRLIVE47
Spatial Weight: 47Q2.gal
Dependent Variable: LE70 Number of Observations: 47
Mean dependent var: 45.7021 Number of Variables: 4
S.D. dependent var: 11.3323 Degrees of Freedom: 43
Lag coeff. (Rho): -0.148402

R-squared: 0.977514 Log likelihood: -91.651
Sq. Correlation: - Akaike info criterion : 191.302
Sigma-square: 2.88768 Schwarz criterion: 198.703
S.E of regression: 1.69932

| Variable | Coefficient | Std.Error | z-value | Probability |
|---|---|---|---|---|
| W_LE70 | -0.1484016 | 0.05470952 | -2.712536 | 0.00668 |
| CONSTANT | 7.793538 | 2.523034 | 3.088954 | 0.00201 |
| LE60 | 1.093388 | 0.02448181 | 44.66126 | 0.00000 |
| CONF70 | -1.019277 | 0.5275425 | -1.932122 | 0.05334 |

REGRESSION DIAGNOSTICS
DIAGNOSTICS FOR HETEROSKEDASTICITY
RANDOM COEFFICIENTS

| TEST | DF | VALUE | PROB |
|---|---|---|---|
| Breusch-Pagan test | 2 | 10.3190 | 0.00574 |

DIAGNOSTICS FOR SPATIAL DEPENDENCE
SPATIAL LAG DEPENDENCE FOR WEIGHT MATRIX : 47Q2.gal

| TEST | DF | VALUE | PROB |
|---|---|---|---|
| Likelihood Ratio Test | 1 | 6.6238 | 0.01006 |

==================== END OF REPORT ====================

SUMMARY OF OUTPUT: SPATIAL ERROR MODEL - MAXIMUM LIKELIHOOD ESTIMATION

Data set: AFRLIVE47
Spatial Weight: 47Q2.gal
Dependent Variable: LE70
Mean dependent var: 45.702128
S.D. dependent var: 11.332339
Lag coeff. (Lambda) : 0.413225

Number of Observations: 47
Number of Variables: 3
Degrees of Freedom: 44

R-squared: 0.975337
Sq. Correlation: -
Sigma-square: 3.16724
S.E of regression: 1.77967

R-squared (BUSE): -
Log likelihood: -94.180445
Akaike info criterion : 194.361
Schwarz criterion: 199.911

| Variable | Coefficient | Std.Error | z-value | Probability |
|---|---|---|---|---|
| CONSTANT | 0.7580858 | 1.147143 | 0.6608467 | 0.50871 |
| LE60 | 1.102914 | 0.02574401 | 42.84157 | 0.00000 |
| CONF70 | -1.366456 | 0.5282616 | -2.586703 | 0.00969 |
| LAMBDA | 0.4132248 | 0.2494152 | 1.656775 | 0.09757 |

REGRESSION DIAGNOSTICS
DIAGNOSTICS FOR HETEROSKEDASTICITY
RANDOM COEFFICIENTS

| *TEST* | *DF* | *VALUE* | *PROB* |
|---|---|---|---|
| Breusch-Pagan test | 2 | 8.2635 | 0.01606 |

DIAGNOSTICS FOR SPATIAL DEPENDENCE
SPATIAL ERROR DEPENDENCE FOR WEIGHT MATRIX : 47Q2.gal

| *TEST* | *DF* | *VALUE* | *PROB* |
|---|---|---|---|
| Likelihood Ratio Test | 1 | 1.5649 | 0.21095 |

==================== END OF REPORT ====================

SUMMARY OF OUTPUT: ORDINARY LEAST SQUARES ESTIMATION

Data set: AFRLIVE47
Dependent Variable: LE70
Mean dependent var: 45.7021
S.D. dependent var: 11.3323

Number of Observations: 47
Number of Variables: 3
Degrees of Freedom: 44

R-squared: 0.974067
Adjusted R-squared: 0.972888
Sum squared residual: 156.529
Sigma-square: 3.55749
S.E. of regression: 1.88613
Sigma-square ML: 3.33041
S.E of regression ML: 1.82494

F-statistic: 826.327
Prob(F-statistic):1.27321e-035
Log likelihood: -94.9629
Akaike info criterion : 195.926
Schwarz criterion: 201.476

| *Variable* | *Coefficient* | *Std.Error* | *t-Statistic* | *Probability* |
|---|---|---|---|---|
| CONSTANT | 1.52844 | 1.123437 | 1.360503 | 0.18060 |
| LE60 | 1.083992 | 0.0268948 | 40.30491 | 0.00000 |
| CONF70 | -1.307219 | 0.5759782 | -2.269563 | 0.02819 |

REGRESSION DIAGNOSTICS
MULTICOLLINEARITY CONDITION NUMBER 9.090302
TEST ON NORMALITY OF ERRORS

| *TEST* | *DF* | *VALUE* | *PROB* |
|---|---|---|---|
| Jarque-Bera | 2 | 5.5875 | 0.06119 |

DIAGNOSTICS FOR HETEROSKEDASTICITY
RANDOM COEFFICIENTS

| *TEST* | *DF* | *VALUE* | *PROB* |
|---|---|---|---|
| Breusch-Pagan test | 2 | 8.9551 | 0.01136 |
| Koenker-Bassett test | 2 | 6.4738 | 0.03929 |

DIAGNOSTICS FOR SPATIAL DEPENDENCE
FOR WEIGHT MATRIX : 47Q3.gal
(row-standardized weights)

| *TEST* | *MI/DF* | *VALUE* | *PROB* |
|---|---|---|---|
| Moran's I (error) | 0.0282 | 1.7405 | 0.08177 |
| Lagrange Multiplier (lag) | 1 | 8.3876 | 0.00378 |
| Robust LM (lag) | 1 | 9.1476 | 0.00249 |
| Lagrange Multiplier (error) | 1 | 0.3845 | 0.53518 |
| Robust LM (error) | 1 | 1.1446 | 0.28469 |
| Lagrange Multiplier (SARMA) | 2 | 9.5321 | 0.00851 |

==================== END OF REPORT ====================

SUMMARY OF OUTPUT: ORDINARY LEAST SQUARES ESTIMATION

Data set: AFRLIVE47
Dependent Variable: LE70
Mean dependent var: 45.7021
S.D. dependent var: 11.3323

Number of Observations: 47
Number of Variables: 3
Degrees of Freedom: 44

R-squared: 0.974067
Adjusted R-squared: 0.972888
Sum squared residual: 156.529
Sigma-square: 3.55749
S.E. of regression: 1.88613
Sigma-square ML: 3.33041
S.E of regression ML: 1.82494

F-statistic: 826.327
Prob(F-statistic):1.27321e-035
Log likelihood: -94.9629
Akaike info criterion : 195.926
Schwarz criterion: 201.476

| *Variable* | *Coefficient* | *Std.Error* | *t-Statistic* | *Probability* |
|---|---|---|---|---|
| CONSTANT | 1.52844 | 1.123437 | 1.360503 | 0.18060 |
| LE60 | 1.083992 | 0.0268948 | 40.30491 | 0.00000 |
| CONF70 | -1.307219 | 0.5759782 | -2.269563 | 0.02819 |

REGRESSION DIAGNOSTICS
MULTICOLLINEARITY CONDITION NUMBER 9.090302
TEST ON NORMALITY OF ERRORS

| TEST | DF | VALUE | PROB |
|---|---|---|---|
| Jarque-Bera | 2 | 5.5875 | 0.06119 |

DIAGNOSTICS FOR HETEROSKEDASTICITY
RANDOM COEFFICIENTS

| TEST | DF | VALUE | PROB |
|---|---|---|---|
| Breusch-Pagan test | 2 | 8.9551 | 0.01136 |
| Koenker-Bassett test | 2 | 6.4738 | 0.03929 |

DIAGNOSTICS FOR SPATIAL DEPENDENCE
FOR WEIGHT MATRIX : 47Q4.gal
(row-standardized weights)

| TEST | MI/DF | VALUE | PROB |
|---|---|---|---|
| Moran's I (error) | 0.0588 | 4.1074 | 0.00004 |
| Lagrange Multiplier (lag) | 1 | 6.2252 | 0.01259 |
| Robust LM (lag) | 1 | 7.7979 | 0.00523 |
| Lagrange Multiplier (error) | 1 | 2.3739 | 0.12338 |
| Robust LM (error) | 1 | 3.9466 | 0.04697 |
| Lagrange Multiplier (SARMA) | 2 | 10.1718 | 0.00618 |

==================== END OF REPORT ====================

SUMMARY OF OUTPUT: SPATIAL LAG MODEL - MAXIMUM LIKELIHOOD ESTIMATION

| | |
|---|---|
| Data set: AFRLIVE47 | |
| Spatial Weight: 47Q4.gal | |
| Dependent Variable: LE70 | Number of Observations: 47 |
| Mean dependent var: 45.7021 | Number of Variables: 4 |
| S.D. dependent var: 11.3323 | Degrees of Freedom: 43 |
| Lag coeff. | (Rho): -0.307816 |
| | |
| R-squared: 0.978664 | Log likelihood: -93.859603 |
| Sq. Correlation: - | Akaike info criterion : 193.719 |
| Sigma-square: 2.74007 | Schwarz criterion: 199.27 |
| S.E of regression: 1.65532 | |

| Variable | Coefficient | Std.Error | z-value | Probability |
|---|---|---|---|---|
| W_LE70 | -0.307816 | 0.09675889 | -3.181268 | 0.00147 |
| CONSTANT | 14.92029 | 4.319126 | 3.45447 | 0.00055 |
| LE60 | 1.102296 | 0.02430398 | 45.35454 | 0.00000 |
| CONF70 | -1.17714 | 0.5070243 | -2.321663 | 0.02025 |

REGRESSION DIAGNOSTICS
DIAGNOSTICS FOR HETEROSKEDASTICITY
RANDOM COEFFICIENTS

| TEST | DF | VALUE | PROB |
|---|---|---|---|
| Breusch-Pagan test | 2 | 7.0401 | 0.02960 |

DIAGNOSTICS FOR SPATIAL DEPENDENCE
SPATIAL LAG DEPENDENCE FOR WEIGHT MATRIX : 47Q4.gal

| TEST | DF | VALUE | PROB |
|---|---|---|---|
| Likelihood Ratio Test | 1 | 9.0412 | 0.00264 |

==================== END OF REPORT ====================

SUMMARY OF OUTPUT: SPATIAL ERROR MODEL - MAXIMUM LIKELIHOOD ESTIMATION

Data set: AFRLIVE47
Spatial Weight: 47Q4.gal
Dependent Variable: LE70
Mean dependent var: 45.702128
S.D. dependent var: 11.332339
Lag coeff. (Lambda) : 0.622313

Number of Observations: 47
Number of Variables: 3
Degrees of Freedom: 44

R-squared: 0.975759
Sq. Correlation: -
Sigma-square: 3.11301
S.E of regression: 1.76437

R-squared (BUSE): -
Log likelihood: -90.4423
Akaike info criterion : 188.885
Schwarz criterion: 196.285

| Variable | Coefficient | Std.Error | z-value | Probability |
|---|---|---|---|---|
| CONSTANT | 0.5838025 | 1.244939 | 0.4689406 | 0.63911 |
| LE60 | 1.104312 | 0.02594425 | 42.56482 | 0.00000 |
| CONF70 | -1.25573 | 0.5273987 | -2.380989 | 0.01727 |
| LAMBDA | 0.6223129 | 0.2465902 | 2.523672 | 0.01161 |

REGRESSION DIAGNOSTICS
DIAGNOSTICS FOR HETEROSKEDASTICITY
RANDOM COEFFICIENTS

| *TEST* | *DF* | *VALUE* | *PROB* |
|---|---|---|---|
| Breusch-Pagan test | 2 | 9.6340 | 0.00809 |

DIAGNOSTICS FOR SPATIAL DEPENDENCE
SPATIAL ERROR DEPENDENCE FOR WEIGHT MATRIX : 47Q4.gal

| *TEST* | *DF* | *VALUE* | *PROB* |
|---|---|---|---|
| Likelihood Ratio Test | 1 | 2.2066 | 0.13742 |

==================== END OF REPORT ====================

SUMMARY OF OUTPUT: ORDINARY LEAST SQUARES ESTIMATION

Data set: AFRLIVE47
Dependent Variable: LE70
Mean dependent var: 45.7021
S.D. dependent var: 11.3323

Number of Observations: 47
Number of Variables: 3
Degrees of Freedom: 44

R-squared: 0.974067
Adjusted R-squared: 0.972888
Sum squared residual: 156.529
Sigma-square: 3.55749
S.E. of regression: 1.88613
Sigma-square ML: 3.33041
S.E of regression ML: 1.82494

F-statistic: 826.327
Prob(F-statistic):1.27321e-035
Log likelihood: -94.9629
Akaike info criterion : 195.926
Schwarz criterion: 201.476

| *Variable* | *Coefficient* | *Std.Error* | *t-Statistic* | *Probability* |
|---|---|---|---|---|
| CONSTANT | 1.52844 | 1.123437 | 1.360503 | 0.18060 |
| LE60 | 1.083992 | 0.0268948 | 40.30491 | 0.00000 |
| CONF70 | -1.307219 | 0.5759782 | -2.269563 | 0.02819 |

REGRESSION DIAGNOSTICS
MULTICOLLINEARITY CONDITION NUMBER 9.090302
TEST ON NORMALITY OF ERRORS

| *TEST* | *DF* | *VALUE* | *PROB* |
|---|---|---|---|
| Jarque-Bera | 2 | 5.5875 | 0.06119 |

DIAGNOSTICS FOR HETEROSKEDASTICITY
RANDOM COEFFICIENTS

| TEST | DF | VALUE | PROB |
|---|---|---|---|
| Breusch-Pagan test | 2 | 8.9551 | 0.01136 |
| Koenker-Bassett test | 2 | 6.4738 | 0.03929 |

DIAGNOSTICS FOR SPATIAL DEPENDENCE
FOR WEIGHT MATRIX : d734.gwt
(row-standardized weights)

| TEST | MI/DF | VALUE | PROB |
|---|---|---|---|
| Moran's I (error) | 0.2271 | 2.4588 | 0.01394 |
| Lagrange Multiplier (lag) | 1 | 0.1661 | 0.68357 |
| Robust LM (lag) | 1 | 0.6741 | 0.41163 |
| Lagrange Multiplier (error) | 1 | 4.5209 | 0.03348 |
| Robust LM (error) | 1 | 5.0288 | 0.02493 |
| Lagrange Multiplier (SARMA) | 2 | 5.1949 | 0.07446 |

=================== END OF REPORT ===================

SUMMARY OF OUTPUT: SPATIAL LAG MODEL - MAXIMUM LIKELIHOOD ESTIMATION

Data set: AFRLIVE47
Spatial Weight: d734.gwt
Dependent Variable: LE70
Mean dependent var: 45.7021
S.D. dependent var: 11.3323
Lag coeff. (Rho): -0.0152297

Number of Observations: 47
Number of Variables: 4
Degrees of Freedom: 43

R-squared: 0.974160
Sq. Correlation: -
Sigma-square: 3.31845
S.E of regression: 1.82166

Log likelihood: -94.8797
Akaike info criterion : 197.759
Schwarz criterion: 205.16

| Variable | Coefficient | Std.Error | z-value | Probability |
|---|---|---|---|---|
| W_LE70 | -0.01522965 | 0.0374704 | -0.4064448 | 0.68442 |
| CONSTANT | 2.153765 | 1.880399 | 1.145377 | 0.25205 |
| LE60 | 1.085832 | 0.026356 | 41.19865 | 0.00000 |
| CONF70 | -1.314719 | 0.5563343 | -2.363182 | 0.01812 |

REGRESSION DIAGNOSTICS
DIAGNOSTICS FOR HETEROSKEDASTICITY
RANDOM COEFFICIENTS

| *TEST* | *DF* | *VALUE* | *PROB* |
|---|---|---|---|
| Breusch-Pagan test | 2 | 9.4164 | 0.00902 |

DIAGNOSTICS FOR SPATIAL DEPENDENCE
SPATIAL LAG DEPENDENCE FOR WEIGHT MATRIX : d734.gwt

| *TEST* | *DF* | *VALUE* | *PROB* |
|---|---|---|---|
| Likelihood Ratio Test | 1 | 0.1664 | 0.68329 |

=================== END OF REPORT ===================

SUMMARY OF OUTPUT: SPATIAL ERROR MODEL - MAXIMUM LIKELIHOOD ESTIMATION

Data set: AFRLIVE47
Spatial Weight: d734.gwt
Dependent Variable: LE70 Number of Observations: 47
Mean dependent var: 45.702128 Number of Variables: 3
S.D. dependent var: 11.332339 Degrees of Freedom: 44
Lag coeff. (Lambda) : 0.332009

R-squared: 0.976787 R-squared (BUSE): -
Sq. Correlation: - Log likelihood: -93.065512
Sigma-square: 2.98111 Akaike info criterion : 192.131
S.E of regression: 1.72659 Schwarz criterion: 197.681

| *Variable* | *Coefficient* | *Std.Error* | *z-value* | *Probability* |
|---|---|---|---|---|
| CONSTANT | 1.225843 | 1.080105 | 1.134929 | 0.25640 |
| LE60 | 1.089085 | 0.02499617 | 43.57008 | 0.00000 |
| CONF70 | -1.109137 | 0.4906296 | -2.26064 | 0.02378 |
| LAMBDA | 0.3320093 | 0.1679233 | 1.977148 | 0.04802 |

REGRESSION DIAGNOSTICS
DIAGNOSTICS FOR HETEROSKEDASTICITY
RANDOM COEFFICIENTS

| *TEST* | *DF* | *VALUE* | *PROB* |
|---|---|---|---|
| Breusch-Pagan test | 2 | 8.0455 | 0.01790 |

DIAGNOSTICS FOR SPATIAL DEPENDENCE
SPATIAL ERROR DEPENDENCE FOR WEIGHT MATRIX : d734.gwt

| *TEST* | *DF* | *VALUE* | *PROB* |
|---|---|---|---|
| Likelihood Ratio Test | 1 | 3.7947 | 0.05141 |

==================== END OF REPORT ====================

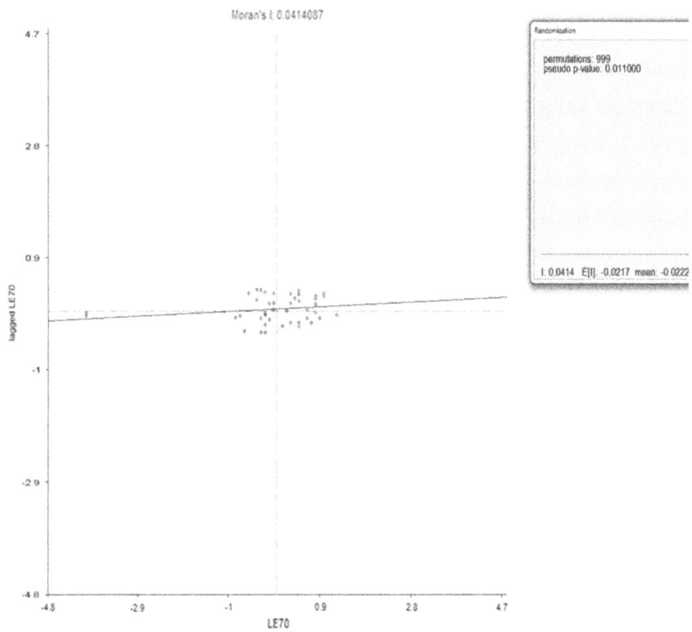


**Figure A Moran Scatterplot of Life Expectancy at Birth in Africa, 1970s.** *Note*: Moran scatterplot of Life expectancy at birth in Africa, 1970s with a Moran's I=0.0414** using queen of order 4 spatial weight matrix. The queen of order 4 spatial weight matrix is used in the analysis because it reveals the highest hotspot and cold spot with a statistical significance at 10%, and 5%.

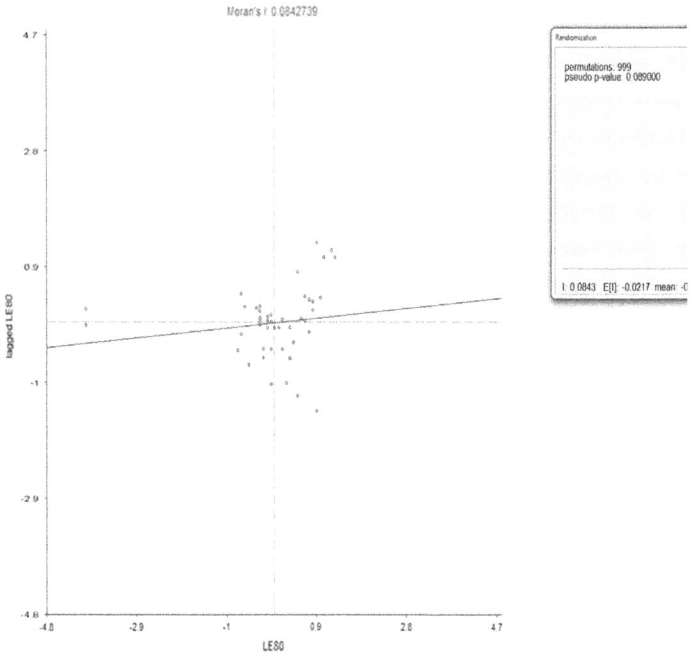


**Figure B Moran Scatterplot of Life Expectancy at Birth in Africa, 1980s.** *Note*: Moran scatterplot of Life expectancy at birth in Africa, 1980s with a Moran's I=0.0843* using 800-mile general distance threshold spatial weight matrix. The 800-mile general distance threshold of spatial weight matrix is used in the analysis because it reveals the highest hotspot and cold spot with a statistical significance at 10%.

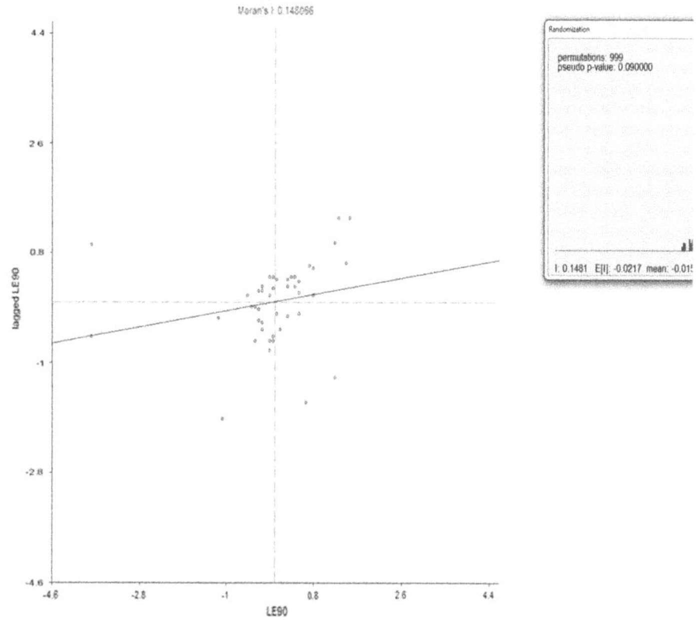


**Figure C Moran Scatterplot of Life Expectancy at Birth in Africa, 1990s.** *Note*: Moran scatterplot of Life expectancy at birth in Africa, 1990s with a Moran's I=0.1481* using k-nearest neighbor of order 2 spatial weight matrix. The 2-nearest neighbor of spatial weight matrix is used in the analysis because it reveals the highest hotspot with a statistical significance at 10%.

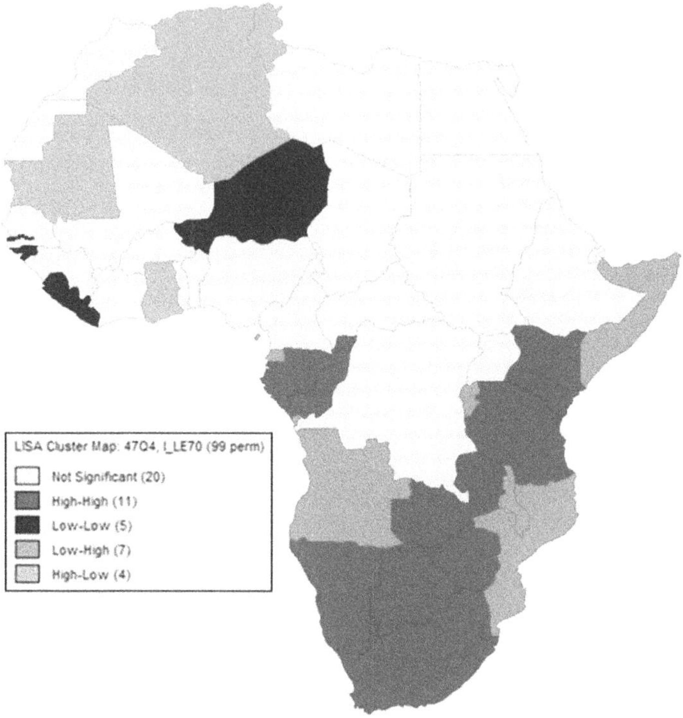


**Figure D Spatial Clusters and Identification of Hotspots and Cold Spots in Life Expectancy at Birth in Africa, 1970s. The spatial weight matrix Queen of order 4 was employed on LISA cluster map.**

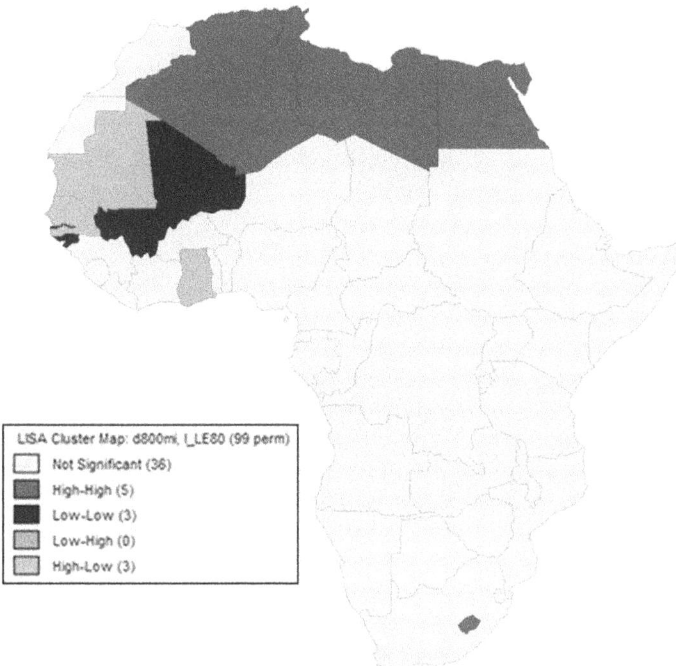


**Figure E Spatial Clusters and Identification of Hotspots and Cold Spots in Life Expectancy at Birth in Africa, 1980s. The spatial weight matrix threshold distance of 800 miles was employed on LISA cluster map.**

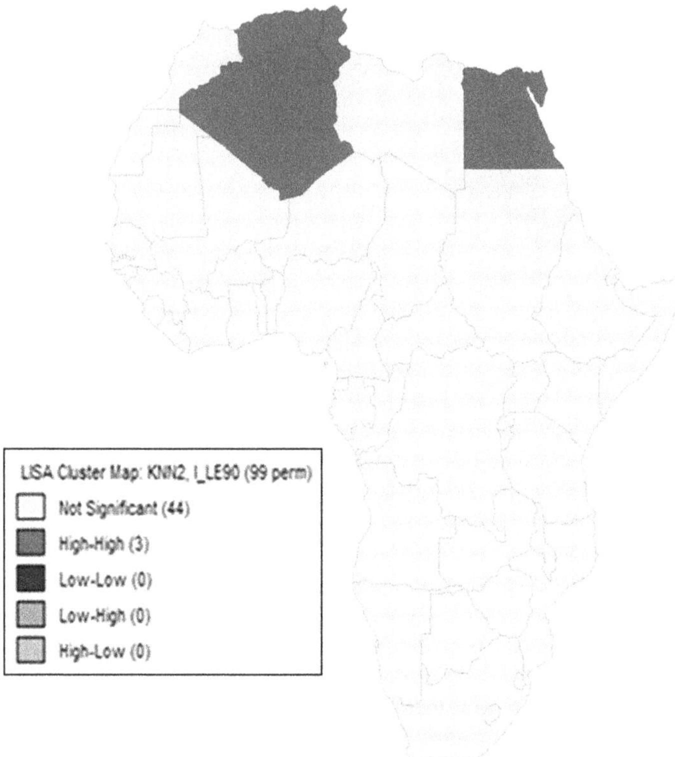


**Figure F Spatial Clusters and Identification of Hotspots and Cold Spots in Life Expectancy at Birth in Africa, 1990s. The spatial weight matrix k-nearest neighbor of order 2 was employed on LISA cluster map.**

# Appendix II

## *Some Selected Development Indicators and Data from World Bank, IMF, and Barro & Lee from 1960 to 2015*

| *Country Name* | *Country Code* | *Year* | *Life Expectancy at Birth* | *GDP Per Capita* |
|---|---|---|---|---|
| Algeria | DZA | 1960 | 46.13512 | 2466.03824 |
| Angola | AGO | 1960 | 33.22602 | |
| Benin | BEN | 1960 | 37.28641 | 520.40418 |
| Botswana | BWA | 1960 | 50.54773 | 390.829725 |
| Burkina Faso | BFA | 1960 | 34.4779 | 238.854562 |
| Burundi | BDI | 1960 | 41.23605 | 214.136954 |
| Cabo Verde | CPV | 1960 | 48.85641 | |
| Cameroon | CMR | 1960 | 41.52376 | 956.456041 |
| Central African Republic | CAF | 1960 | 36.48263 | 601.852493 |
| Chad | TCD | 1960 | 38.0082 | 696.276928 |
| Comoros | COM | 1960 | 41.44244 | |
| Congo, Dem. Rep. | COD | 1960 | 41.01805 | 988.981572 |
| Congo, Rep. | COG | 1960 | 48.58112 | 1429.99798 |
| Cote d'Ivoire | CIV | 1960 | 36.87241 | 1205.26063 |
| Djibouti | DJI | 1960 | 44.02127 | |
| Egypt, Arab Rep. | EGY | 1960 | 48.01371 | 631.12839 |
| Equatorial Guinea | GNQ | 1960 | 36.73305 | |
| Eritrea | ERI | 1960 | 38.40422 | |
| Ethiopia | ETH | 1960 | 38.40571 | |
| Gabon | GAB | 1960 | 39.57012 | 4377.37613 |
| Gambia, The | GMB | 1960 | 32.04222 | |
| Ghana | GHA | 1960 | 45.83146 | 1053.26722 |
| Guinea | GIN | 1960 | 34.88639 | |
| Guinea-Bissau | GNB | 1960 | 37.84044 | |
| Kenya | KEN | 1960 | 46.36241 | 538.442994 |
| Lesotho | LSO | 1960 | 46.50095 | 257.216739 |
| Liberia | LBR | 1960 | 34.78317 | 1273.4841 |
| Libya | LBY | 1960 | 42.6412 | |
| Madagascar | MDG | 1960 | 39.97468 | 716.081771 |

| Country Name | Country Code | Year | Life Expectancy at Birth | GDP Per Capita |
|---|---|---|---|---|
| Malawi | MWI | 1960 | 37.77363 | 241.186085 |
| Mali | MLI | 1960 | 28.21161 | |
| Mauritania | MRT | 1960 | 43.4831 | 791.08535 |
| Mauritius | MUS | 1960 | 58.74522 | |
| Morocco | MAR | 1960 | 48.44663 | |
| Mozambique | MOZ | 1960 | 35.00371 | |
| Namibia | NAM | 1960 | 46.88141 | |
| Niger | NER | 1960 | 34.99773 | 612.255192 |
| Nigeria | NGA | 1960 | 36.975 | 1299.94925 |
| Rwanda | RWA | 1960 | 42.24929 | 331.644434 |
| Sao Tome and Principe | STP | 1960 | 50.45137 | |
| Senegal | SEN | 1960 | 38.206 | 1080.32335 |
| Seychelles | SYC | 1960 | | 2829.64066 |
| Sierra Leone | SLE | 1960 | 30.33154 | 376.270866 |
| Somalia | SOM | 1960 | 36.96588 | |
| South Africa | ZAF | 1960 | 52.22624 | 4542.9931 |
| Sudan | SDN | 1960 | 48.18763 | 887.794108 |
| Swaziland | SWZ | 1960 | 44.23878 | |
| Tanzania | TZA | 1960 | 43.65388 | |
| Togo | TGO | 1960 | 40.27283 | 349.049555 |
| Tunisia | TUN | 1960 | 42.00976 | |
| Uganda | UGA | 1960 | 43.98356 | |
| Zambia | ZMB | 1960 | 45.1098 | 1508.44269 |
| Zimbabwe | ZWE | 1960 | 51.54198 | 897.523519 |
| Algeria | DZA | 1961 | 46.59032 | 2078.22193 |
| Angola | AGO | 1961 | 33.54776 | |
| Benin | BEN | 1961 | 37.73885 | 529.297339 |
| Botswana | BWA | 1961 | 50.90763 | 405.798638 |
| Burkina Faso | BFA | 1961 | 34.93863 | 245.198583 |
| Burundi | BDI | 1961 | 41.54546 | 181.217677 |
| Cabo Verde | CPV | 1961 | 49.04798 | |
| Cameroon | CMR | 1961 | 41.96534 | 947.825238 |
| Central African Republic | CAF | 1961 | 36.89571 | 621.042039 |
| Chad | TCD | 1961 | 38.26449 | 692.452985 |
| Comoros | COM | 1961 | 41.83954 | |
| Congo, Dem. Rep. | COD | 1961 | 41.23354 | 859.704266 |
| Congo, Rep. | COG | 1961 | 49.23005 | 1510.25819 |
| Cote d'Ivoire | CIV | 1961 | 37.56307 | 1276.47651 |
| Djibouti | DJI | 1961 | 44.45134 | |
| Egypt, Arab Rep. | EGY | 1961 | 48.58159 | 641.132204 |
| Equatorial Guinea | GNQ | 1961 | 37.03249 | |
| Eritrea | ERI | 1961 | 39.06071 | |
| Ethiopia | ETH | 1961 | 39.06863 | |
| Gabon | GAB | 1961 | 39.92805 | 4974.12325 |
| Gambia, The | GMB | 1961 | 32.32563 | |
| Ghana | GHA | 1961 | 46.26671 | 1055.39932 |
| Guinea | GIN | 1961 | 35.08112 | |

| Country Name | Country Code | Year | Life Expectancy at Birth | GDP Per Capita |
|---|---|---|---|---|
| Guinea-Bissau | GNB | 1961 | 38.14329 | |
| Kenya | KEN | 1961 | 47.013 | 481.377269 |
| Lesotho | LSO | 1961 | 46.98498 | 257.516396 |
| Liberia | LBR | 1961 | 35.04627 | 1276.44537 |
| Libya | LBY | 1961 | 44.24668 | |
| Madagascar | MDG | 1961 | 40.45724 | 713.377383 |
| Malawi | MWI | 1961 | 37.99815 | 253.898345 |
| Mali | MLI | 1961 | 28.35873 | |
| Mauritania | MRT | 1961 | 44.16393 | 888.015853 |
| Mauritius | MUS | 1961 | 59.74837 | |
| Morocco | MAR | 1961 | 48.86412 | |
| Mozambique | MOZ | 1961 | 35.46676 | |
| Namibia | NAM | 1961 | 47.50437 | |
| Niger | NER | 1961 | 35.08515 | 622.183833 |
| Nigeria | NGA | 1961 | 37.42929 | 1276.28521 |
| Rwanda | RWA | 1961 | 42.54876 | 310.753183 |
| Sao Tome and Principe | STP | 1961 | 51.0311 | |
| Senegal | SEN | 1961 | 38.36324 | 1082.76521 |
| Seychelles | SYC | 1961 | | 2616.87435 |
| Sierra Leone | SLE | 1961 | 30.54044 | 377.799358 |
| Somalia | SOM | 1961 | 37.36229 | |
| South Africa | ZAF | 1961 | 52.56873 | 4597.75552 |
| Sudan | SDN | 1961 | 48.61154 | 864.851245 |
| Swaziland | SWZ | 1961 | 44.53488 | |
| Tanzania | TZA | 1961 | 43.90729 | |
| Togo | TGO | 1961 | 40.91649 | 387.356905 |
| Tunisia | TUN | 1961 | 42.64551 | |
| Uganda | UGA | 1961 | 44.56002 | |
| Zambia | ZMB | 1961 | 45.48751 | 1482.51983 |
| Zimbabwe | ZWE | 1961 | 51.91495 | 923.795352 |
| Algeria | DZA | 1962 | 47.045 | 1628.38872 |
| Angola | AGO | 1962 | 33.888 | |
| Benin | BEN | 1962 | 38.19371 | 503.599084 |
| Botswana | BWA | 1962 | 51.25502 | 422.172033 |
| Burkina Faso | BFA | 1962 | 35.40588 | 256.777174 |
| Burundi | BDI | 1962 | 41.86039 | 193.95324 |
| Cabo Verde | CPV | 1962 | 49.32251 | |
| Cameroon | CMR | 1962 | 42.40595 | 955.910378 |
| Central African Republic | CAF | 1962 | 37.31878 | 587.439246 |
| Chad | TCD | 1962 | 38.51939 | 715.343302 |
| Comoros | COM | 1962 | 42.23776 | |
| Congo, Dem. Rep. | COD | 1962 | 41.45151 | 1015.75609 |
| Congo, Rep. | COG | 1962 | 49.84395 | 1547.83496 |
| Cote d'Ivoire | CIV | 1962 | 38.23383 | 1242.73298 |
| Djibouti | DJI | 1962 | 44.87444 | |
| Egypt, Arab Rep. | EGY | 1962 | 49.10651 | 666.791874 |
| Equatorial Guinea | GNQ | 1962 | 37.33241 | |

| Country Name | Country Code | Year | Life Expectancy at Birth | GDP Per Capita |
|---|---|---|---|---|
| Eritrea | ERI | 1962 | 39.67934 | |
| Ethiopia | ETH | 1962 | 39.69866 | |
| Gabon | GAB | 1962 | 40.374 | 5285.5386 |
| Gambia, The | GMB | 1962 | 32.6611 | |
| Ghana | GHA | 1962 | 46.68254 | 1064.8179 |
| Guinea | GIN | 1962 | 35.26039 | |
| Guinea-Bissau | GNB | 1962 | 38.46722 | |
| Kenya | KEN | 1962 | 47.65224 | 510.566849 |
| Lesotho | LSO | 1962 | 47.39249 | 291.709952 |
| Liberia | LBR | 1962 | 35.35412 | 1265.43269 |
| Libya | LBY | 1962 | 45.8712 | |
| Madagascar | MDG | 1962 | 40.9378 | 712.004056 |
| Malawi | MWI | 1962 | 38.21417 | 249.893982 |
| Mali | MLI | 1962 | 28.54846 | |
| Mauritania | MRT | 1962 | 44.82522 | 868.935037 |
| Mauritius | MUS | 1962 | 60.6269 | |
| Morocco | MAR | 1962 | 49.28759 | |
| Mozambique | MOZ | 1962 | 35.91227 | |
| Namibia | NAM | 1962 | 48.11298 | |
| Niger | NER | 1962 | 35.1671 | 666.658207 |
| Nigeria | NGA | 1962 | 37.86907 | 1301.35336 |
| Rwanda | RWA | 1962 | 42.83771 | 339.791493 |
| Sao Tome and Principe | STP | 1962 | 51.59729 | |
| Senegal | SEN | 1962 | 38.446 | 1052.05546 |
| Seychelles | SYC | 1962 | | 2762.64714 |
| Sierra Leone | SLE | 1962 | 30.75278 | 389.304251 |
| Somalia | SOM | 1962 | 37.76122 | |
| South Africa | ZAF | 1962 | 52.90134 | 4755.96262 |
| Sudan | SDN | 1962 | 49.02746 | 900.161084 |
| Swaziland | SWZ | 1962 | 44.81946 | |
| Tanzania | TZA | 1962 | 44.16224 | |
| Togo | TGO | 1962 | 41.5551 | 398.178627 |
| Tunisia | TUN | 1962 | 43.34168 | |
| Uganda | UGA | 1962 | 45.14705 | |
| Zambia | ZMB | 1962 | 45.85366 | 1400.83957 |
| Zimbabwe | ZWE | 1962 | 52.2779 | 906.901732 |
| Algeria | DZA | 1963 | 47.4962 | 2133.31861 |
| Angola | AGO | 1963 | 34.24473 | |
| Benin | BEN | 1963 | 38.6539 | 519.130656 |
| Botswana | BWA | 1963 | 51.59341 | 435.689893 |
| Burkina Faso | BFA | 1963 | 35.87966 | 250.117852 |
| Burundi | BDI | 1963 | 42.1778 | 198.122222 |
| Cabo Verde | CPV | 1963 | 49.69051 | |
| Cameroon | CMR | 1963 | 42.84356 | 970.055061 |
| Central African Republic | CAF | 1963 | 37.76034 | 572.581494 |
| Chad | TCD | 1963 | 38.77537 | 690.119083 |
| Comoros | COM | 1963 | 42.635 | |

| Country Name | Country Code | Year | Life Expectancy at Birth | GDP Per Capita |
|---|---|---|---|---|
| Congo, Dem. Rep. | COD | 1963 | 41.678 | 1041.40758 |
| Congo, Rep. | COG | 1963 | 50.41885 | 1446.47787 |
| Cote d'Ivoire | CIV | 1963 | 38.88017 | 1367.32366 |
| Djibouti | DJI | 1963 | 45.29105 | |
| Egypt, Arab Rep. | EGY | 1963 | 49.60195 | 707.925292 |
| Equatorial Guinea | GNQ | 1963 | 37.63183 | |
| Eritrea | ERI | 1963 | 40.24559 | |
| Ethiopia | ETH | 1963 | 40.2778 | |
| Gabon | GAB | 1963 | 40.92495 | 5537.40039 |
| Gambia, The | GMB | 1963 | 33.0621 | |
| Ghana | GHA | 1963 | 47.07844 | 1078.55426 |
| Guinea | GIN | 1963 | 35.42517 | |
| Guinea-Bissau | GNB | 1963 | 38.81371 | |
| Kenya | KEN | 1963 | 48.26927 | 537.96413 |
| Lesotho | LSO | 1963 | 47.71649 | 316.758808 |
| Liberia | LBR | 1963 | 35.71522 | 1265.65695 |
| Libya | LBY | 1963 | 47.45622 | |
| Madagascar | MDG | 1963 | 41.4149 | 688.181696 |
| Malawi | MWI | 1963 | 38.42171 | 240.837956 |
| Mali | MLI | 1963 | 28.79639 | |
| Mauritania | MRT | 1963 | 45.46002 | 827.273378 |
| Mauritius | MUS | 1963 | 61.35766 | |
| Morocco | MAR | 1963 | 49.71476 | |
| Mozambique | MOZ | 1963 | 36.33878 | |
| Namibia | NAM | 1963 | 48.70622 | |
| Niger | NER | 1963 | 35.24459 | 708.635298 |
| Nigeria | NGA | 1963 | 38.28883 | 1383.48257 |
| Rwanda | RWA | 1963 | 43.11312 | 301.251051 |
| Sao Tome and Principe | STP | 1963 | 52.146 | |
| Senegal | SEN | 1963 | 38.46324 | 1042.46641 |
| Seychelles | SYC | 1963 | | 2966.28182 |
| Sierra Leone | SLE | 1963 | 30.97756 | 390.077448 |
| Somalia | SOM | 1963 | 38.16217 | |
| South Africa | ZAF | 1963 | 53.23405 | 4974.27087 |
| Sudan | SDN | 1963 | 49.43793 | 850.99319 |
| Swaziland | SWZ | 1963 | 45.10056 | |
| Tanzania | TZA | 1963 | 44.42371 | |
| Togo | TGO | 1963 | 42.18917 | 413.215904 |
| Tunisia | TUN | 1963 | 44.10078 | |
| Uganda | UGA | 1963 | 45.73812 | |
| Zambia | ZMB | 1963 | 46.20922 | 1401.46217 |
| Zimbabwe | ZWE | 1963 | 52.62932 | 932.444933 |
| Algeria | DZA | 1964 | 47.9419 | 2200.81388 |
| Angola | AGO | 1964 | 34.61746 | |
| Benin | BEN | 1964 | 39.12239 | 544.427763 |
| Botswana | BWA | 1964 | 51.92876 | 453.078975 |
| Burkina Faso | BFA | 1964 | 36.35895 | 252.261832 |

| Country Name | Country Code | Year | Life Expectancy at Birth | GDP Per Capita |
|---|---|---|---|---|
| Burundi | BDI | 1964 | 42.49222 | 206.289436 |
| Cabo Verde | CPV | 1964 | 50.152 | |
| Cameroon | CMR | 1964 | 43.27866 | 982.052248 |
| Central African Republic | CAF | 1964 | 38.22537 | 573.373508 |
| Chad | TCD | 1964 | 39.03837 | 659.744315 |
| Comoros | COM | 1964 | 43.03271 | |
| Congo, Dem. Rep. | COD | 1964 | 41.918 | 989.429321 |
| Congo, Rep. | COG | 1964 | 50.95229 | 1461.71235 |
| Cote d'Ivoire | CIV | 1964 | 39.5051 | 1545.87327 |
| Djibouti | DJI | 1964 | 45.70863 | |
| Egypt, Arab Rep. | EGY | 1964 | 50.07539 | 745.458024 |
| Equatorial Guinea | GNQ | 1964 | 37.93173 | |
| Eritrea | ERI | 1964 | 40.75446 | |
| Ethiopia | ETH | 1964 | 40.79756 | |
| Gabon | GAB | 1964 | 41.58541 | 5706.43366 |
| Gambia, The | GMB | 1964 | 33.53763 | |
| Ghana | GHA | 1964 | 47.45337 | 1071.5919 |
| Guinea | GIN | 1964 | 35.58093 | |
| Guinea-Bissau | GNB | 1964 | 39.18127 | |
| Kenya | KEN | 1964 | 48.86061 | 546.765581 |
| Lesotho | LSO | 1964 | 47.96149 | 336.464422 |
| Liberia | LBR | 1964 | 36.13 | 1301.02058 |
| Libya | LBY | 1964 | 48.95771 | |
| Madagascar | MDG | 1964 | 41.89054 | 697.791666 |
| Malawi | MWI | 1964 | 38.62578 | 241.551465 |
| Mali | MLI | 1964 | 29.11105 | |
| Mauritania | MRT | 1964 | 46.06234 | 1025.95706 |
| Mauritius | MUS | 1964 | 61.93495 | |
| Morocco | MAR | 1964 | 50.142 | |
| Mozambique | MOZ | 1964 | 36.74876 | |
| Namibia | NAM | 1964 | 49.28351 | |
| Niger | NER | 1964 | 35.31761 | 689.266914 |
| Nigeria | NGA | 1964 | 38.68707 | 1421.37894 |
| Rwanda | RWA | 1964 | 43.37054 | 258.799983 |
| Sao Tome and Principe | STP | 1964 | 52.67476 | |
| Senegal | SEN | 1964 | 38.43598 | 1053.14099 |
| Seychelles | SYC | 1964 | | 3064.13408 |
| Sierra Leone | SLE | 1964 | 31.23039 | 409.867968 |
| Somalia | SOM | 1964 | 38.56512 | |
| South Africa | ZAF | 1964 | 53.57366 | 5230.67009 |
| Sudan | SDN | 1964 | 49.84388 | 818.463055 |
| Swaziland | SWZ | 1964 | 45.38866 | |
| Tanzania | TZA | 1964 | 44.69771 | |
| Togo | TGO | 1964 | 42.81922 | 463.636221 |
| Tunisia | TUN | 1964 | 44.92385 | |
| Uganda | UGA | 1964 | 46.32127 | |
| Zambia | ZMB | 1964 | 46.55868 | 1523.54145 |

| *Country Name* | *Country Code* | *Year* | *Life Expectancy at Birth* | *GDP Per Capita* |
|---|---|---|---|---|
| Zimbabwe | ZWE | 1964 | 52.97166 | 892.520512 |
| Algeria | DZA | 1965 | 48.3761 | 2276.147 |
| Angola | AGO | 1965 | 35.00222 | |
| Benin | BEN | 1965 | 39.59954 | 563.146439 |
| Botswana | BWA | 1965 | 52.27254 | 466.26218 |
| Burkina Faso | BFA | 1965 | 36.83776 | 257.915078 |
| Burundi | BDI | 1965 | 42.79015 | 209.803506 |
| Cabo Verde | CPV | 1965 | 50.68698 | |
| Cameroon | CMR | 1965 | 43.71517 | 979.142277 |
| Central African Republic | CAF | 1965 | 38.72585 | 567.462107 |
| Chad | TCD | 1965 | 39.32176 | 651.095409 |
| Comoros | COM | 1965 | 43.43427 | |
| Congo, Dem. Rep. | COD | 1965 | 42.18049 | 972.490489 |
| Congo, Rep. | COG | 1965 | 51.44137 | 1474.62735 |
| Cote d'Ivoire | CIV | 1965 | 40.12441 | 1441.02482 |
| Djibouti | DJI | 1965 | 46.14715 | |
| Egypt, Arab Rep. | EGY | 1965 | 50.52039 | 763.349667 |
| Equatorial Guinea | GNQ | 1965 | 38.23163 | |
| Eritrea | ERI | 1965 | 41.20785 | |
| Ethiopia | ETH | 1965 | 41.25546 | |
| Gabon | GAB | 1965 | 42.34439 | 6080.71542 |
| Gambia, The | GMB | 1965 | 34.0932 | |
| Ghana | GHA | 1965 | 47.80763 | 1058.472 |
| Guinea | GIN | 1965 | 35.73161 | |
| Guinea-Bissau | GNB | 1965 | 39.56588 | |
| Kenya | KEN | 1965 | 49.42827 | 539.879388 |
| Lesotho | LSO | 1965 | 48.14049 | 337.147248 |
| Liberia | LBR | 1965 | 36.59337 | 1332.23792 |
| Libya | LBY | 1965 | 50.34954 | |
| Madagascar | MDG | 1965 | 42.36568 | 677.291224 |
| Malawi | MWI | 1965 | 38.84139 | 268.001215 |
| Mali | MLI | 1965 | 29.50193 | |
| Mauritania | MRT | 1965 | 46.63073 | 1157.16553 |
| Mauritius | MUS | 1965 | 62.35829 | |
| Morocco | MAR | 1965 | 50.56488 | |
| Mozambique | MOZ | 1965 | 37.14922 | |
| Namibia | NAM | 1965 | 49.84117 | |
| Niger | NER | 1965 | 35.38763 | 716.006771 |
| Nigeria | NGA | 1965 | 39.0678 | 1459.25359 |
| Rwanda | RWA | 1965 | 43.60141 | 270.84063 |
| Sao Tome and Principe | STP | 1965 | 53.18971 | |
| Senegal | SEN | 1965 | 38.39568 | 1037.4513 |
| Seychelles | SYC | 1965 | | 2956.45217 |
| Sierra Leone | SLE | 1965 | 31.54263 | 432.531725 |
| Somalia | SOM | 1965 | 38.9691 | |
| South Africa | ZAF | 1965 | 53.9289 | 5409.23558 |
| Sudan | SDN | 1965 | 50.24837 | 849.701698 |

| Country Name | Country Code | Year | Life Expectancy at Birth | GDP Per Capita |
|---|---|---|---|---|
| Swaziland | SWZ | 1965 | 45.70076 | |
| Tanzania | TZA | 1965 | 44.98873 | |
| Togo | TGO | 1965 | 43.44471 | 520.72676 |
| Tunisia | TUN | 1965 | 45.81441 | 1113.19282 |
| Uganda | UGA | 1965 | 46.87949 | |
| Zambia | ZMB | 1965 | 46.91202 | 1722.08031 |
| Zimbabwe | ZWE | 1965 | 53.30446 | 906.550349 |
| Algeria | DZA | 1966 | 48.7908 | 2107.80039 |
| Angola | AGO | 1966 | 35.39651 | |
| Benin | BEN | 1966 | 40.08622 | 572.453223 |
| Botswana | BWA | 1966 | 52.63571 | 481.785854 |
| Burkina Faso | BFA | 1966 | 37.30905 | 255.281531 |
| Burundi | BDI | 1966 | 43.05507 | 214.271136 |
| Cabo Verde | CPV | 1966 | 51.26293 | |
| Cameroon | CMR | 1966 | 44.15851 | 1000.55475 |
| Central African Republic | CAF | 1966 | 39.27276 | 559.564776 |
| Chad | TCD | 1966 | 39.64039 | 627.461752 |
| Comoros | COM | 1966 | 43.84561 | |
| Congo, Dem. Rep. | COD | 1966 | 42.47249 | 1009.77966 |
| Congo, Rep. | COG | 1966 | 51.88866 | 1454.05902 |
| Cote d'Ivoire | CIV | 1966 | 40.76193 | 1548.58657 |
| Djibouti | DJI | 1966 | 46.63351 | |
| Egypt, Arab Rep. | EGY | 1966 | 50.92049 | 751.419523 |
| Equatorial Guinea | GNQ | 1966 | 38.53156 | |
| Eritrea | ERI | 1966 | 41.61766 | |
| Ethiopia | ETH | 1966 | 41.65598 | |
| Gabon | GAB | 1966 | 43.17937 | 6237.16807 |
| Gambia, The | GMB | 1966 | 34.73224 | 422.352686 |
| Ghana | GHA | 1966 | 48.14098 | 990.225831 |
| Guinea | GIN | 1966 | 35.88161 | |
| Guinea-Bissau | GNB | 1966 | 39.96002 | |
| Kenya | KEN | 1966 | 49.98168 | 599.356019 |
| Lesotho | LSO | 1966 | 48.273 | 329.238333 |
| Liberia | LBR | 1966 | 37.0962 | 1401.47669 |
| Libya | LBY | 1966 | 51.62954 | |
| Madagascar | MDG | 1966 | 42.84283 | 673.827468 |
| Malawi | MWI | 1966 | 39.08605 | 296.249689 |
| Mali | MLI | 1966 | 29.97098 | |
| Mauritania | MRT | 1966 | 47.16468 | 1126.33856 |
| Mauritius | MUS | 1966 | 62.63871 | |
| Morocco | MAR | 1966 | 50.97805 | 815.500859 |
| Mozambique | MOZ | 1966 | 37.54868 | |
| Namibia | NAM | 1966 | 50.37244 | |
| Niger | NER | 1966 | 35.45763 | 693.111187 |
| Nigeria | NGA | 1966 | 39.43702 | 1367.48827 |
| Rwanda | RWA | 1966 | 43.79727 | 282.301129 |
| Sao Tome and Principe | STP | 1966 | 53.69949 | |

| Country Name | Country Code | Year | Life Expectancy at Birth | GDP Per Capita |
|---|---|---|---|---|
| Senegal | SEN | 1966 | 38.37585 | 1037.34522 |
| Seychelles | SYC | 1966 | | 3284.39083 |
| Sierra Leone | SLE | 1966 | 31.94822 | 432.994441 |
| Somalia | SOM | 1966 | 39.37207 | |
| South Africa | ZAF | 1966 | 54.30688 | 5507.20512 |
| Sudan | SDN | 1966 | 50.65337 | 796.279434 |
| Swaziland | SWZ | 1966 | 46.05232 | |
| Tanzania | TZA | 1966 | 45.2968 | |
| Togo | TGO | 1966 | 44.06863 | 548.717919 |
| Tunisia | TUN | 1966 | 46.77495 | 1128.57679 |
| Uganda | UGA | 1966 | 47.39424 | |
| Zambia | ZMB | 1966 | 47.28527 | 1576.2662 |
| Zimbabwe | ZWE | 1966 | 53.62771 | 891.409882 |
| Algeria | DZA | 1967 | 49.18751 | 2242.45042 |
| Angola | AGO | 1967 | 35.79785 | |
| Benin | BEN | 1967 | 40.58041 | 567.383629 |
| Botswana | BWA | 1967 | 53.02824 | 495.385282 |
| Burkina Faso | BFA | 1967 | 37.76832 | 273.300218 |
| Burundi | BDI | 1967 | 43.28002 | 237.755603 |
| Cabo Verde | CPV | 1967 | 51.84737 | |
| Cameroon | CMR | 1967 | 44.61363 | 870.27322 |
| Central African Republic | CAF | 1967 | 39.86856 | 573.560064 |
| Chad | TCD | 1967 | 40.00163 | 620.744772 |
| Comoros | COM | 1967 | 44.2712 | |
| Congo, Dem. Rep. | COD | 1967 | 42.79198 | 971.735922 |
| Congo, Rep. | COG | 1967 | 52.29822 | 1444.12831 |
| Cote d'Ivoire | CIV | 1967 | 41.43695 | 1560.95153 |
| Djibouti | DJI | 1967 | 47.18166 | |
| Egypt, Arab Rep. | EGY | 1967 | 51.26824 | 736.684131 |
| Equatorial Guinea | GNQ | 1967 | 38.83205 | |
| Eritrea | ERI | 1967 | 42.00329 | |
| Ethiopia | ETH | 1967 | 42.01505 | |
| Gabon | GAB | 1967 | 44.05234 | 6361.73788 |
| Gambia, The | GMB | 1967 | 35.44327 | 414.075835 |
| Ghana | GHA | 1967 | 48.45524 | 999.593528 |
| Guinea | GIN | 1967 | 36.03844 | |
| Guinea-Bissau | GNB | 1967 | 40.35717 | |
| Kenya | KEN | 1967 | 50.53273 | 599.248123 |
| Lesotho | LSO | 1967 | 48.39007 | 357.908421 |
| Liberia | LBR | 1967 | 37.62388 | 1460.57702 |
| Libya | LBY | 1967 | 52.83115 | |
| Madagascar | MDG | 1967 | 43.32393 | 692.941343 |
| Malawi | MWI | 1967 | 39.37173 | 310.074766 |
| Mali | MLI | 1967 | 30.50563 | 340.694161 |
| Mauritania | MRT | 1967 | 47.67317 | 1132.81205 |
| Mauritius | MUS | 1967 | 62.81532 | |
| Morocco | MAR | 1967 | 51.38139 | 875.531126 |

| Country Name | Country Code | Year | Life Expectancy at Birth | GDP Per Capita |
|---|---|---|---|---|
| Mozambique | MOZ | 1967 | 37.95466 | |
| Namibia | NAM | 1967 | 50.87868 | |
| Niger | NER | 1967 | 35.53256 | 674.432392 |
| Nigeria | NGA | 1967 | 39.80424 | 1127.44303 |
| Rwanda | RWA | 1967 | 43.95961 | 293.06303 |
| Sao Tome and Principe | STP | 1967 | 54.21563 | |
| Senegal | SEN | 1967 | 38.41598 | 995.777705 |
| Seychelles | SYC | 1967 | | 3220.81029 |
| Sierra Leone | SLE | 1967 | 32.46283 | 426.21763 |
| Somalia | SOM | 1967 | 39.77254 | |
| South Africa | ZAF | 1967 | 54.70334 | 5756.66623 |
| Sudan | SDN | 1967 | 51.05785 | 784.587859 |
| Swaziland | SWZ | 1967 | 46.45232 | |
| Tanzania | TZA | 1967 | 45.62088 | |
| Togo | TGO | 1967 | 44.68946 | 553.49852 |
| Tunisia | TUN | 1967 | 47.80051 | 1106.69902 |
| Uganda | UGA | 1967 | 47.85151 | |
| Zambia | ZMB | 1967 | 47.68398 | 1649.19771 |
| Zimbabwe | ZWE | 1967 | 53.94544 | 935.862046 |
| Algeria | DZA | 1968 | 49.57271 | 2414.0167 |
| Angola | AGO | 1968 | 36.20227 | |
| Benin | BEN | 1968 | 41.08215 | 577.305495 |
| Botswana | BWA | 1968 | 53.45763 | 531.213925 |
| Burkina Faso | BFA | 1968 | 38.21654 | 276.974204 |
| Burundi | BDI | 1968 | 43.46798 | 231.170921 |
| Cabo Verde | CPV | 1968 | 52.42232 | |
| Cameroon | CMR | 1968 | 45.08456 | 903.180544 |
| Central African Republic | CAF | 1968 | 40.51276 | 569.439779 |
| Chad | TCD | 1968 | 40.40598 | 606.510125 |
| Comoros | COM | 1968 | 44.71205 | |
| Congo, Dem. Rep. | COD | 1968 | 43.13346 | 985.160335 |
| Congo, Rep. | COG | 1968 | 52.67659 | 1511.09974 |
| Cote d'Ivoire | CIV | 1968 | 42.161 | 1692.16358 |
| Djibouti | DJI | 1968 | 47.79163 | |
| Egypt, Arab Rep. | EGY | 1968 | 51.56868 | 737.614383 |
| Equatorial Guinea | GNQ | 1968 | 39.13305 | |
| Eritrea | ERI | 1968 | 42.38222 | |
| Ethiopia | ETH | 1968 | 42.34417 | |
| Gabon | GAB | 1968 | 44.93332 | 6382.47232 |
| Gambia, The | GMB | 1968 | 36.21124 | 443.949143 |
| Ghana | GHA | 1968 | 48.75641 | 983.318069 |
| Guinea | GIN | 1968 | 36.21159 | |
| Guinea-Bissau | GNB | 1968 | 40.75085 | |
| Kenya | KEN | 1968 | 51.0918 | 625.657332 |
| Lesotho | LSO | 1968 | 48.52117 | 349.408925 |
| Liberia | LBR | 1968 | 38.16829 | 1493.23837 |
| Libya | LBY | 1968 | 53.97737 | |

| *Country Name* | *Country Code* | *Year* | *Life Expectancy at Birth* | *GDP Per Capita* |
|---|---|---|---|---|
| Madagascar | MDG | 1968 | 43.80898 | 721.151433 |
| Malawi | MWI | 1968 | 39.70544 | 296.552215 |
| Mali | MLI | 1968 | 31.09378 | 348.766696 |
| Mauritania | MRT | 1968 | 48.16271 | 1212.26355 |
| Mauritius | MUS | 1968 | 62.93168 | |
| Morocco | MAR | 1968 | 51.77522 | 939.69873 |
| Mozambique | MOZ | 1968 | 38.37117 | |
| Namibia | NAM | 1968 | 51.36383 | |
| Niger | NER | 1968 | 35.61939 | 658.067813 |
| Nigeria | NGA | 1968 | 40.17846 | 1089.14462 |
| Rwanda | RWA | 1968 | 44.09146 | 303.931166 |
| Sao Tome and Principe | STP | 1968 | 54.74715 | |
| Senegal | SEN | 1968 | 38.55056 | 1028.27698 |
| Seychelles | SYC | 1968 | | 3381.23324 |
| Sierra Leone | SLE | 1968 | 33.08695 | 427.619497 |
| Somalia | SOM | 1968 | 40.16851 | |
| South Africa | ZAF | 1968 | 55.10927 | 5846.77729 |
| Sudan | SDN | 1968 | 51.45783 | 776.894137 |
| Swaziland | SWZ | 1968 | 46.90429 | |
| Tanzania | TZA | 1968 | 45.95795 | |
| Togo | TGO | 1968 | 45.30822 | 554.315972 |
| Tunisia | TUN | 1968 | 48.87912 | 1195.52309 |
| Uganda | UGA | 1968 | 48.24329 | |
| Zambia | ZMB | 1968 | 48.10915 | 1618.48133 |
| Zimbabwe | ZWE | 1968 | 54.26015 | 924.520651 |
| Algeria | DZA | 1969 | 49.9559 | 2543.56327 |
| Angola | AGO | 1969 | 36.60722 | |
| Benin | BEN | 1969 | 41.58995 | 581.610374 |
| Botswana | BWA | 1969 | 53.92788 | 592.671386 |
| Burkina Faso | BFA | 1969 | 38.65773 | 277.774091 |
| Burundi | BDI | 1969 | 43.62744 | 222.724813 |
| Cabo Verde | CPV | 1969 | 52.98873 | |
| Cameroon | CMR | 1969 | 45.57178 | 924.184379 |
| Central African Republic | CAF | 1969 | 41.20237 | 597.274394 |
| Chad | TCD | 1969 | 40.84541 | 635.706782 |
| Comoros | COM | 1969 | 45.16822 | |
| Congo, Dem. Rep. | COD | 1969 | 43.48895 | 1046.8594 |
| Congo, Rep. | COG | 1969 | 53.02871 | 1579.01468 |
| Cote d'Ivoire | CIV | 1969 | 42.9321 | 1782.17739 |
| Djibouti | DJI | 1969 | 48.45293 | |
| Egypt, Arab Rep. | EGY | 1969 | 51.84178 | 768.532854 |
| Equatorial Guinea | GNQ | 1969 | 39.43559 | |
| Eritrea | ERI | 1969 | 42.76195 | |
| Ethiopia | ETH | 1969 | 42.64929 | |
| Gabon | GAB | 1969 | 45.8038 | 6752.36583 |
| Gambia, The | GMB | 1969 | 37.02417 | 444.025946 |
| Ghana | GHA | 1969 | 49.04807 | 1020.49008 |

| Country Name | Country Code | Year | Life Expectancy at Birth | GDP Per Capita |
|---|---|---|---|---|
| Guinea | GIN | 1969 | 36.41007 | |
| Guinea-Bissau | GNB | 1969 | 41.13951 | |
| Kenya | KEN | 1969 | 51.65988 | 652.739898 |
| Lesotho | LSO | 1969 | 48.6848 | 347.620367 |
| Liberia | LBR | 1969 | 38.7249 | 1562.45008 |
| Libya | LBY | 1969 | 55.07229 | |
| Madagascar | MDG | 1969 | 44.29549 | 728.421871 |
| Malawi | MWI | 1969 | 40.08663 | 306.029078 |
| Mali | MLI | 1969 | 31.72641 | 344.766763 |
| Mauritania | MRT | 1969 | 48.63932 | 1191.97261 |
| Mauritius | MUS | 1969 | 63.0202 | |
| Morocco | MAR | 1969 | 52.16015 | 995.366825 |
| Mozambique | MOZ | 1969 | 38.79971 | |
| Namibia | NAM | 1969 | 51.83441 | |
| Niger | NER | 1969 | 35.72215 | 604.663288 |
| Nigeria | NGA | 1969 | 40.56468 | 1322.7572 |
| Rwanda | RWA | 1969 | 44.19983 | 326.883502 |
| Sao Tome and Principe | STP | 1969 | 55.29598 | |
| Senegal | SEN | 1969 | 38.80859 | 933.143936 |
| Seychelles | SYC | 1969 | | 3301.74698 |
| Sierra Leone | SLE | 1969 | 33.81039 | 455.990753 |
| Somalia | SOM | 1969 | 40.56046 | |
| South Africa | ZAF | 1969 | 55.51673 | 5968.57887 |
| Sudan | SDN | 1969 | 51.84829 | 764.702182 |
| Swaziland | SWZ | 1969 | 47.40973 | |
| Tanzania | TZA | 1969 | 46.31051 | |
| Togo | TGO | 1969 | 45.92341 | 587.445116 |
| Tunisia | TUN | 1969 | 49.9978 | 1224.96614 |
| Uganda | UGA | 1969 | 48.56354 | |
| Zambia | ZMB | 1969 | 48.55629 | 1560.80535 |
| Zimbabwe | ZWE | 1969 | 54.57685 | 1006.62167 |
| Algeria | DZA | 1970 | 50.34363 | 2691.80232 |
| Angola | AGO | 1970 | 37.01422 | |
| Benin | BEN | 1970 | 42.10746 | 581.235119 |
| Botswana | BWA | 1970 | 54.44346 | 672.227359 |
| Burkina Faso | BFA | 1970 | 39.09688 | 273.331516 |
| Burundi | BDI | 1970 | 43.78193 | 265.22918 |
| Cabo Verde | CPV | 1970 | 53.57817 | |
| Cameroon | CMR | 1970 | 46.0769 | 928.959998 |
| Central African Republic | CAF | 1970 | 41.93541 | 599.012402 |
| Chad | TCD | 1970 | 41.30561 | 634.169057 |
| Comoros | COM | 1970 | 45.63178 | |
| Congo, Dem. Rep. | COD | 1970 | 43.84293 | 1015.53637 |
| Congo, Rep. | COG | 1970 | 53.35856 | 1630.60765 |
| Cote d'Ivoire | CIV | 1970 | 43.74344 | 1886.62157 |
| Djibouti | DJI | 1970 | 49.1361 | |
| Egypt, Arab Rep. | EGY | 1970 | 52.12249 | 792.351949 |

| *Country Name* | *Country Code* | *Year* | *Life Expectancy at Birth* | *GDP Per Capita* |
|---|---|---|---|---|
| Equatorial Guinea | GNQ | 1970 | 39.73115 | |
| Eritrea | ERI | 1970 | 43.1471 | |
| Ethiopia | ETH | 1970 | 42.93441 | |
| Gabon | GAB | 1970 | 46.65527 | 7189.07612 |
| Gambia, The | GMB | 1970 | 37.87056 | 459.245578 |
| Ghana | GHA | 1970 | 49.33498 | 1093.71549 |
| Guinea | GIN | 1970 | 36.64349 | |
| Guinea-Bissau | GNB | 1970 | 41.52168 | 488.413509 |
| Kenya | KEN | 1970 | 52.23646 | 601.070778 |
| Lesotho | LSO | 1970 | 48.89846 | 347.955953 |
| Liberia | LBR | 1970 | 39.30215 | 1624.33188 |
| Libya | LBY | 1970 | 56.11859 | |
| Madagascar | MDG | 1970 | 44.78241 | 746.521973 |
| Malawi | MWI | 1970 | 40.50883 | 299.528548 |
| Mali | MLI | 1970 | 32.393 | 360.53465 |
| Mauritania | MRT | 1970 | 49.10695 | 1296.36165 |
| Mauritius | MUS | 1970 | 63.11805 | |
| Morocco | MAR | 1970 | 52.53729 | 1019.55188 |
| Mozambique | MOZ | 1970 | 39.24329 | |
| Namibia | NAM | 1970 | 52.30659 | |
| Niger | NER | 1970 | 35.8458 | 605.909763 |
| Nigeria | NGA | 1970 | 40.9659 | 1616.18743 |
| Rwanda | RWA | 1970 | 44.29027 | 335.98489 |
| Sao Tome and Principe | STP | 1970 | 55.86846 | |
| Senegal | SEN | 1970 | 39.22054 | 983.378031 |
| Seychelles | SYC | 1970 | | 3511.84863 |
| Sierra Leone | SLE | 1970 | 34.6091 | 486.165028 |
| Somalia | SOM | 1970 | 40.94793 | |
| South Africa | ZAF | 1970 | 55.90949 | 6120.95857 |
| Sudan | SDN | 1970 | 52.22122 | 786.138327 |
| Swaziland | SWZ | 1970 | 47.96017 | 1186.00263 |
| Tanzania | TZA | 1970 | 46.68305 | |
| Togo | TGO | 1970 | 46.5351 | 579.323494 |
| Tunisia | TUN | 1970 | 51.14273 | 1254.2347 |
| Uganda | UGA | 1970 | 48.81224 | |
| Zambia | ZMB | 1970 | 49.01895 | 1582.77318 |
| Zimbabwe | ZWE | 1970 | 54.8991 | 1194.17139 |
| Algeria | DZA | 1971 | 50.74393 | 2321.3504 |
| Angola | AGO | 1971 | 37.42576 | |
| Benin | BEN | 1971 | 42.63724 | 560.180111 |
| Botswana | BWA | 1971 | 55.00841 | 818.684568 |
| Burkina Faso | BFA | 1971 | 39.53851 | 272.41046 |
| Burundi | BDI | 1971 | 43.95993 | 268.644208 |
| Cabo Verde | CPV | 1971 | 54.23807 | |
| Cameroon | CMR | 1971 | 46.6 | 936.870276 |
| Central African Republic | CAF | 1971 | 42.70895 | 594.122608 |
| Chad | TCD | 1971 | 41.76571 | 606.18267 |

| *Country Name* | *Country Code* | *Year* | *Life Expectancy at Birth* | *GDP Per Capita* |
|---|---|---|---|---|
| Comoros | COM | 1971 | 46.09337 | |
| Congo, Dem. Rep. | COD | 1971 | 44.1769 | 1047.57218 |
| Congo, Rep. | COG | 1971 | 53.67002 | 1704.77839 |
| Cote d'Ivoire | CIV | 1971 | 44.57983 | 1975.73434 |
| Djibouti | DJI | 1971 | 49.80176 | |
| Egypt, Arab Rep. | EGY | 1971 | 52.45524 | 800.942228 |
| Equatorial Guinea | GNQ | 1971 | 40.01371 | |
| Eritrea | ERI | 1971 | 43.53678 | |
| Ethiopia | ETH | 1971 | 43.20349 | |
| Gabon | GAB | 1971 | 47.48676 | 7773.6064 |
| Gambia, The | GMB | 1971 | 38.73741 | 446.069131 |
| Ghana | GHA | 1971 | 49.62195 | 1120.74336 |
| Guinea | GIN | 1971 | 36.92044 | |
| Guinea-Bissau | GNB | 1971 | 41.8999 | 459.987693 |
| Kenya | KEN | 1971 | 52.8151 | 708.837672 |
| Lesotho | LSO | 1971 | 49.17012 | 358.325555 |
| Liberia | LBR | 1971 | 39.91354 | 1659.86276 |
| Libya | LBY | 1971 | 57.11798 | |
| Madagascar | MDG | 1971 | 45.26734 | 755.01272 |
| Malawi | MWI | 1971 | 40.95954 | 338.90726 |
| Mali | MLI | 1971 | 33.08151 | 363.955118 |
| Mauritania | MRT | 1971 | 49.56759 | 1282.25462 |
| Mauritius | MUS | 1971 | 63.25334 | |
| Morocco | MAR | 1971 | 52.90368 | 1053.88866 |
| Mozambique | MOZ | 1971 | 39.70695 | |
| Namibia | NAM | 1971 | 52.8021 | |
| Niger | NER | 1971 | 35.9919 | 622.738758 |
| Nigeria | NGA | 1971 | 41.38661 | 1803.95614 |
| Rwanda | RWA | 1971 | 44.3648 | 330.035993 |
| Sao Tome and Principe | STP | 1971 | 56.47298 | |
| Senegal | SEN | 1971 | 39.8079 | 952.693778 |
| Seychelles | SYC | 1971 | | 3987.0864 |
| Sierra Leone | SLE | 1971 | 35.4519 | 493.210464 |
| Somalia | SOM | 1971 | 41.33288 | |
| South Africa | ZAF | 1971 | 56.26841 | 6215.9436 |
| Sudan | SDN | 1971 | 52.57015 | 779.926088 |
| Swaziland | SWZ | 1971 | 48.54461 | 1311.12729 |
| Tanzania | TZA | 1971 | 47.08405 | |
| Togo | TGO | 1971 | 47.14229 | 560.732445 |
| Tunisia | TUN | 1971 | 52.29754 | 1356.58082 |
| Uganda | UGA | 1971 | 48.99493 | |
| Zambia | ZMB | 1971 | 49.48915 | 1528.73609 |
| Zimbabwe | ZWE | 1971 | 55.22937 | 1257.98687 |
| Algeria | DZA | 1972 | 51.1718 | 2877.74526 |
| Angola | AGO | 1972 | 37.84332 | |
| Benin | BEN | 1972 | 43.179 | 583.056243 |
| Botswana | BWA | 1972 | 55.61273 | 1000.80926 |

| Country Name | Country Code | Year | Life Expectancy at Birth | GDP Per Capita |
|---|---|---|---|---|
| Burkina Faso | BFA | 1972 | 39.99517 | 273.836955 |
| Burundi | BDI | 1972 | 44.18495 | 248.697791 |
| Cabo Verde | CPV | 1972 | 55.00049 | |
| Cameroon | CMR | 1972 | 47.13571 | 937.088877 |
| Central African Republic | CAF | 1972 | 43.50851 | 582.950223 |
| Chad | TCD | 1972 | 42.20541 | 598.845713 |
| Comoros | COM | 1972 | 46.54759 | |
| Congo, Dem. Rep. | COD | 1972 | 44.47639 | 1021.47247 |
| Congo, Rep. | COG | 1972 | 53.966 | 1795.67901 |
| Cote d'Ivoire | CIV | 1972 | 45.41602 | 1966.84828 |
| Djibouti | DJI | 1972 | 50.41549 | |
| Egypt, Arab Rep. | EGY | 1972 | 52.86995 | 799.137639 |
| Equatorial Guinea | GNQ | 1972 | 40.28224 | |
| Eritrea | ERI | 1972 | 43.92612 | |
| Ethiopia | ETH | 1972 | 43.45502 | |
| Gabon | GAB | 1972 | 48.31073 | 8494.08741 |
| Gambia, The | GMB | 1972 | 39.61376 | 433.630335 |
| Ghana | GHA | 1972 | 49.91229 | 1062.02716 |
| Guinea | GIN | 1972 | 37.242 | |
| Guinea-Bissau | GNB | 1972 | 42.27917 | 479.258311 |
| Kenya | KEN | 1972 | 53.38983 | 800.687279 |
| Lesotho | LSO | 1972 | 49.49427 | 350.327544 |
| Liberia | LBR | 1972 | 40.56615 | 1682.86309 |
| Libya | LBY | 1972 | 58.0732 | |
| Madagascar | MDG | 1972 | 45.74673 | 725.148377 |
| Malawi | MWI | 1972 | 41.4212 | 350.327467 |
| Mali | MLI | 1972 | 33.785 | 378.774828 |
| Mauritania | MRT | 1972 | 50.02371 | 1236.29234 |
| Mauritius | MUS | 1972 | 63.43995 | |
| Morocco | MAR | 1972 | 53.26673 | 1057.36821 |
| Mozambique | MOZ | 1972 | 40.18117 | |
| Namibia | NAM | 1972 | 53.3292 | |
| Niger | NER | 1972 | 36.163 | 574.433949 |
| Nigeria | NGA | 1972 | 41.82283 | 1821.18208 |
| Rwanda | RWA | 1972 | 44.43798 | 321.321638 |
| Sao Tome and Principe | STP | 1972 | 57.0998 | |
| Senegal | SEN | 1972 | 40.55622 | 982.898872 |
| Seychelles | SYC | 1972 | | 4137.68674 |
| Sierra Leone | SLE | 1972 | 36.29524 | 487.485987 |
| Somalia | SOM | 1972 | 41.71685 | |
| South Africa | ZAF | 1972 | 56.58098 | 6151.1771 |
| Sudan | SDN | 1972 | 52.88754 | 718.189247 |
| Swaziland | SWZ | 1972 | 49.14561 | 1342.36546 |
| Tanzania | TZA | 1972 | 47.511 | |
| Togo | TGO | 1972 | 47.74305 | 586.863288 |
| Tunisia | TUN | 1972 | 53.45024 | 1562.58033 |
| Uganda | UGA | 1972 | 49.1261 | |

| Country Name | Country Code | Year | Life Expectancy at Birth | GDP Per Capita |
|---|---|---|---|---|
| Zambia | ZMB | 1972 | 49.94934 | 1612.68811 |
| Zimbabwe | ZWE | 1972 | 55.57068 | 1317.31164 |
| Algeria | DZA | 1973 | 51.64571 | 2906.7005 |
| Angola | AGO | 1973 | 38.26185 | |
| Benin | BEN | 1973 | 43.72985 | 591.050532 |
| Botswana | BWA | 1973 | 56.245 | 1173.45171 |
| Burkina Faso | BFA | 1973 | 40.48034 | 270.182896 |
| Burundi | BDI | 1973 | 44.47146 | 263.272084 |
| Cabo Verde | CPV | 1973 | 55.87388 | |
| Cameroon | CMR | 1973 | 47.67759 | 961.355583 |
| Central African Republic | CAF | 1973 | 44.31612 | 582.761162 |
| Chad | TCD | 1973 | 42.61032 | 535.665476 |
| Comoros | COM | 1973 | 46.99154 | |
| Congo, Dem. Rep. | COD | 1973 | 44.73737 | 1075.60936 |
| Congo, Rep. | COG | 1973 | 54.24941 | 1884.33893 |
| Cote d'Ivoire | CIV | 1973 | 46.23122 | 1987.8344 |
| Djibouti | DJI | 1973 | 50.95485 | |
| Egypt, Arab Rep. | EGY | 1973 | 53.38359 | 787.289808 |
| Equatorial Guinea | GNQ | 1973 | 40.54473 | |
| Eritrea | ERI | 1973 | 44.30822 | |
| Ethiopia | ETH | 1973 | 43.68354 | |
| Gabon | GAB | 1973 | 49.13471 | 9186.71225 |
| Gambia, The | GMB | 1973 | 40.49012 | 458.924725 |
| Ghana | GHA | 1973 | 50.20729 | 1061.51436 |
| Guinea | GIN | 1973 | 37.60924 | |
| Guinea-Bissau | GNB | 1973 | 42.66246 | 475.101044 |
| Kenya | KEN | 1973 | 53.95317 | 817.674503 |
| Lesotho | LSO | 1973 | 49.86539 | 433.607775 |
| Liberia | LBR | 1973 | 41.2601 | 1600.41427 |
| Libya | LBY | 1973 | 58.98541 | |
| Madagascar | MDG | 1973 | 46.21615 | 686.782163 |
| Malawi | MWI | 1973 | 41.87734 | 348.537823 |
| Mali | MLI | 1973 | 34.49446 | 366.776112 |
| Mauritania | MRT | 1973 | 50.48137 | 1145.80653 |
| Mauritius | MUS | 1973 | 63.68554 | |
| Morocco | MAR | 1973 | 53.63632 | 1072.54736 |
| Mozambique | MOZ | 1973 | 40.64946 | |
| Namibia | NAM | 1973 | 53.89159 | |
| Niger | NER | 1973 | 36.3621 | 463.48817 |
| Nigeria | NGA | 1973 | 42.27002 | 1873.16322 |
| Rwanda | RWA | 1973 | 44.52976 | 322.758317 |
| Sao Tome and Principe | STP | 1973 | 57.73376 | |
| Senegal | SEN | 1973 | 41.44046 | 900.300665 |
| Seychelles | SYC | 1973 | | 4443.8728 |
| Sierra Leone | SLE | 1973 | 37.09973 | 487.919336 |
| Somalia | SOM | 1973 | 42.09985 | |
| South Africa | ZAF | 1973 | 56.84105 | 6261.45963 |

| *Country Name* | *Country Code* | *Year* | *Life Expectancy at Birth* | *GDP Per Capita* |
|---|---|---|---|---|
| Sudan | SDN | 1973 | 53.17044 | 700.78356 |
| Swaziland | SWZ | 1973 | 49.75317 | 1420.32569 |
| Tanzania | TZA | 1973 | 47.95739 | |
| Togo | TGO | 1973 | 48.33741 | 594.631144 |
| Tunisia | TUN | 1973 | 54.58878 | 1518.51686 |
| Uganda | UGA | 1973 | 49.21971 | |
| Zambia | ZMB | 1973 | 50.37851 | 1542.14233 |
| Zimbabwe | ZWE | 1973 | 55.92654 | 1306.50634 |
| Algeria | DZA | 1974 | 52.18807 | 3039.42057 |
| Angola | AGO | 1974 | 38.67532 | |
| Benin | BEN | 1974 | 44.28446 | 596.657708 |
| Botswana | BWA | 1974 | 56.89473 | 1232.45501 |
| Burkina Faso | BFA | 1974 | 41.00659 | 287.264562 |
| Burundi | BDI | 1974 | 44.81846 | 258.462588 |
| Cabo Verde | CPV | 1974 | 56.83729 | |
| Cameroon | CMR | 1974 | 48.21966 | 1036.10148 |
| Central African Republic | CAF | 1974 | 45.11376 | 607.569031 |
| Chad | TCD | 1974 | 42.97393 | 549.328078 |
| Comoros | COM | 1974 | 47.43073 | |
| Congo, Dem. Rep. | COD | 1974 | 44.96037 | 1079.82454 |
| Congo, Rep. | COG | 1974 | 54.5232 | 1971.46356 |
| Cote d'Ivoire | CIV | 1974 | 47.00946 | 1978.00372 |
| Djibouti | DJI | 1974 | 51.4139 | |
| Egypt, Arab Rep. | EGY | 1974 | 53.99661 | 789.299269 |
| Equatorial Guinea | GNQ | 1974 | 40.81368 | |
| Eritrea | ERI | 1974 | 44.68261 | |
| Ethiopia | ETH | 1974 | 43.88402 | |
| Gabon | GAB | 1974 | 49.95868 | 12571.2541 |
| Gambia, The | GMB | 1974 | 41.35698 | 470.860041 |
| Ghana | GHA | 1974 | 50.50951 | 1104.23819 |
| Guinea | GIN | 1974 | 38.02468 | |
| Guinea-Bissau | GNB | 1974 | 43.05168 | 488.580068 |
| Kenya | KEN | 1974 | 54.50412 | 820.296127 |
| Lesotho | LSO | 1974 | 50.28395 | 470.67637 |
| Liberia | LBR | 1974 | 41.98439 | 1630.06137 |
| Libya | LBY | 1974 | 59.85766 | |
| Madagascar | MDG | 1974 | 46.67154 | 681.190406 |
| Malawi | MWI | 1974 | 42.3199 | 363.067001 |
| Mali | MLI | 1974 | 35.20541 | 354.807745 |
| Mauritania | MRT | 1974 | 50.94607 | 1248.41135 |
| Mauritius | MUS | 1974 | 63.99998 | |
| Morocco | MAR | 1974 | 54.02437 | 1108.75935 |
| Mozambique | MOZ | 1974 | 41.09432 | |
| Namibia | NAM | 1974 | 54.48134 | |
| Niger | NER | 1974 | 36.59273 | 490.292753 |
| Nigeria | NGA | 1974 | 42.72322 | 2029.44666 |
| Rwanda | RWA | 1974 | 44.66215 | 317.669496 |

| Country Name | Country Code | Year | Life Expectancy at Birth | GDP Per Capita |
|---|---|---|---|---|
| Sao Tome and Principe | STP | 1974 | 58.35824 | |
| Senegal | SEN | 1974 | 42.43915 | 911.181257 |
| Seychelles | SYC | 1974 | | 4420.57211 |
| Sierra Leone | SLE | 1974 | 37.83678 | 494.00226 |
| Somalia | SOM | 1974 | 42.48185 | |
| South Africa | ZAF | 1974 | 57.05034 | 6469.938 |
| Sudan | SDN | 1974 | 53.41632 | 756.832427 |
| Swaziland | SWZ | 1974 | 50.36027 | 1457.12744 |
| Tanzania | TZA | 1974 | 48.41124 | |
| Togo | TGO | 1974 | 48.92337 | 609.276048 |
| Tunisia | TUN | 1974 | 55.70398 | 1605.08224 |
| Uganda | UGA | 1974 | 49.28376 | |
| Zambia | ZMB | 1974 | 50.75666 | 1584.67268 |
| Zimbabwe | ZWE | 1974 | 56.30088 | 1347.44433 |
| Algeria | DZA | 1975 | 52.83624 | 3104.49357 |
| Angola | AGO | 1975 | 39.07212 | |
| Benin | BEN | 1975 | 44.8289 | 553.936648 |
| Botswana | BWA | 1975 | 57.55049 | 1288.41151 |
| Burkina Faso | BFA | 1975 | 41.60639 | 290.373109 |
| Burundi | BDI | 1975 | 45.2189 | 256.515815 |
| Cabo Verde | CPV | 1975 | 57.84224 | |
| Cameroon | CMR | 1975 | 48.75593 | 1121.25235 |
| Central African Republic | CAF | 1975 | 45.88339 | 597.374356 |
| Chad | TCD | 1975 | 43.29663 | 585.869438 |
| Comoros | COM | 1975 | 47.87571 | |
| Congo, Dem. Rep. | COD | 1975 | 45.15685 | 998.192913 |
| Congo, Rep. | COG | 1975 | 54.79483 | 2060.64291 |
| Cote d'Ivoire | CIV | 1975 | 47.74222 | 2042.96719 |
| Djibouti | DJI | 1975 | 51.80361 | |
| Egypt, Arab Rep. | EGY | 1975 | 54.69351 | 840.861156 |
| Equatorial Guinea | GNQ | 1975 | 41.11607 | |
| Eritrea | ERI | 1975 | 45.04576 | |
| Ethiopia | ETH | 1975 | 44.03402 | |
| Gabon | GAB | 1975 | 50.78515 | 14683.4261 |
| Gambia, The | GMB | 1975 | 42.21037 | 513.414532 |
| Ghana | GHA | 1975 | 50.81395 | 944.624033 |
| Guinea | GIN | 1975 | 38.48327 | |
| Guinea-Bissau | GNB | 1975 | 43.44873 | 520.464977 |
| Kenya | KEN | 1975 | 55.04766 | 797.525924 |
| Lesotho | LSO | 1975 | 50.75298 | 397.597305 |
| Liberia | LBR | 1975 | 42.72566 | 1528.91976 |
| Libya | LBY | 1975 | 60.69141 | |
| Madagascar | MDG | 1975 | 47.11144 | 670.571834 |
| Malawi | MWI | 1975 | 42.74539 | 374.133634 |
| Mali | MLI | 1975 | 35.91985 | 389.093423 |
| Mauritania | MRT | 1975 | 51.42793 | 1150.53495 |
| Mauritius | MUS | 1975 | 64.39054 | |

| Country Name | Country Code | Year | Life Expectancy at Birth | GDP Per Capita |
|---|---|---|---|---|
| Morocco | MAR | 1975 | 54.44871 | 1166.44917 |
| Mozambique | MOZ | 1975 | 41.48127 | |
| Namibia | NAM | 1975 | 55.08044 | |
| Niger | NER | 1975 | 36.86493 | 463.34692 |
| Nigeria | NGA | 1975 | 43.1799 | 1871.75787 |
| Rwanda | RWA | 1975 | 44.88459 | 301.517436 |
| Sao Tome and Principe | STP | 1975 | 58.94059 | |
| Senegal | SEN | 1975 | 43.51876 | 953.273195 |
| Seychelles | SYC | 1975 | | 4456.79835 |
| Sierra Leone | SLE | 1975 | 38.49307 | 491.107719 |
| Somalia | SOM | 1975 | 42.86337 | |
| South Africa | ZAF | 1975 | 57.21146 | 6411.18738 |
| Sudan | SDN | 1975 | 53.62373 | 848.104055 |
| Swaziland | SWZ | 1975 | 50.96893 | 1609.99335 |
| Tanzania | TZA | 1975 | 48.8561 | |
| Togo | TGO | 1975 | 49.50241 | 610.208834 |
| Tunisia | TUN | 1975 | 56.79502 | 1681.6917 |
| Uganda | UGA | 1975 | 49.32976 | |
| Zambia | ZMB | 1975 | 51.06671 | 1495.65805 |
| Zimbabwe | ZWE | 1975 | 56.70922 | 1279.40997 |
| Algeria | DZA | 1976 | 53.63051 | 3270.68036 |
| Angola | AGO | 1976 | 39.4412 | |
| Benin | BEN | 1976 | 45.34571 | 545.143577 |
| Botswana | BWA | 1976 | 58.20432 | 1372.39063 |
| Burkina Faso | BFA | 1976 | 42.31329 | 309.153851 |
| Burundi | BDI | 1976 | 45.65322 | 271.842957 |
| Cabo Verde | CPV | 1976 | 58.82324 | |
| Cameroon | CMR | 1976 | 49.28385 | 1030.33584 |
| Central African Republic | CAF | 1976 | 46.61044 | 616.074445 |
| Chad | TCD | 1976 | 43.58627 | 591.14508 |
| Comoros | COM | 1976 | 48.34293 | |
| Congo, Dem. Rep. | COD | 1976 | 45.34537 | 918.849692 |
| Congo, Rep. | COG | 1976 | 55.06734 | 2018.7081 |
| Cote d'Ivoire | CIV | 1976 | 48.42488 | 2202.09099 |
| Djibouti | DJI | 1976 | 52.14998 | |
| Egypt, Arab Rep. | EGY | 1976 | 55.44183 | 942.185688 |
| Equatorial Guinea | GNQ | 1976 | 41.48688 | |
| Eritrea | ERI | 1976 | 45.39605 | |
| Ethiopia | ETH | 1976 | 44.10607 | |
| Gabon | GAB | 1976 | 51.61461 | 19492.7977 |
| Gambia, The | GMB | 1976 | 43.05327 | 535.396069 |
| Ghana | GHA | 1976 | 51.11546 | 893.81562 |
| Guinea | GIN | 1976 | 38.97695 | |
| Guinea-Bissau | GNB | 1976 | 43.85693 | 542.233419 |
| Kenya | KEN | 1976 | 55.59576 | 785.01448 |
| Lesotho | LSO | 1976 | 51.27341 | 430.641741 |
| Liberia | LBR | 1976 | 43.46793 | 1564.58796 |

| Country Name | Country Code | Year | Life Expectancy at Birth | GDP Per Capita |
|---|---|---|---|---|
| Libya | LBY | 1976 | 61.48861 | |
| Madagascar | MDG | 1976 | 47.5378 | 631.812662 |
| Malawi | MWI | 1976 | 43.15778 | 381.172481 |
| Mali | MLI | 1976 | 36.64229 | 434.428121 |
| Mauritania | MRT | 1976 | 51.93954 | 1213.35833 |
| Mauritius | MUS | 1976 | 64.85563 | 2343.41252 |
| Morocco | MAR | 1976 | 54.93068 | 1263.06424 |
| Mozambique | MOZ | 1976 | 41.77283 | |
| Namibia | NAM | 1976 | 55.65927 | |
| Niger | NER | 1976 | 37.18768 | 453.363882 |
| Nigeria | NGA | 1976 | 43.64056 | 1983.03689 |
| Rwanda | RWA | 1976 | 45.25254 | 349.082342 |
| Sao Tome and Principe | STP | 1976 | 59.44717 | |
| Senegal | SEN | 1976 | 44.64032 | 1011.97333 |
| Seychelles | SYC | 1976 | | 5078.45063 |
| Sierra Leone | SLE | 1976 | 39.06802 | 477.875394 |
| Somalia | SOM | 1976 | 43.24688 | |
| South Africa | ZAF | 1976 | 57.33249 | 6392.43502 |
| Sudan | SDN | 1976 | 53.79415 | 957.682019 |
| Swaziland | SWZ | 1976 | 51.58507 | 1528.02232 |
| Tanzania | TZA | 1976 | 49.27049 | |
| Togo | TGO | 1976 | 50.07749 | 584.591766 |
| Tunisia | TUN | 1976 | 57.87054 | 1773.57929 |
| Uganda | UGA | 1976 | 49.36573 | |
| Zambia | ZMB | 1976 | 51.2951 | 1534.84991 |
| Zimbabwe | ZWE | 1976 | 57.16905 | 1246.04643 |
| Algeria | DZA | 1977 | 54.57827 | 3345.37802 |
| Angola | AGO | 1977 | 39.77246 | |
| Benin | BEN | 1977 | 45.82834 | 557.932227 |
| Botswana | BWA | 1977 | 58.84527 | 1478.52106 |
| Burkina Faso | BFA | 1977 | 43.13024 | 304.242227 |
| Burundi | BDI | 1977 | 46.09241 | 296.556107 |
| Cabo Verde | CPV | 1977 | 59.71785 | |
| Cameroon | CMR | 1977 | 49.79783 | 1139.00371 |
| Central African Republic | CAF | 1977 | 47.28437 | 624.962672 |
| Chad | TCD | 1977 | 43.85915 | 592.739632 |
| Comoros | COM | 1977 | 48.84529 | |
| Congo, Dem. Rep. | COD | 1977 | 45.54537 | 899.552161 |
| Congo, Rep. | COG | 1977 | 55.3418 | 1785.01904 |
| Cote d'Ivoire | CIV | 1977 | 49.06166 | 2256.93426 |
| Djibouti | DJI | 1977 | 52.4869 | |
| Egypt, Arab Rep. | EGY | 1977 | 56.20012 | 1038.84114 |
| Equatorial Guinea | GNQ | 1977 | 41.94261 | |
| Eritrea | ERI | 1977 | 45.73139 | |
| Ethiopia | ETH | 1977 | 44.09368 | |
| Gabon | GAB | 1977 | 52.44707 | 16663.5301 |
| Gambia, The | GMB | 1977 | 43.88868 | 538.347736 |

| Country Name | Country Code | Year | Life Expectancy at Birth | GDP Per Capita |
|---|---|---|---|---|
| Ghana | GHA | 1977 | 51.40983 | 899.212474 |
| Guinea | GIN | 1977 | 39.49963 | |
| Guinea-Bissau | GNB | 1977 | 44.2732 | 501.692737 |
| Kenya | KEN | 1977 | 56.15088 | 827.789077 |
| Lesotho | LSO | 1977 | 51.83832 | 511.097337 |
| Liberia | LBR | 1977 | 44.19027 | 1544.9151 |
| Libya | LBY | 1977 | 62.24802 | |
| Madagascar | MDG | 1977 | 47.94961 | 628.577779 |
| Malawi | MWI | 1977 | 43.56156 | 387.636702 |
| Mali | MLI | 1977 | 37.38073 | 454.049861 |
| Mauritania | MRT | 1977 | 52.48193 | 1156.83529 |
| Mauritius | MUS | 1977 | 65.37244 | 2456.54853 |
| Morocco | MAR | 1977 | 55.47817 | 1308.01176 |
| Mozambique | MOZ | 1977 | 41.952 | |
| Namibia | NAM | 1977 | 56.19615 | |
| Niger | NER | 1977 | 37.56349 | 474.68501 |
| Nigeria | NGA | 1977 | 44.09771 | 2040.26382 |
| Rwanda | RWA | 1977 | 45.77641 | 344.697356 |
| Sao Tome and Principe | STP | 1977 | 59.86007 | |
| Senegal | SEN | 1977 | 45.76734 | 961.127308 |
| Seychelles | SYC | 1977 | | 4665.23288 |
| Sierra Leone | SLE | 1977 | 39.57227 | 467.141286 |
| Somalia | SOM | 1977 | 43.6299 | |
| South Africa | ZAF | 1977 | 57.43415 | 6231.40436 |
| Sudan | SDN | 1977 | 53.93259 | 984.251208 |
| Swaziland | SWZ | 1977 | 52.2182 | 1496.02209 |
| Tanzania | TZA | 1977 | 49.63995 | |
| Togo | TGO | 1977 | 50.64756 | 611.840091 |
| Tunisia | TUN | 1977 | 58.93673 | 1792.77309 |
| Uganda | UGA | 1977 | 49.39263 | |
| Zambia | ZMB | 1977 | 51.43483 | 1415.59827 |
| Zimbabwe | ZWE | 1977 | 57.68034 | 1126.00339 |
| Algeria | DZA | 1978 | 55.66754 | 3548.90007 |
| Angola | AGO | 1978 | 40.06149 | |
| Benin | BEN | 1978 | 46.27934 | 550.426504 |
| Botswana | BWA | 1978 | 59.46029 | 1625.44945 |
| Burkina Faso | BFA | 1978 | 44.03978 | 311.834179 |
| Burundi | BDI | 1978 | 46.51298 | 286.818183 |
| Cabo Verde | CPV | 1978 | 60.48005 | |
| Cameroon | CMR | 1978 | 50.2908 | 1350.003 |
| Central African Republic | CAF | 1978 | 47.89317 | 617.369294 |
| Chad | TCD | 1978 | 44.12763 | 578.844903 |
| Comoros | COM | 1978 | 49.3892 | |
| Congo, Dem. Rep. | COD | 1978 | 45.77088 | 827.341609 |
| Congo, Rep. | COG | 1978 | 55.61273 | 1844.32811 |
| Cote d'Ivoire | CIV | 1978 | 49.6559 | 2391.92388 |
| Djibouti | DJI | 1978 | 52.83988 | |

| Country Name | Country Code | Year | Life Expectancy at Birth | GDP Per Capita |
|---|---|---|---|---|
| Egypt, Arab Rep. | EGY | 1978 | 56.93644 | 1073.29316 |
| Equatorial Guinea | GNQ | 1978 | 42.48532 | |
| Eritrea | ERI | 1978 | 46.0512 | |
| Ethiopia | ETH | 1978 | 44.00737 | |
| Gabon | GAB | 1978 | 53.28102 | 12365.3731 |
| Gambia, The | GMB | 1978 | 44.7201 | 556.210675 |
| Ghana | GHA | 1978 | 51.69729 | 959.922415 |
| Guinea | GIN | 1978 | 40.05027 | |
| Guinea-Bissau | GNB | 1978 | 44.69602 | 566.292001 |
| Kenya | KEN | 1978 | 56.70744 | 852.4623 |
| Lesotho | LSO | 1978 | 52.43366 | 588.881979 |
| Liberia | LBR | 1978 | 44.86866 | 1572.9093 |
| Libya | LBY | 1978 | 62.96851 | |
| Madagascar | MDG | 1978 | 48.34137 | 594.595029 |
| Malawi | MWI | 1978 | 43.95922 | 412.275682 |
| Mali | MLI | 1978 | 38.1342 | 439.618172 |
| Mauritania | MRT | 1978 | 53.05215 | 1118.43301 |
| Mauritius | MUS | 1978 | 65.91332 | 2517.53795 |
| Morocco | MAR | 1978 | 56.0942 | 1304.97864 |
| Mozambique | MOZ | 1978 | 42.01924 | |
| Namibia | NAM | 1978 | 56.67493 | |
| Niger | NER | 1978 | 37.98585 | 523.253733 |
| Nigeria | NGA | 1978 | 44.54034 | 1865.00944 |
| Rwanda | RWA | 1978 | 46.43671 | 364.013127 |
| Sao Tome and Principe | STP | 1978 | 60.17095 | |
| Senegal | SEN | 1978 | 46.86983 | 901.289618 |
| Seychelles | SYC | 1978 | | 5618.90592 |
| Sierra Leone | SLE | 1978 | 40.01227 | 467.282582 |
| Somalia | SOM | 1978 | 44.00839 | |
| South Africa | ZAF | 1978 | 57.53873 | 6265.07405 |
| Sudan | SDN | 1978 | 54.04907 | 895.487603 |
| Swaziland | SWZ | 1978 | 52.87224 | 1469.29359 |
| Tanzania | TZA | 1978 | 49.95246 | |
| Togo | TGO | 1978 | 51.21163 | 664.151341 |
| Tunisia | TUN | 1978 | 59.99249 | 1864.14439 |
| Uganda | UGA | 1978 | 49.40593 | |
| Zambia | ZMB | 1978 | 51.48085 | 1375.87752 |
| Zimbabwe | ZWE | 1978 | 58.23002 | 1062.62602 |
| Algeria | DZA | 1979 | 56.87488 | 3702.77745 |
| Angola | AGO | 1979 | 40.30778 | |
| Benin | BEN | 1979 | 46.70578 | 571.072511 |
| Botswana | BWA | 1979 | 60.03593 | 1753.75607 |
| Burkina Faso | BFA | 1979 | 45.01339 | 316.437747 |
| Burundi | BDI | 1979 | 46.90244 | 284.36119 |
| Cabo Verde | CPV | 1979 | 61.09583 | |
| Cameroon | CMR | 1979 | 50.75427 | 1390.01137 |
| Central African Republic | CAF | 1979 | 48.4249 | 586.862677 |

| Country Name | Country Code | Year | Life Expectancy at Birth | GDP Per Capita |
|---|---|---|---|---|
| Chad | TCD | 1979 | 44.39724 | 445.983483 |
| Comoros | COM | 1979 | 49.97412 | |
| Congo, Dem. Rep. | COD | 1979 | 46.02488 | 808.000712 |
| Congo, Rep. | COG | 1979 | 55.87463 | 1967.48494 |
| Cote d'Ivoire | CIV | 1979 | 50.20405 | 2341.66109 |
| Djibouti | DJI | 1979 | 53.21737 | |
| Egypt, Arab Rep. | EGY | 1979 | 57.63932 | 1111.04456 |
| Equatorial Guinea | GNQ | 1979 | 43.10249 | |
| Eritrea | ERI | 1979 | 46.35693 | |
| Ethiopia | ETH | 1979 | 43.87261 | |
| Gabon | GAB | 1979 | 54.11298 | 12130.6738 |
| Gambia, The | GMB | 1979 | 45.54202 | 532.572992 |
| Ghana | GHA | 1979 | 51.98178 | 918.372428 |
| Guinea | GIN | 1979 | 40.6308 | |
| Guinea-Bissau | GNB | 1979 | 45.12046 | 574.69334 |
| Kenya | KEN | 1979 | 57.24939 | 883.416727 |
| Lesotho | LSO | 1979 | 53.04746 | 590.113837 |
| Liberia | LBR | 1979 | 45.48661 | 1574.80631 |
| Libya | LBY | 1979 | 63.64946 | |
| Madagascar | MDG | 1979 | 48.70907 | 634.723338 |
| Malawi | MWI | 1979 | 44.34571 | 417.495359 |
| Mali | MLI | 1979 | 38.89822 | 476.579133 |
| Mauritania | MRT | 1979 | 53.64266 | 1138.83473 |
| Mauritius | MUS | 1979 | 66.45578 | 2561.10373 |
| Morocco | MAR | 1979 | 56.77534 | 1334.25169 |
| Mozambique | MOZ | 1979 | 41.98605 | |
| Namibia | NAM | 1979 | 57.09661 | |
| Niger | NER | 1979 | 38.44876 | 544.640934 |
| Nigeria | NGA | 1979 | 44.95695 | 1932.56837 |
| Rwanda | RWA | 1979 | 47.19288 | 393.749855 |
| Sao Tome and Principe | STP | 1979 | 60.38293 | |
| Senegal | SEN | 1979 | 47.9268 | 940.879578 |
| Seychelles | SYC | 1979 | | 6450.74195 |
| Sierra Leone | SLE | 1979 | 40.37673 | 476.932363 |
| Somalia | SOM | 1979 | 44.37739 | |
| South Africa | ZAF | 1979 | 57.6631 | 6345.18049 |
| Sudan | SDN | 1979 | 54.14907 | 822.359002 |
| Swaziland | SWZ | 1979 | 53.54771 | 1468.91392 |
| Tanzania | TZA | 1979 | 50.20346 | |
| Togo | TGO | 1979 | 51.76473 | 614.011077 |
| Tunisia | TUN | 1979 | 61.02885 | 1938.45424 |
| Uganda | UGA | 1979 | 49.39902 | |
| Zambia | ZMB | 1979 | 51.4232 | 1289.66047 |
| Zimbabwe | ZWE | 1979 | 58.79598 | 1062.9942 |
| Algeria | DZA | 1980 | 58.16402 | 3620.70354 |
| Angola | AGO | 1980 | 40.51093 | |
| Benin | BEN | 1980 | 47.12973 | 593.619562 |

| Country Name | Country Code | Year | Life Expectancy at Birth | GDP Per Capita |
|---|---|---|---|---|
| Botswana | BWA | 1980 | 60.56563 | 1891.40967 |
| Burkina Faso | BFA | 1980 | 45.99756 | 311.891569 |
| Burundi | BDI | 1980 | 47.26232 | 279.958965 |
| Cabo Verde | CPV | 1980 | 61.5702 | 673.82264 |
| Cameroon | CMR | 1980 | 51.18368 | 1322.60836 |
| Central African Republic | CAF | 1980 | 48.87012 | 545.519599 |
| Chad | TCD | 1980 | 44.67205 | 410.53086 |
| Comoros | COM | 1980 | 50.596 | 873.145314 |
| Congo, Dem. Rep. | COD | 1980 | 46.30288 | 803.944318 |
| Congo, Rep. | COG | 1980 | 56.12251 | 2248.05702 |
| Cote d'Ivoire | CIV | 1980 | 50.70907 | 1994.71511 |
| Djibouti | DJI | 1980 | 53.61734 | |
| Egypt, Arab Rep. | EGY | 1980 | 58.31327 | 1192.58146 |
| Equatorial Guinea | GNQ | 1980 | 43.76371 | 645.544406 |
| Eritrea | ERI | 1980 | 46.64715 | |
| Ethiopia | ETH | 1980 | 43.7399 | |
| Gabon | GAB | 1980 | 54.94895 | 12139.6407 |
| Gambia, The | GMB | 1980 | 46.35095 | 547.974525 |
| Ghana | GHA | 1980 | 52.27178 | 901.242606 |
| Guinea | GIN | 1980 | 41.25878 | |
| Guinea-Bissau | GNB | 1980 | 45.53861 | 477.953095 |
| Kenya | KEN | 1980 | 57.75815 | 898.062967 |
| Lesotho | LSO | 1980 | 53.65973 | 559.261058 |
| Liberia | LBR | 1980 | 46.02207 | 1461.13118 |
| Libya | LBY | 1980 | 64.28688 | |
| Madagascar | MDG | 1980 | 49.03076 | 621.715477 |
| Malawi | MWI | 1980 | 44.71049 | 407.171658 |
| Mali | MLI | 1980 | 39.66334 | 447.37473 |
| Mauritania | MRT | 1980 | 54.24244 | 1143.86 |
| Mauritius | MUS | 1980 | 66.96539 | 2264.914 |
| Morocco | MAR | 1980 | 57.5128 | 1349.20785 |
| Mozambique | MOZ | 1980 | 41.88137 | 190.479472 |
| Namibia | NAM | 1980 | 57.47522 | 4357.69083 |
| Niger | NER | 1980 | 38.93466 | 517.331794 |
| Nigeria | NGA | 1980 | 45.32756 | 1957.09878 |
| Rwanda | RWA | 1980 | 48.03744 | 414.589704 |
| Sao Tome and Principe | STP | 1980 | 60.51178 | |
| Senegal | SEN | 1980 | 48.94276 | 886.219353 |
| Seychelles | SYC | 1980 | | 6120.53884 |
| Sierra Leone | SLE | 1980 | 40.65024 | 488.25596 |
| Somalia | SOM | 1980 | 44.73537 | |
| South Africa | ZAF | 1980 | 57.83607 | 6598.60441 |
| Sudan | SDN | 1980 | 54.24112 | 807.0409 |
| Swaziland | SWZ | 1980 | 54.25356 | 1602.42667 |
| Tanzania | TZA | 1980 | 50.39639 | |
| Togo | TGO | 1980 | 52.30441 | 683.348901 |
| Tunisia | TUN | 1980 | 62.02451 | 2028.98009 |

| Country Name | Country Code | Year | Life Expectancy at Birth | GDP Per Capita |
|---|---|---|---|---|
| Uganda | UGA | 1980 | 49.35473 | |
| Zambia | ZMB | 1980 | 51.24829 | 1284.25129 |
| Zimbabwe | ZWE | 1980 | 59.35556 | 1175.13524 |
| Algeria | DZA | 1981 | 59.48676 | 3616.01631 |
| Angola | AGO | 1981 | 40.67559 | |
| Benin | BEN | 1981 | 47.57932 | 635.117493 |
| Botswana | BWA | 1981 | 61.04988 | 1988.88484 |
| Burkina Faso | BFA | 1981 | 46.92832 | 317.607545 |
| Burundi | BDI | 1981 | 47.60468 | 306.101524 |
| Cabo Verde | CPV | 1981 | 61.93015 | 718.37873 |
| Cameroon | CMR | 1981 | 51.57651 | 1502.40773 |
| Central African Republic | CAF | 1981 | 49.22393 | 521.765929 |
| Chad | TCD | 1981 | 44.95368 | 405.983296 |
| Comoros | COM | 1981 | 51.24434 | 878.974461 |
| Congo, Dem. Rep. | COD | 1981 | 46.59288 | 802.087018 |
| Congo, Rep. | COG | 1981 | 56.35034 | 2567.76337 |
| Cote d'Ivoire | CIV | 1981 | 51.17449 | 1976.28253 |
| Djibouti | DJI | 1981 | 54.02885 | |
| Egypt, Arab Rep. | EGY | 1981 | 58.97685 | 1206.7987 |
| Equatorial Guinea | GNQ | 1981 | 44.42549 | 645.52713 |
| Eritrea | ERI | 1981 | 46.92095 | |
| Ethiopia | ETH | 1981 | 43.66966 | 227.783444 |
| Gabon | GAB | 1981 | 55.79793 | 12443.7062 |
| Gambia, The | GMB | 1981 | 47.14485 | 547.128568 |
| Ghana | GHA | 1981 | 52.57832 | 844.985554 |
| Guinea | GIN | 1981 | 41.95571 | |
| Guinea-Bissau | GNB | 1981 | 45.94363 | 555.318264 |
| Kenya | KEN | 1981 | 58.21263 | 897.06566 |
| Lesotho | LSO | 1981 | 54.24951 | 549.075738 |
| Liberia | LBR | 1981 | 46.45893 | 1379.40262 |
| Libya | LBY | 1981 | 64.87422 | |
| Madagascar | MDG | 1981 | 49.28493 | 545.472014 |
| Malawi | MWI | 1981 | 45.045 | 375.607059 |
| Mali | MLI | 1981 | 40.41915 | 445.0742 |
| Mauritania | MRT | 1981 | 54.83595 | 1149.71163 |
| Mauritius | MUS | 1981 | 67.40739 | 2362.86655 |
| Morocco | MAR | 1981 | 58.29185 | 1293.49722 |
| Mozambique | MOZ | 1981 | 41.74663 | 195.309704 |
| Namibia | NAM | 1981 | 57.83888 | 4308.16572 |
| Niger | NER | 1981 | 39.42559 | 505.696485 |
| Nigeria | NGA | 1981 | 45.63166 | 1654.63342 |
| Rwanda | RWA | 1981 | 48.96593 | 422.791244 |
| Sao Tome and Principe | STP | 1981 | 60.58629 | |
| Senegal | SEN | 1981 | 49.93671 | 905.611484 |
| Seychelles | SYC | 1981 | | 5549.82339 |
| Sierra Leone | SLE | 1981 | 40.81771 | 490.684541 |
| Somalia | SOM | 1981 | 45.08285 | |

| Country Name | Country Code | Year | Life Expectancy at Birth | GDP Per Capita |
|---|---|---|---|---|
| South Africa | ZAF | 1981 | 58.08198 | 6777.12923 |
| Sudan | SDN | 1981 | 54.33168 | 837.910028 |
| Swaziland | SWZ | 1981 | 55.0008 | 1784.10486 |
| Tanzania | TZA | 1981 | 50.54312 | |
| Togo | TGO | 1981 | 52.8282 | 639.266977 |
| Tunisia | TUN | 1981 | 62.9548 | 2083.01008 |
| Uganda | UGA | 1981 | 49.25388 | |
| Zambia | ZMB | 1981 | 50.94317 | 1317.60386 |
| Zimbabwe | ZWE | 1981 | 59.88605 | 1274.68338 |
| Algeria | DZA | 1982 | 60.78634 | 3729.25718 |
| Angola | AGO | 1982 | 40.81437 | |
| Benin | BEN | 1982 | 48.07754 | 631.527136 |
| Botswana | BWA | 1982 | 61.4861 | 2153.10404 |
| Burkina Faso | BFA | 1982 | 47.74963 | 339.563292 |
| Burundi | BDI | 1982 | 47.9391 | 295.17478 |
| Cabo Verde | CPV | 1982 | 62.23163 | 724.552421 |
| Cameroon | CMR | 1982 | 51.93032 | 1566.73192 |
| Central African Republic | CAF | 1982 | 49.49244 | 545.283965 |
| Chad | TCD | 1982 | 45.23883 | 418.16294 |
| Comoros | COM | 1982 | 51.90312 | 908.371928 |
| Congo, Dem. Rep. | COD | 1982 | 46.88037 | 778.889585 |
| Congo, Rep. | COG | 1982 | 56.54807 | 3081.76606 |
| Cote d'Ivoire | CIV | 1982 | 51.6029 | 1896.96078 |
| Djibouti | DJI | 1982 | 54.43241 | |
| Egypt, Arab Rep. | EGY | 1982 | 59.65307 | 1293.09573 |
| Equatorial Guinea | GNQ | 1982 | 45.04539 | 613.079211 |
| Eritrea | ERI | 1982 | 47.1819 | |
| Ethiopia | ETH | 1982 | 43.70788 | 223.57766 |
| Gabon | GAB | 1982 | 56.65495 | 11755.284 |
| Gambia, The | GMB | 1982 | 47.91824 | 523.848713 |
| Ghana | GHA | 1982 | 52.91044 | 761.117017 |
| Guinea | GIN | 1982 | 42.73117 | |
| Guinea-Bissau | GNB | 1982 | 46.32973 | 566.021548 |
| Kenya | KEN | 1982 | 58.58985 | 876.470647 |
| Lesotho | LSO | 1982 | 54.80629 | 559.53426 |
| Liberia | LBR | 1982 | 46.80007 | 1296.56604 |
| Libya | LBY | 1982 | 65.41056 | |
| Madagascar | MDG | 1982 | 49.46563 | 520.355915 |
| Malawi | MWI | 1982 | 45.34124 | 375.69538 |
| Mali | MLI | 1982 | 41.15461 | 403.677529 |
| Mauritania | MRT | 1982 | 55.40754 | 1090.89903 |
| Mauritius | MUS | 1982 | 67.76537 | 2462.46847 |
| Morocco | MAR | 1982 | 59.09173 | 1375.28472 |
| Mozambique | MOZ | 1982 | 41.6278 | 177.786616 |
| Namibia | NAM | 1982 | 58.21368 | 4201.2358 |
| Niger | NER | 1982 | 39.90498 | 499.293729 |
| Nigeria | NGA | 1982 | 45.86276 | 1595.1456 |

| Country Name | Country Code | Year | Life Expectancy at Birth | GDP Per Capita |
|---|---|---|---|---|
| Rwanda | RWA | 1982 | 49.88737 | 416.780325 |
| Sao Tome and Principe | STP | 1982 | 60.64217 | |
| Senegal | SEN | 1982 | 50.93315 | 948.640102 |
| Seychelles | SYC | 1982 | 68.68293 | 5455.59002 |
| Sierra Leone | SLE | 1982 | 40.87037 | 502.4628 |
| Somalia | SOM | 1982 | 45.41434 | |
| South Africa | ZAF | 1982 | 58.40571 | 6578.60699 |
| Sudan | SDN | 1982 | 54.42478 | 857.944815 |
| Swaziland | SWZ | 1982 | 55.78046 | 1754.30791 |
| Tanzania | TZA | 1982 | 50.66005 | |
| Togo | TGO | 1982 | 53.32966 | 594.581679 |
| Tunisia | TUN | 1982 | 63.80366 | 2014.57033 |
| Uganda | UGA | 1982 | 49.08285 | 303.281887 |
| Zambia | ZMB | 1982 | 50.51437 | 1237.59119 |
| Zimbabwe | ZWE | 1982 | 60.35088 | 1259.19598 |
| Algeria | DZA | 1983 | 62.00895 | 3809.80376 |
| Angola | AGO | 1983 | 40.93783 | |
| Benin | BEN | 1983 | 48.63793 | 587.287626 |
| Botswana | BWA | 1983 | 61.86473 | 2353.79727 |
| Burkina Faso | BFA | 1983 | 48.422 | 332.26018 |
| Burundi | BDI | 1983 | 48.26312 | 298.20417 |
| Cabo Verde | CPV | 1983 | 62.51863 | 777.623629 |
| Cameroon | CMR | 1983 | 52.23861 | 1623.54003 |
| Central African Republic | CAF | 1983 | 49.67922 | 486.04333 |
| Chad | TCD | 1983 | 45.52061 | 472.316579 |
| Comoros | COM | 1983 | 52.55737 | 926.242711 |
| Congo, Dem. Rep. | COD | 1983 | 47.15234 | 770.766055 |
| Congo, Rep. | COG | 1983 | 56.70573 | 3168.04877 |
| Cote d'Ivoire | CIV | 1983 | 51.98839 | 1747.9398 |
| Djibouti | DJI | 1983 | 54.811 | |
| Egypt, Arab Rep. | EGY | 1983 | 60.3539 | 1353.34791 |
| Equatorial Guinea | GNQ | 1983 | 45.5939 | 594.920486 |
| Eritrea | ERI | 1983 | 47.43502 | |
| Ethiopia | ETH | 1983 | 43.88149 | 234.726716 |
| Gabon | GAB | 1983 | 57.506 | 12096.5711 |
| Gambia, The | GMB | 1983 | 48.66163 | 559.266552 |
| Ghana | GHA | 1983 | 53.27368 | 701.52682 |
| Guinea | GIN | 1983 | 43.5832 | |
| Guinea-Bissau | GNB | 1983 | 46.69454 | 533.057837 |
| Kenya | KEN | 1983 | 58.87076 | 854.841093 |
| Lesotho | LSO | 1983 | 55.32256 | 557.258486 |
| Liberia | LBR | 1983 | 47.05302 | 1228.98995 |
| Libya | LBY | 1983 | 65.89841 | |
| Madagascar | MDG | 1983 | 49.58137 | 510.125927 |
| Malawi | MWI | 1983 | 45.59473 | 379.318009 |
| Mali | MLI | 1983 | 41.85876 | 402.523439 |
| Mauritania | MRT | 1983 | 55.94163 | 1099.59489 |

| Country Name | Country Code | Year | Life Expectancy at Birth | GDP Per Capita |
|---|---|---|---|---|
| Mauritius | MUS | 1983 | 68.03761 | 2449.29007 |
| Morocco | MAR | 1983 | 59.88961 | 1361.16615 |
| Mozambique | MOZ | 1983 | 41.56485 | 146.932154 |
| Namibia | NAM | 1983 | 58.61617 | 4030.33366 |
| Niger | NER | 1983 | 40.36385 | 462.061718 |
| Nigeria | NGA | 1983 | 46.01834 | 1476.66534 |
| Rwanda | RWA | 1983 | 50.6628 | 427.357647 |
| Sao Tome and Principe | STP | 1983 | 60.70859 | |
| Senegal | SEN | 1983 | 51.93861 | 871.548108 |
| Seychelles | SYC | 1983 | | 5368.84191 |
| Sierra Leone | SLE | 1983 | 40.80695 | 480.535567 |
| Somalia | SOM | 1983 | 45.71934 | |
| South Africa | ZAF | 1983 | 58.80222 | 6292.93495 |
| Sudan | SDN | 1983 | 54.52437 | 846.653927 |
| Swaziland | SWZ | 1983 | 56.57354 | 1723.93662 |
| Tanzania | TZA | 1983 | 50.75617 | |
| Togo | TGO | 1983 | 53.80241 | 541.730963 |
| Tunisia | TUN | 1983 | 64.56685 | 2049.11915 |
| Uganda | UGA | 1983 | 48.83368 | 311.085749 |
| Zambia | ZMB | 1983 | 49.97998 | 1173.09858 |
| Zimbabwe | ZWE | 1983 | 60.71159 | 1230.39367 |
| Algeria | DZA | 1984 | 63.11712 | 3900.85048 |
| Angola | AGO | 1984 | 41.05302 | |
| Benin | BEN | 1984 | 49.26144 | 616.037501 |
| Botswana | BWA | 1984 | 62.17071 | 2471.15711 |
| Burkina Faso | BFA | 1984 | 48.92437 | 318.102432 |
| Burundi | BDI | 1984 | 48.56229 | 290.660219 |
| Cabo Verde | CPV | 1984 | 62.81363 | 791.316956 |
| Cameroon | CMR | 1984 | 52.49046 | 1691.65181 |
| Central African Republic | CAF | 1984 | 49.78485 | 517.057823 |
| Chad | TCD | 1984 | 45.79454 | 469.836916 |
| Comoros | COM | 1984 | 53.19756 | 938.15886 |
| Congo, Dem. Rep. | COD | 1984 | 47.40732 | 793.457435 |
| Congo, Rep. | COG | 1984 | 56.81085 | 3292.42655 |
| Cote d'Ivoire | CIV | 1984 | 52.32249 | 1632.64566 |
| Djibouti | DJI | 1984 | 55.15863 | |
| Egypt, Arab Rep. | EGY | 1984 | 61.07237 | 1398.34516 |
| Equatorial Guinea | GNQ | 1984 | 46.06302 | 558.969581 |
| Eritrea | ERI | 1984 | 47.68822 | |
| Ethiopia | ETH | 1984 | 44.196 | 220.927145 |
| Gabon | GAB | 1984 | 58.3291 | 12665.8006 |
| Gambia, The | GMB | 1984 | 49.36802 | 556.023683 |
| Ghana | GHA | 1984 | 53.67049 | 736.434964 |
| Guinea | GIN | 1984 | 44.49637 | |
| Guinea-Bissau | GNB | 1984 | 47.03963 | 566.518935 |
| Kenya | KEN | 1984 | 59.04039 | 837.769634 |
| Lesotho | LSO | 1984 | 55.79685 | 575.145846 |

| Country Name | Country Code | Year | Life Expectancy at Birth | GDP Per Capita |
|---|---|---|---|---|
| Liberia | LBR | 1984 | 47.22678 | 1171.78766 |
| Libya | LBY | 1984 | 66.34278 | |
| Madagascar | MDG | 1984 | 49.65212 | 504.150291 |
| Malawi | MWI | 1984 | 45.80598 | 386.056202 |
| Mali | MLI | 1984 | 42.52502 | 393.54682 |
| Mauritania | MRT | 1984 | 56.43066 | 1034.2349 |
| Mauritius | MUS | 1984 | 68.23037 | 2537.6904 |
| Morocco | MAR | 1984 | 60.66949 | 1415.04943 |
| Mozambique | MOZ | 1984 | 41.57727 | 135.285941 |
| Namibia | NAM | 1984 | 59.04532 | 3912.04241 |
| Niger | NER | 1984 | 40.8012 | 373.426876 |
| Nigeria | NGA | 1984 | 46.10193 | 1410.67882 |
| Rwanda | RWA | 1984 | 51.13271 | 394.742435 |
| Sao Tome and Principe | STP | 1984 | 60.80261 | |
| Senegal | SEN | 1984 | 52.9381 | 877.046539 |
| Seychelles | SYC | 1984 | | 5577.91764 |
| Sierra Leone | SLE | 1984 | 40.62832 | 487.938364 |
| Somalia | SOM | 1984 | 45.98437 | |
| South Africa | ZAF | 1984 | 59.26049 | 6450.54454 |
| Sudan | SDN | 1984 | 54.63544 | 778.653045 |
| Swaziland | SWZ | 1984 | 57.35402 | 1771.87406 |
| Tanzania | TZA | 1984 | 50.83149 | |
| Togo | TGO | 1984 | 54.23905 | 551.068271 |
| Tunisia | TUN | 1984 | 65.24905 | 2106.86267 |
| Uganda | UGA | 1984 | 48.50941 | 300.407674 |
| Zambia | ZMB | 1984 | 49.3581 | 1131.45991 |
| Zimbabwe | ZWE | 1984 | 60.93276 | 1161.40584 |
| Algeria | DZA | 1985 | 64.07376 | 3924.70927 |
| Angola | AGO | 1985 | 41.16134 | 2574.05124 |
| Benin | BEN | 1985 | 49.95161 | 643.587476 |
| Botswana | BWA | 1985 | 62.3929 | 2563.03352 |
| Burkina Faso | BFA | 1985 | 49.25122 | 336.411586 |
| Burundi | BDI | 1985 | 48.78917 | 315.872851 |
| Cabo Verde | CPV | 1985 | 63.12512 | 844.226526 |
| Cameroon | CMR | 1985 | 52.66944 | 1772.07232 |
| Central African Republic | CAF | 1985 | 49.80785 | 523.404809 |
| Chad | TCD | 1985 | 46.05256 | 556.775298 |
| Comoros | COM | 1985 | 53.8192 | 932.896713 |
| Congo, Dem. Rep. | COD | 1985 | 47.65276 | 776.843298 |
| Congo, Rep. | COG | 1985 | 56.85295 | 3162.20222 |
| Cote d'Ivoire | CIV | 1985 | 52.59412 | 1639.95874 |
| Djibouti | DJI | 1985 | 55.47273 | |
| Egypt, Arab Rep. | EGY | 1985 | 61.78644 | 1450.99547 |
| Equatorial Guinea | GNQ | 1985 | 46.4572 | 594.511974 |
| Eritrea | ERI | 1985 | 47.94834 | |
| Ethiopia | ETH | 1985 | 44.6299 | 190.14025 |
| Gabon | GAB | 1985 | 59.09276 | 12042.4298 |

| Country Name | Country Code | Year | Life Expectancy at Birth | GDP Per Capita |
|---|---|---|---|---|
| Gambia, The | GMB | 1985 | 50.01944 | 528.160205 |
| Ghana | GHA | 1985 | 54.10971 | 749.27816 |
| Guinea | GIN | 1985 | 45.45473 | |
| Guinea-Bissau | GNB | 1985 | 47.368 | 575.272558 |
| Kenya | KEN | 1985 | 59.08473 | 842.072992 |
| Lesotho | LSO | 1985 | 56.26556 | 578.140484 |
| Liberia | LBR | 1985 | 47.31983 | 1144.17104 |
| Libya | LBY | 1985 | 66.75415 | |
| Madagascar | MDG | 1985 | 49.71032 | 495.655446 |
| Malawi | MWI | 1985 | 45.97849 | 386.058057 |
| Mali | MLI | 1985 | 43.15129 | 465.029651 |
| Mauritania | MRT | 1985 | 56.86605 | 1035.63975 |
| Mauritius | MUS | 1985 | 68.37068 | 2692.08034 |
| Morocco | MAR | 1985 | 61.42078 | 1466.72404 |
| Mozambique | MOZ | 1985 | 41.67056 | 135.26419 |
| Namibia | NAM | 1985 | 59.501 | 3802.98221 |
| Niger | NER | 1985 | 41.21949 | 390.888844 |
| Nigeria | NGA | 1985 | 46.12198 | 1489.42397 |
| Rwanda | RWA | 1985 | 50.90595 | 396.081731 |
| Sao Tome and Principe | STP | 1985 | 60.93022 | |
| Senegal | SEN | 1985 | 53.90415 | 878.547412 |
| Seychelles | SYC | 1985 | | 6148.43451 |
| Sierra Leone | SLE | 1985 | 40.3248 | 449.852281 |
| Somalia | SOM | 1985 | 46.1679 | |
| South Africa | ZAF | 1985 | 59.77002 | 6222.07399 |
| Sudan | SDN | 1985 | 54.75798 | 707.752357 |
| Swaziland | SWZ | 1985 | 58.09793 | 1773.57916 |
| Tanzania | TZA | 1985 | 50.87254 | |
| Togo | TGO | 1985 | 54.63473 | 561.520547 |
| Tunisia | TUN | 1985 | 65.86768 | 2166.91358 |
| Uganda | UGA | 1985 | 48.1112 | 281.111193 |
| Zambia | ZMB | 1985 | 48.66737 | 1113.95656 |
| Zimbabwe | ZWE | 1985 | 60.97202 | 1196.6352 |
| Algeria | DZA | 1986 | 64.8572 | 3825.90402 |
| Angola | AGO | 1986 | 41.26071 | 2570.52951 |
| Benin | BEN | 1986 | 50.70395 | 638.749043 |
| Botswana | BWA | 1986 | 62.52617 | 2687.31788 |
| Burkina Faso | BFA | 1986 | 49.41754 | 353.888019 |
| Burundi | BDI | 1986 | 48.88476 | 316.742305 |
| Cabo Verde | CPV | 1986 | 63.45161 | 854.596841 |
| Cameroon | CMR | 1986 | 52.75859 | 1833.98994 |
| Central African Republic | CAF | 1986 | 49.74571 | 529.518474 |
| Chad | TCD | 1986 | 46.28656 | 518.620833 |
| Comoros | COM | 1986 | 54.42229 | 923.234882 |
| Congo, Dem. Rep. | COD | 1986 | 47.90371 | 792.21739 |
| Congo, Rep. | COG | 1986 | 56.82156 | 2864.09216 |
| Cote d'Ivoire | CIV | 1986 | 52.79168 | 1629.99567 |

| Country Name | Country Code | Year | Life Expectancy at Birth | GDP Per Capita |
|---|---|---|---|---|
| Djibouti | DJI | 1986 | 55.75673 | |
| Egypt, Arab Rep. | EGY | 1986 | 62.46659 | 1448.91489 |
| Equatorial Guinea | GNQ | 1986 | 46.79785 | 554.207467 |
| Eritrea | ERI | 1986 | 48.22115 | |
| Ethiopia | ETH | 1986 | 45.14368 | 201.974533 |
| Gabon | GAB | 1986 | 59.76095 | 11624.3809 |
| Gambia, The | GMB | 1986 | 50.60044 | 525.030584 |
| Ghana | GHA | 1986 | 54.60268 | 764.891721 |
| Guinea | GIN | 1986 | 46.43534 | 552.322695 |
| Guinea-Bissau | GNB | 1986 | 47.68802 | 557.010085 |
| Kenya | KEN | 1986 | 58.99676 | 870.298659 |
| Lesotho | LSO | 1986 | 56.77963 | 594.060509 |
| Liberia | LBR | 1986 | 47.33117 | 1120.22467 |
| Libya | LBY | 1986 | 67.14451 | |
| Madagascar | MDG | 1986 | 49.79488 | 491.275875 |
| Malawi | MWI | 1986 | 46.11827 | 364.303498 |
| Mali | MLI | 1986 | 43.74046 | 470.150897 |
| Mauritania | MRT | 1986 | 57.24578 | 1064.72662 |
| Mauritius | MUS | 1986 | 68.49937 | 2931.8434 |
| Morocco | MAR | 1986 | 62.13876 | 1568.68403 |
| Mozambique | MOZ | 1986 | 41.83322 | 131.646381 |
| Namibia | NAM | 1986 | 59.97656 | 3833.09994 |
| Niger | NER | 1986 | 41.63124 | 404.018052 |
| Nigeria | NGA | 1986 | 46.09546 | 1324.11519 |
| Rwanda | RWA | 1986 | 49.54037 | 399.007723 |
| Sao Tome and Principe | STP | 1986 | 61.08829 | |
| Senegal | SEN | 1986 | 54.80078 | 878.609291 |
| Seychelles | SYC | 1986 | | 6099.42159 |
| Sierra Leone | SLE | 1986 | 39.88627 | 442.272363 |
| Somalia | SOM | 1986 | 46.21998 | |
| South Africa | ZAF | 1986 | 60.3159 | 6084.72475 |
| Sudan | SDN | 1986 | 54.88946 | 724.888764 |
| Swaziland | SWZ | 1986 | 58.7852 | 1912.02955 |
| Tanzania | TZA | 1986 | 50.85737 | |
| Togo | TGO | 1986 | 54.98817 | 551.602673 |
| Tunisia | TUN | 1986 | 66.44961 | 2082.13092 |
| Uganda | UGA | 1986 | 47.64166 | 272.749704 |
| Zambia | ZMB | 1986 | 47.92439 | 1088.30907 |
| Zimbabwe | ZWE | 1986 | 60.79505 | 1178.55863 |
| Algeria | DZA | 1987 | 65.48715 | 3691.64756 |
| Angola | AGO | 1987 | 41.35149 | 2700.11403 |
| Benin | BEN | 1987 | 51.49085 | 611.028136 |
| Botswana | BWA | 1987 | 62.55702 | 2917.43605 |
| Burkina Faso | BFA | 1987 | 49.47227 | 343.970455 |
| Burundi | BDI | 1987 | 48.82805 | 324.379639 |
| Cabo Verde | CPV | 1987 | 63.7791 | 878.498948 |
| Cameroon | CMR | 1987 | 52.753 | 1739.59313 |

| Country Name | Country Code | Year | Life Expectancy at Birth | GDP Per Capita |
|---|---|---|---|---|
| Central African Republic | CAF | 1987 | 49.60188 | 492.721522 |
| Chad | TCD | 1987 | 46.49095 | 490.779323 |
| Comoros | COM | 1987 | 55.00937 | 911.217186 |
| Congo, Dem. Rep. | COD | 1987 | 48.17015 | 791.640596 |
| Congo, Rep. | COG | 1987 | 56.71324 | 2791.56319 |
| Cote d'Ivoire | CIV | 1987 | 52.90417 | 1565.43783 |
| Djibouti | DJI | 1987 | 56.01666 | |
| Egypt, Arab Rep. | EGY | 1987 | 63.0888 | 1444.59226 |
| Equatorial Guinea | GNQ | 1987 | 47.12144 | 557.807079 |
| Eritrea | ERI | 1987 | 48.513 | |
| Ethiopia | ETH | 1987 | 45.67841 | 222.709599 |
| Gabon | GAB | 1987 | 60.31068 | 9369.45057 |
| Gambia, The | GMB | 1987 | 51.10751 | 512.807006 |
| Ghana | GHA | 1987 | 55.13732 | 779.145577 |
| Guinea | GIN | 1987 | 47.4052 | 554.467139 |
| Guinea-Bissau | GNB | 1987 | 48.00761 | 559.805802 |
| Kenya | KEN | 1987 | 58.78754 | 889.634127 |
| Lesotho | LSO | 1987 | 57.35605 | 588.35376 |
| Liberia | LBR | 1987 | 47.2829 | 1114.47607 |
| Libya | LBY | 1987 | 67.52439 | |
| Madagascar | MDG | 1987 | 49.94327 | 483.262598 |
| Malawi | MWI | 1987 | 46.23637 | 347.665134 |
| Mali | MLI | 1987 | 44.29844 | 462.944299 |
| Mauritania | MRT | 1987 | 57.57785 | 1055.37224 |
| Mauritius | MUS | 1987 | 68.65551 | 3168.7207 |
| Morocco | MAR | 1987 | 62.82668 | 1531.86548 |
| Mozambique | MOZ | 1987 | 42.0408 | 151.155233 |
| Namibia | NAM | 1987 | 60.44337 | 3802.39644 |
| Niger | NER | 1987 | 42.05446 | 392.879429 |
| Nigeria | NGA | 1987 | 46.0429 | 1151.12561 |
| Rwanda | RWA | 1987 | 46.93741 | 379.686028 |
| Sao Tome and Principe | STP | 1987 | 61.2601 | |
| Senegal | SEN | 1987 | 55.59702 | 904.065967 |
| Seychelles | SYC | 1987 | 69.73195 | 6103.37376 |
| Sierra Leone | SLE | 1987 | 39.33066 | 459.886764 |
| Somalia | SOM | 1987 | 46.13156 | |
| South Africa | ZAF | 1987 | 60.86532 | 6081.03866 |
| Sudan | SDN | 1987 | 55.02737 | 805.660605 |
| Swaziland | SWZ | 1987 | 59.38383 | 2098.52708 |
| Tanzania | TZA | 1987 | 50.7741 | |
| Togo | TGO | 1987 | 55.29639 | 536.852636 |
| Tunisia | TUN | 1987 | 67.02307 | 2168.95351 |
| Uganda | UGA | 1987 | 47.12507 | 273.783978 |
| Zambia | ZMB | 1987 | 47.15778 | 1084.89525 |
| Zimbabwe | ZWE | 1987 | 60.39959 | 1151.44671 |
| Algeria | DZA | 1988 | 65.48715 | 3554.62274 |
| Angola | AGO | 1988 | 41.35149 | 2778.09323 |

| Country Name | Country Code | Year | Life Expectancy at Birth | GDP Per Capita |
|---|---|---|---|---|
| Benin | BEN | 1988 | 51.49085 | 613.23118 |
| Botswana | BWA | 1988 | 62.55702 | 3384.48086 |
| Burkina Faso | BFA | 1988 | 49.47227 | 354.488976 |
| Burundi | BDI | 1988 | 48.82805 | 330.866922 |
| Cabo Verde | CPV | 1988 | 63.7791 | 917.685424 |
| Cameroon | CMR | 1988 | 52.753 | 1554.722 |
| Central African Republic | CAF | 1988 | 49.60188 | 490.990353 |
| Chad | TCD | 1988 | 46.49095 | 548.875442 |
| Comoros | COM | 1988 | 55.00937 | 908.430773 |
| Congo, Dem. Rep. | COD | 1988 | 48.17015 | 772.949569 |
| Congo, Rep. | COG | 1988 | 56.71324 | 2764.4173 |
| Cote d'Ivoire | CIV | 1988 | 52.90417 | 1527.15612 |
| Djibouti | DJI | 1988 | 56.01666 | |
| Egypt, Arab Rep. | EGY | 1988 | 63.0888 | 1479.86357 |
| Equatorial Guinea | GNQ | 1988 | 47.12144 | 555.321325 |
| Eritrea | ERI | 1988 | 48.513 | |
| Ethiopia | ETH | 1988 | 45.67841 | 216.663971 |
| Gabon | GAB | 1988 | 60.31068 | 10284.5206 |
| Gambia, The | GMB | 1988 | 51.10751 | 511.027363 |
| Ghana | GHA | 1988 | 55.13732 | 800.850879 |
| Guinea | GIN | 1988 | 47.4052 | 571.043735 |
| Guinea-Bissau | GNB | 1988 | 48.00761 | 572.141851 |
| Kenya | KEN | 1988 | 58.78754 | 912.328923 |
| Lesotho | LSO | 1988 | 57.35605 | 628.740962 |
| Liberia | LBR | 1988 | 47.2829 | 1104.79599 |
| Libya | LBY | 1988 | 67.52439 | |
| Madagascar | MDG | 1988 | 49.94327 | 485.810599 |
| Malawi | MWI | 1988 | 46.23637 | 337.245849 |
| Mali | MLI | 1988 | 44.29844 | 490.289242 |
| Mauritania | MRT | 1988 | 57.57785 | 1044.48609 |
| Mauritius | MUS | 1988 | 68.65551 | 3360.70459 |
| Morocco | MAR | 1988 | 62.82668 | 1680.34999 |
| Mozambique | MOZ | 1988 | 42.0408 | 163.780238 |
| Namibia | NAM | 1988 | 60.44337 | 3666.32576 |
| Niger | NER | 1988 | 42.05446 | 407.937854 |
| Nigeria | NGA | 1988 | 46.0429 | 1205.80462 |
| Rwanda | RWA | 1988 | 46.93741 | 379.946282 |
| Sao Tome and Principe | STP | 1988 | 61.2601 | |
| Senegal | SEN | 1988 | 55.59702 | 871.642402 |
| Seychelles | SYC | 1988 | 69.73195 | 6408.80583 |
| Sierra Leone | SLE | 1988 | 39.33066 | 415.1525 |
| Somalia | SOM | 1988 | 46.13156 | |
| South Africa | ZAF | 1988 | 60.86532 | 6204.5707 |
| Sudan | SDN | 1988 | 55.02737 | 782.144918 |
| Swaziland | SWZ | 1988 | 59.38383 | 2142.10513 |
| Tanzania | TZA | 1988 | 50.7741 | 473.70255 |
| Togo | TGO | 1988 | 55.29639 | 555.274641 |

| Country Name | Country Code | Year | Life Expectancy at Birth | GDP Per Capita |
|---|---|---|---|---|
| Tunisia | TUN | 1988 | 67.02307 | 2121.10365 |
| Uganda | UGA | 1988 | 47.12507 | 286.080943 |
| Zambia | ZMB | 1988 | 47.15778 | 1120.50951 |
| Zimbabwe | ZWE | 1988 | 60.39959 | 1198.30453 |
| Algeria | DZA | 1989 | 66.38205 | 3613.14659 |
| Angola | AGO | 1989 | 41.54359 | 2715.32769 |
| Benin | BEN | 1989 | 53.03461 | 577.539883 |
| Botswana | BWA | 1989 | 62.22078 | 3718.48569 |
| Burkina Faso | BFA | 1989 | 49.41988 | 352.67786 |
| Burundi | BDI | 1989 | 48.32502 | 326.182284 |
| Cabo Verde | CPV | 1989 | 64.41759 | 954.020839 |
| Cameroon | CMR | 1989 | 52.46361 | 1480.75685 |
| Central African Republic | CAF | 1989 | 49.09846 | 490.166814 |
| Chad | TCD | 1989 | 46.80656 | 557.347597 |
| Comoros | COM | 1989 | 56.13051 | 853.854632 |
| Congo, Dem. Rep. | COD | 1989 | 48.73702 | 739.873713 |
| Congo, Rep. | COG | 1989 | 56.27254 | 2760.26451 |
| Cote d'Ivoire | CIV | 1989 | 52.82744 | 1517.06964 |
| Djibouti | DJI | 1989 | 56.47361 | |
| Egypt, Arab Rep. | EGY | 1989 | 64.1208 | 1512.97214 |
| Equatorial Guinea | GNQ | 1989 | 47.82129 | 532.851308 |
| Eritrea | ERI | 1989 | 49.18427 | |
| Ethiopia | ETH | 1989 | 46.66632 | 208.786874 |
| Gabon | GAB | 1989 | 61.00532 | 10860.2046 |
| Gambia, The | GMB | 1989 | 51.91695 | 517.764145 |
| Ghana | GHA | 1989 | 56.24717 | 819.133649 |
| Guinea | GIN | 1989 | 49.1782 | 571.698666 |
| Guinea-Bissau | GNB | 1989 | 48.67239 | 593.05471 |
| Kenya | KEN | 1989 | 58.05793 | 922.981426 |
| Lesotho | LSO | 1989 | 58.58205 | 654.305737 |
| Liberia | LBR | 1989 | 47.15944 | 822.921638 |
| Libya | LBY | 1989 | 68.26956 | |
| Madagascar | MDG | 1989 | 50.53605 | 491.435526 |
| Malawi | MWI | 1989 | 46.43356 | 324.578888 |
| Mali | MLI | 1989 | 45.30861 | 502.853259 |
| Mauritania | MRT | 1989 | 58.13061 | 1065.01874 |
| Mauritius | MUS | 1989 | 69.12402 | 3483.97829 |
| Morocco | MAR | 1989 | 64.10478 | 1695.42985 |
| Mozambique | MOZ | 1989 | 42.53939 | 173.66386 |
| Namibia | NAM | 1989 | 61.21868 | 3577.41763 |
| Niger | NER | 1989 | 42.98688 | 399.624644 |
| Nigeria | NGA | 1989 | 45.93266 | 1250.68277 |
| Rwanda | RWA | 1989 | 38.76734 | 370.025519 |
| Sao Tome and Principe | STP | 1989 | 61.60424 | |
| Senegal | SEN | 1989 | 56.8009 | 879.0309 |
| Seychelles | SYC | 1989 | | 7084.06687 |
| Sierra Leone | SLE | 1989 | 38.01859 | 408.688282 |

| *Country Name* | *Country Code* | *Year* | *Life Expectancy at Birth* | *GDP Per Capita* |
|---|---|---|---|---|
| Somalia | SOM | 1989 | 45.64627 | |
| South Africa | ZAF | 1989 | 61.81415 | 6217.22056 |
| Sudan | SDN | 1989 | 55.32139 | 830.221385 |
| Swaziland | SWZ | 1989 | 60.15485 | 2325.06834 |
| Tanzania | TZA | 1989 | 50.42185 | 476.604598 |
| Togo | TGO | 1989 | 55.74424 | 561.447726 |
| Tunisia | TUN | 1989 | 68.21007 | 2110.04297 |
| Uganda | UGA | 1989 | 46.0648 | 293.74079 |
| Zambia | ZMB | 1989 | 45.68137 | 1078.70477 |
| Zimbabwe | ZWE | 1989 | 58.98141 | 1222.64726 |
| Algeria | DZA | 1990 | 66.69302 | 3550.03267 |
| Angola | AGO | 1990 | 41.66949 | 2630.62357 |
| Benin | BEN | 1990 | 53.71395 | 609.345624 |
| Botswana | BWA | 1990 | 61.76151 | 3860.0086 |
| Burkina Faso | BFA | 1990 | 49.36561 | 341.352617 |
| Burundi | BDI | 1990 | 48.00012 | 329.157781 |
| Cabo Verde | CPV | 1990 | 64.73659 | 941.801425 |
| Cameroon | CMR | 1990 | 52.18385 | 1349.63265 |
| Central African Republic | CAF | 1990 | 48.74688 | 468.690673 |
| Chad | TCD | 1990 | 46.92385 | 517.13464 |
| Comoros | COM | 1990 | 56.65361 | 871.249029 |
| Congo, Dem. Rep. | COD | 1990 | 48.99298 | 668.327408 |
| Congo, Rep. | COG | 1990 | 55.93232 | 2713.10129 |
| Cote d'Ivoire | CIV | 1990 | 52.60693 | 1448.03364 |
| Djibouti | DJI | 1990 | 56.66317 | 1560.99938 |
| Egypt, Arab Rep. | EGY | 1990 | 64.54959 | 1560.08335 |
| Equatorial Guinea | GNQ | 1990 | 48.22161 | 507.895779 |
| Eritrea | ERI | 1990 | 49.58193 | |
| Ethiopia | ETH | 1990 | 47.09956 | 207.219781 |
| Gabon | GAB | 1990 | 61.14576 | 11117.078 |
| Gambia, The | GMB | 1990 | 52.24573 | 515.329318 |
| Ghana | GHA | 1990 | 56.75163 | 823.581673 |
| Guinea | GIN | 1990 | 49.91885 | 569.719339 |
| Guinea-Bissau | GNB | 1990 | 49.02429 | 614.461883 |
| Kenya | KEN | 1990 | 57.54683 | 930.053026 |
| Lesotho | LSO | 1990 | 59.07634 | 681.785188 |
| Liberia | LBR | 1990 | 47.20244 | 409.566918 |
| Libya | LBY | 1990 | 68.6299 | |
| Madagascar | MDG | 1990 | 51.0081 | 492.398909 |
| Malawi | MWI | 1990 | 46.51295 | 330.59112 |
| Mali | MLI | 1990 | 45.73185 | 481.254852 |
| Mauritania | MRT | 1990 | 58.36424 | 1018.27052 |
| Mauritius | MUS | 1990 | 69.40488 | 3707.85678 |
| Morocco | MAR | 1990 | 64.67898 | 1720.78049 |
| Mozambique | MOZ | 1990 | 42.8459 | 172.910866 |
| Namibia | NAM | 1990 | 61.45385 | 3509.35624 |
| Niger | NER | 1990 | 43.50915 | 382.485945 |

| Country Name | Country Code | Year | Life Expectancy at Birth | GDP Per Capita |
|---|---|---|---|---|
| Nigeria | NGA | 1990 | 45.89463 | 1374.43676 |
| Rwanda | RWA | 1990 | 34.2118 | 360.160785 |
| Sao Tome and Principe | STP | 1990 | 61.77144 | |
| Senegal | SEN | 1990 | 57.1831 | 846.858807 |
| Seychelles | SYC | 1990 | | 7542.55943 |
| Sierra Leone | SLE | 1990 | 37.35341 | 416.230302 |
| Somalia | SOM | 1990 | 45.38934 | |
| South Africa | ZAF | 1990 | 62.13568 | 6057.93507 |
| Sudan | SDN | 1990 | 55.48695 | 764.731509 |
| Swaziland | SWZ | 1990 | 60.22524 | 2720.02953 |
| Tanzania | TZA | 1990 | 50.18366 | 494.202502 |
| Togo | TGO | 1990 | 55.84844 | 545.206096 |
| Tunisia | TUN | 1990 | 68.8271 | 2227.47056 |
| Uganda | UGA | 1990 | 45.57107 | 302.126107 |
| Zambia | ZMB | 1990 | 45.02763 | 1044.97061 |
| Zimbabwe | ZWE | 1990 | 57.96573 | 1272.05103 |
| Algeria | DZA | 1991 | 66.955 | 3422.63862 |
| Angola | AGO | 1991 | 41.82846 | 2519.96606 |
| Benin | BEN | 1991 | 54.26785 | 614.005294 |
| Botswana | BWA | 1991 | 61.01244 | 4034.26086 |
| Burkina Faso | BFA | 1991 | 49.31646 | 362.47892 |
| Burundi | BDI | 1991 | 47.76268 | 337.708351 |
| Cabo Verde | CPV | 1991 | 65.06161 | 933.053237 |
| Cameroon | CMR | 1991 | 51.81088 | 1261.03936 |
| Central African Republic | CAF | 1991 | 48.32859 | 454.529078 |
| Chad | TCD | 1991 | 47.02559 | 543.638836 |
| Comoros | COM | 1991 | 57.14522 | 800.364752 |
| Congo, Dem. Rep. | COD | 1991 | 49.17493 | 589.888934 |
| Congo, Rep. | COG | 1991 | 55.49946 | 2703.519 |
| Cote d'Ivoire | CIV | 1991 | 52.23273 | 1398.22024 |
| Djibouti | DJI | 1991 | 56.81615 | 1453.73099 |
| Egypt, Arab Rep. | EGY | 1991 | 64.95585 | 1540.94382 |
| Equatorial Guinea | GNQ | 1991 | 48.65993 | 486.984678 |
| Eritrea | ERI | 1991 | 50.0341 | |
| Ethiopia | ETH | 1991 | 47.50537 | 185.7299 |
| Gabon | GAB | 1991 | 61.16178 | 11482.9374 |
| Gambia, The | GMB | 1991 | 52.55151 | 513.050121 |
| Ghana | GHA | 1991 | 57.15727 | 843.371561 |
| Guinea | GIN | 1991 | 50.52734 | 554.046551 |
| Guinea-Bissau | GNB | 1991 | 49.39351 | 630.310664 |
| Kenya | KEN | 1991 | 56.93061 | 913.110171 |
| Lesotho | LSO | 1991 | 59.33083 | 715.638863 |
| Liberia | LBR | 1991 | 47.42273 | 357.608221 |
| Libya | LBY | 1991 | 68.96873 | |
| Madagascar | MDG | 1991 | 51.59824 | 448.035509 |
| Malawi | MWI | 1991 | 46.57176 | 351.861643 |
| Mali | MLI | 1991 | 46.06149 | 526.136353 |

| Country Name | Country Code | Year | Life Expectancy at Birth | GDP Per Capita |
|---|---|---|---|---|
| Mauritania | MRT | 1991 | 58.5802 | 1009.10877 |
| Mauritius | MUS | 1991 | 69.9561 | 3830.74132 |
| Morocco | MAR | 1991 | 65.19661 | 1811.40162 |
| Mozambique | MOZ | 1991 | 43.21534 | 176.788568 |
| Namibia | NAM | 1991 | 61.53307 | 3663.71454 |
| Niger | NER | 1991 | 44.07549 | 379.737074 |
| Nigeria | NGA | 1991 | 45.86978 | 1331.612 |
| Rwanda | RWA | 1991 | 30.43561 | 360.268222 |
| Sao Tome and Principe | STP | 1991 | 61.93454 | |
| Senegal | SEN | 1991 | 57.40949 | 842.409326 |
| Seychelles | SYC | 1991 | | 7648.21345 |
| Sierra Leone | SLE | 1991 | 36.74834 | 423.564968 |
| Somalia | SOM | 1991 | 45.27088 | |
| South Africa | ZAF | 1991 | 62.30598 | 5853.25503 |
| Sudan | SDN | 1991 | 55.67485 | 801.060519 |
| Swaziland | SWZ | 1991 | 60.00756 | 2692.12171 |
| Tanzania | TZA | 1991 | 49.9329 | 488.076716 |
| Togo | TGO | 1991 | 55.83502 | 528.095748 |
| Tunisia | TUN | 1991 | 69.44556 | 2263.60845 |
| Uganda | UGA | 1991 | 45.12624 | 308.273027 |
| Zambia | ZMB | 1991 | 44.45493 | 1017.65597 |
| Zimbabwe | ZWE | 1991 | 56.74966 | 1309.00499 |
| Algeria | DZA | 1992 | 67.20066 | 3403.90345 |
| Angola | AGO | 1992 | 42.03466 | 2271.0295 |
| Benin | BEN | 1992 | 54.67817 | 610.550902 |
| Botswana | BWA | 1992 | 59.96227 | 4040.42667 |
| Burkina Faso | BFA | 1992 | 49.27795 | 353.668786 |
| Burundi | BDI | 1992 | 47.69866 | 333.943219 |
| Cabo Verde | CPV | 1992 | 65.39815 | 1008.71436 |
| Cameroon | CMR | 1992 | 51.36763 | 1187.65853 |
| Central African Republic | CAF | 1992 | 47.85056 | 414.176125 |
| Chad | TCD | 1992 | 47.12137 | 568.734343 |
| Comoros | COM | 1992 | 57.59934 | 843.613797 |
| Congo, Dem. Rep. | COD | 1992 | 49.26141 | 507.716404 |
| Congo, Rep. | COG | 1992 | 54.98651 | 2699.5731 |
| Cote d'Ivoire | CIV | 1992 | 51.71161 | 1346.79807 |
| Djibouti | DJI | 1992 | 56.92959 | 1434.06828 |
| Egypt, Arab Rep. | EGY | 1992 | 65.37015 | 1574.84393 |
| Equatorial Guinea | GNQ | 1992 | 49.12529 | 635.249742 |
| Eritrea | ERI | 1992 | 50.54056 | 378.195429 |
| Ethiopia | ETH | 1992 | 47.91324 | 163.623281 |
| Gabon | GAB | 1992 | 61.08544 | 10835.0964 |
| Gambia, The | GMB | 1992 | 52.85622 | 514.021748 |
| Ghana | GHA | 1992 | 57.43678 | 852.048913 |
| Guinea | GIN | 1992 | 51.0041 | 539.61853 |
| Guinea-Bissau | GNB | 1992 | 49.77524 | 621.867599 |
| Kenya | KEN | 1992 | 56.22588 | 877.349813 |

| Country Name | Country Code | Year | Life Expectancy at Birth | GDP Per Capita |
|---|---|---|---|---|
| Lesotho | LSO | 1992 | 59.25617 | 750.451918 |
| Liberia | LBR | 1992 | 47.85149 | 236.446998 |
| Libya | LBY | 1992 | 69.27507 | |
| Madagascar | MDG | 1992 | 52.28012 | 440.13721 |
| Malawi | MWI | 1992 | 46.60507 | 323.091773 |
| Mali | MLI | 1992 | 46.29012 | 496.813829 |
| Mauritania | MRT | 1992 | 58.78451 | 1001.02076 |
| Mauritius | MUS | 1992 | 70.05854 | 4026.8923 |
| Morocco | MAR | 1992 | 65.65832 | 1741.92089 |
| Mozambique | MOZ | 1992 | 43.66071 | 161.833816 |
| Namibia | NAM | 1992 | 61.44059 | 3802.63236 |
| Niger | NER | 1992 | 44.67846 | 343.512962 |
| Nigeria | NGA | 1992 | 45.85266 | 1304.09028 |
| Rwanda | RWA | 1992 | 28.10705 | 401.340273 |
| Sao Tome and Principe | STP | 1992 | 62.0951 | |
| Senegal | SEN | 1992 | 57.50661 | 827.378247 |
| Seychelles | SYC | 1992 | 70.67073 | 8158.41126 |
| Sierra Leone | SLE | 1992 | 36.24659 | 343.500766 |
| Somalia | SOM | 1992 | 45.37232 | |
| South Africa | ZAF | 1992 | 62.31202 | 5586.70482 |
| Sudan | SDN | 1992 | 55.88859 | 831.791579 |
| Swaziland | SWZ | 1992 | 59.49283 | 2716.37079 |
| Tanzania | TZA | 1992 | 49.70066 | 474.644596 |
| Togo | TGO | 1992 | 55.69768 | 495.453391 |
| Tunisia | TUN | 1992 | 70.04312 | 2387.671 |
| Uganda | UGA | 1992 | 44.74729 | 308.343027 |
| Zambia | ZMB | 1992 | 43.96912 | 974.893858 |
| Zimbabwe | ZWE | 1992 | 55.37273 | 1164.25359 |
| Algeria | DZA | 1993 | 67.46061 | 3259.84368 |
| Angola | AGO | 1993 | 42.3031 | 1654.53709 |
| Benin | BEN | 1993 | 54.9458 | 623.953655 |
| Botswana | BWA | 1993 | 58.64173 | 4010.78715 |
| Burkina Faso | BFA | 1993 | 49.25966 | 356.128863 |
| Burundi | BDI | 1993 | 47.85449 | 307.123481 |
| Cabo Verde | CPV | 1993 | 65.75468 | 1067.06634 |
| Cameroon | CMR | 1993 | 50.88802 | 1063.4615 |
| Central African Republic | CAF | 1993 | 47.32878 | 404.406949 |
| Chad | TCD | 1993 | 47.21732 | 464.285496 |
| Comoros | COM | 1993 | 58.01346 | 844.164635 |
| Congo, Dem. Rep. | COD | 1993 | 49.25341 | 422.504043 |
| Congo, Rep. | COG | 1993 | 54.41741 | 2600.98948 |
| Cote d'Ivoire | CIV | 1993 | 51.06751 | 1298.84419 |
| Djibouti | DJI | 1993 | 57.00359 | 1331.67012 |
| Egypt, Arab Rep. | EGY | 1993 | 65.81095 | 1587.73138 |
| Equatorial Guinea | GNQ | 1993 | 49.6058 | 682.16415 |
| Eritrea | ERI | 1993 | 51.09498 | 431.785458 |
| Ethiopia | ETH | 1993 | 48.34722 | 178.608647 |

| *Country Name* | *Country Code* | *Year* | *Life Expectancy at Birth* | *GDP Per Capita* |
|---|---|---|---|---|
| Gabon | GAB | 1993 | 60.94722 | 10969.7818 |
| Gambia, The | GMB | 1993 | 53.17934 | 514.46529 |
| Ghana | GHA | 1993 | 57.5798 | 869.062575 |
| Guinea | GIN | 1993 | 51.35554 | 534.837045 |
| Guinea-Bissau | GNB | 1993 | 50.16107 | 619.896601 |
| Kenya | KEN | 1993 | 55.46368 | 853.435579 |
| Lesotho | LSO | 1993 | 58.80295 | 761.605254 |
| Liberia | LBR | 1993 | 48.48366 | 160.258822 |
| Libya | LBY | 1993 | 69.5409 | |
| Madagascar | MDG | 1993 | 53.0228 | 436.101667 |
| Malawi | MWI | 1993 | 46.614 | 353.455712 |
| Mali | MLI | 1993 | 46.42937 | 499.220412 |
| Mauritania | MRT | 1993 | 58.98173 | 1031.7071 |
| Mauritius | MUS | 1993 | 70.10732 | 4181.67106 |
| Morocco | MAR | 1993 | 66.06929 | 1699.40366 |
| Mozambique | MOZ | 1993 | 44.18202 | 169.218234 |
| Namibia | NAM | 1993 | 61.17356 | 3631.58074 |
| Niger | NER | 1993 | 45.31002 | 336.944783 |
| Nigeria | NGA | 1993 | 45.8408 | 1298.44095 |
| Rwanda | RWA | 1993 | 27.61271 | 392.326522 |
| Sao Tome and Principe | STP | 1993 | 62.25515 | |
| Senegal | SEN | 1993 | 57.51137 | 813.575966 |
| Seychelles | SYC | 1993 | | 8485.29143 |
| Sierra Leone | SLE | 1993 | 35.88576 | 350.165295 |
| Somalia | SOM | 1993 | 45.73322 | |
| South Africa | ZAF | 1993 | 62.14778 | 5516.75949 |
| Sudan | SDN | 1993 | 56.13268 | 847.276733 |
| Swaziland | SWZ | 1993 | 58.69517 | 2746.21316 |
| Tanzania | TZA | 1993 | 49.52188 | 464.533054 |
| Togo | TGO | 1993 | 55.4502 | 411.18144 |
| Tunisia | TUN | 1993 | 70.6019 | 2389.50095 |
| Uganda | UGA | 1993 | 44.45717 | 323.228929 |
| Zambia | ZMB | 1993 | 43.5811 | 1015.11139 |
| Zimbabwe | ZWE | 1993 | 53.89239 | 1152.45044 |
| Algeria | DZA | 1994 | 67.75537 | 3164.89858 |
| Angola | AGO | 1994 | 42.65029 | 1658.31009 |
| Benin | BEN | 1994 | 55.07976 | 615.120446 |
| Botswana | BWA | 1994 | 57.1129 | 4053.43604 |
| Burkina Faso | BFA | 1994 | 49.27771 | 351.104459 |
| Burundi | BDI | 1994 | 48.23468 | 290.319818 |
| Cabo Verde | CPV | 1994 | 66.13822 | 1237.73976 |
| Cameroon | CMR | 1994 | 50.41193 | 1056.98901 |
| Central African Republic | CAF | 1994 | 46.78217 | 412.999642 |
| Chad | TCD | 1994 | 47.31449 | 494.999868 |
| Comoros | COM | 1994 | 58.38259 | 777.128894 |
| Congo, Dem. Rep. | COD | 1994 | 49.17241 | 391.507717 |
| Congo, Rep. | COG | 1994 | 53.82207 | 2391.31033 |

| Country Name | Country Code | Year | Life Expectancy at Birth | GDP Per Capita |
|---|---|---|---|---|
| Cote d'Ivoire | CIV | 1994 | 50.3361 | 1266.5316 |
| Djibouti | DJI | 1994 | 57.04366 | 1310.9827 |
| Egypt, Arab Rep. | EGY | 1994 | 66.2788 | 1618.58478 |
| Equatorial Guinea | GNQ | 1994 | 50.09349 | 768.866811 |
| Eritrea | ERI | 1994 | 51.68983 | 525.724217 |
| Ethiopia | ETH | 1994 | 48.81278 | 177.994873 |
| Gabon | GAB | 1994 | 60.76868 | 11085.1951 |
| Gambia, The | GMB | 1994 | 53.5299 | 501.110487 |
| Ghana | GHA | 1994 | 57.59483 | 873.896927 |
| Guinea | GIN | 1994 | 51.58759 | 527.984005 |
| Guinea-Bissau | GNB | 1994 | 50.5441 | 625.386789 |
| Kenya | KEN | 1994 | 54.68407 | 849.696268 |
| Lesotho | LSO | 1994 | 57.96924 | 792.286752 |
| Liberia | LBR | 1994 | 49.28695 | 124.595577 |
| Libya | LBY | 1994 | 69.76568 | |
| Madagascar | MDG | 1994 | 53.80729 | 422.746161 |
| Malawi | MWI | 1994 | 46.60556 | 315.929624 |
| Mali | MLI | 1994 | 46.50376 | 504.358538 |
| Mauritania | MRT | 1994 | 59.17388 | 972.880754 |
| Mauritius | MUS | 1994 | 70.15854 | 4294.08812 |
| Morocco | MAR | 1994 | 66.44056 | 1848.78324 |
| Mozambique | MOZ | 1994 | 44.77034 | 172.792562 |
| Namibia | NAM | 1994 | 60.73463 | 3586.94271 |
| Niger | NER | 1994 | 45.96422 | 338.592438 |
| Nigeria | NGA | 1994 | 45.83971 | 1277.99293 |
| Rwanda | RWA | 1994 | 28.99993 | 204.772683 |
| Sao Tome and Principe | STP | 1994 | 62.41471 | |
| Senegal | SEN | 1994 | 57.45624 | 790.499967 |
| Seychelles | SYC | 1994 | | 8196.09255 |
| Sierra Leone | SLE | 1994 | 35.70139 | 345.2441 |
| Somalia | SOM | 1994 | 46.34805 | |
| South Africa | ZAF | 1994 | 61.80785 | 5563.3322 |
| Sudan | SDN | 1994 | 56.40568 | 833.417574 |
| Swaziland | SWZ | 1994 | 57.64022 | 2759.14267 |
| Tanzania | TZA | 1994 | 49.42607 | 456.893124 |
| Togo | TGO | 1994 | 55.11344 | 461.577032 |
| Tunisia | TUN | 1994 | 71.11395 | 2418.1837 |
| Uganda | UGA | 1994 | 44.28585 | 333.005141 |
| Zambia | ZMB | 1994 | 43.30929 | 903.891525 |
| Zimbabwe | ZWE | 1994 | 52.36559 | 1234.96618 |
| Algeria | DZA | 1995 | 68.09837 | 3223.55756 |
| Angola | AGO | 1995 | 43.09812 | 1775.89946 |
| Benin | BEN | 1995 | 55.11012 | 631.171224 |
| Botswana | BWA | 1995 | 55.45498 | 4237.5673 |
| Burkina Faso | BFA | 1995 | 49.34032 | 361.121422 |
| Burundi | BDI | 1995 | 48.7972 | 263.27085 |
| Cabo Verde | CPV | 1995 | 66.56876 | 1377.41961 |

| Country Name | Country Code | Year | Life Expectancy at Birth | GDP Per Capita |
|---|---|---|---|---|
| Cameroon | CMR | 1995 | 49.99327 | 1065.11953 |
| Central African Republic | CAF | 1995 | 46.22717 | 431.498671 |
| Chad | TCD | 1995 | 47.40651 | 484.758088 |
| Comoros | COM | 1995 | 58.69717 | 782.96773 |
| Congo, Dem. Rep. | COD | 1995 | 49.06593 | 381.717822 |
| Congo, Rep. | COG | 1995 | 53.2269 | 2418.42675 |
| Cote d'Ivoire | CIV | 1995 | 49.56066 | 1314.11994 |
| Djibouti | DJI | 1995 | 57.05341 | 1249.15124 |
| Egypt, Arab Rep. | EGY | 1995 | 66.76068 | 1661.33176 |
| Equatorial Guinea | GNQ | 1995 | 50.58085 | 871.588666 |
| Eritrea | ERI | 1995 | 52.308 | 539.926148 |
| Ethiopia | ETH | 1995 | 49.30451 | 182.708878 |
| Gabon | GAB | 1995 | 60.55785 | 11342.2074 |
| Gambia, The | GMB | 1995 | 53.91095 | 491.59291 |
| Ghana | GHA | 1995 | 57.50271 | 886.476947 |
| Guinea | GIN | 1995 | 51.69671 | 529.374823 |
| Guinea-Bissau | GNB | 1995 | 50.91249 | 639.364254 |
| Kenya | KEN | 1995 | 53.92356 | 861.249091 |
| Lesotho | LSO | 1995 | 56.75968 | 804.839088 |
| Liberia | LBR | 1995 | 50.16283 | 115.794136 |
| Libya | LBY | 1995 | 69.9509 | |
| Madagascar | MDG | 1995 | 54.61405 | 416.938321 |
| Malawi | MWI | 1995 | 46.57485 | 364.608506 |
| Mali | MLI | 1995 | 46.55634 | 495.698186 |
| Mauritania | MRT | 1995 | 59.35749 | 1038.26412 |
| Mauritius | MUS | 1995 | 70.32585 | 4439.86281 |
| Morocco | MAR | 1995 | 66.78471 | 1722.19331 |
| Mozambique | MOZ | 1995 | 45.39927 | 170.581709 |
| Namibia | NAM | 1995 | 60.12193 | 3617.29004 |
| Niger | NER | 1995 | 46.62951 | 335.480748 |
| Nigeria | NGA | 1995 | 45.85132 | 1242.73805 |
| Rwanda | RWA | 1995 | 31.96439 | 280.499456 |
| Sao Tome and Principe | STP | 1995 | 62.57027 | |
| Senegal | SEN | 1995 | 57.37861 | 810.574264 |
| Seychelles | SYC | 1995 | | 8009.7945 |
| Sierra Leone | SLE | 1995 | 35.72478 | 318.279426 |
| Somalia | SOM | 1995 | 47.16183 | |
| South Africa | ZAF | 1995 | 61.27385 | 5616.42349 |
| Sudan | SDN | 1995 | 56.70561 | 860.004008 |
| Swaziland | SWZ | 1995 | 56.34524 | 2835.03905 |
| Tanzania | TZA | 1995 | 49.44017 | 459.174973 |
| Togo | TGO | 1995 | 54.72488 | 484.935503 |
| Tunisia | TUN | 1995 | 71.57534 | 2432.31251 |
| Uganda | UGA | 1995 | 44.27224 | 359.764248 |
| Zambia | ZMB | 1995 | 43.17215 | 905.554642 |
| Zimbabwe | ZWE | 1995 | 50.84178 | 1214.69346 |
| Algeria | DZA | 1996 | 68.49102 | 3297.86337 |

| Country Name | Country Code | Year | Life Expectancy at Birth | GDP Per Capita |
|---|---|---|---|---|
| Angola | AGO | 1996 | 43.66595 | 1919.21177 |
| Benin | BEN | 1996 | 55.08012 | 638.076331 |
| Botswana | BWA | 1996 | 53.76402 | 4386.85154 |
| Burkina Faso | BFA | 1996 | 49.4508 | 389.965446 |
| Burundi | BDI | 1996 | 49.46005 | 239.039633 |
| Cabo Verde | CPV | 1996 | 67.06727 | 1496.60967 |
| Cameroon | CMR | 1996 | 49.68539 | 1083.28482 |
| Central African Republic | CAF | 1996 | 45.67424 | 404.224952 |
| Chad | TCD | 1996 | 47.48193 | 479.042125 |
| Comoros | COM | 1996 | 58.94717 | 751.923935 |
| Congo, Dem. Rep. | COD | 1996 | 48.99695 | 367.434633 |
| Congo, Rep. | COG | 1996 | 52.65727 | 2452.13807 |
| Cote d'Ivoire | CIV | 1996 | 48.79024 | 1372.7902 |
| Djibouti | DJI | 1996 | 57.03841 | 1173.0054 |
| Egypt, Arab Rep. | EGY | 1996 | 67.2321 | 1711.46506 |
| Equatorial Guinea | GNQ | 1996 | 51.05995 | 1398.89266 |
| Eritrea | ERI | 1996 | 52.9292 | 584.953705 |
| Ethiopia | ETH | 1996 | 49.80944 | 199.005022 |
| Gabon | GAB | 1996 | 60.31329 | 11459.4584 |
| Gambia, The | GMB | 1996 | 54.31859 | 488.555139 |
| Ghana | GHA | 1996 | 57.34078 | 904.337547 |
| Guinea | GIN | 1996 | 51.68388 | 535.220157 |
| Guinea-Bissau | GNB | 1996 | 51.24898 | 700.025225 |
| Kenya | KEN | 1996 | 53.2151 | 871.429954 |
| Lesotho | LSO | 1996 | 55.20988 | 837.563559 |
| Liberia | LBR | 1996 | 50.97951 | 122.85611 |
| Libya | LBY | 1996 | 70.10102 | |
| Madagascar | MDG | 1996 | 55.427 | 412.808337 |
| Malawi | MWI | 1996 | 46.5129 | 383.517887 |
| Mali | MLI | 1996 | 46.64061 | 517.086961 |
| Mauritania | MRT | 1996 | 59.5241 | 1066.51937 |
| Mauritius | MUS | 1996 | 70.32293 | 4640.25303 |
| Morocco | MAR | 1996 | 67.11817 | 1907.78645 |
| Mozambique | MOZ | 1996 | 46.0349 | 209.861657 |
| Namibia | NAM | 1996 | 59.33805 | 3620.88906 |
| Niger | NER | 1996 | 47.29539 | 334.845581 |
| Nigeria | NGA | 1996 | 45.87705 | 1272.72925 |
| Rwanda | RWA | 1996 | 35.89959 | 306.575546 |
| Sao Tome and Principe | STP | 1996 | 62.71832 | |
| Senegal | SEN | 1996 | 57.31634 | 805.924536 |
| Seychelles | SYC | 1996 | | 8281.2801 |
| Sierra Leone | SLE | 1996 | 35.97415 | 323.291931 |
| Somalia | SOM | 1996 | 48.07761 | |
| South Africa | ZAF | 1996 | 60.53444 | 5749.57955 |
| Sudan | SDN | 1996 | 57.02802 | 886.475756 |
| Swaziland | SWZ | 1996 | 54.83654 | 2881.07517 |
| Tanzania | TZA | 1996 | 49.58656 | 466.813007 |

| Country Name | Country Code | Year | Life Expectancy at Birth | GDP Per Capita |
|---|---|---|---|---|
| Togo | TGO | 1996 | 54.32761 | 512.879839 |
| Tunisia | TUN | 1996 | 71.98561 | 2566.12859 |
| Uganda | UGA | 1996 | 44.45266 | 380.338653 |
| Zambia | ZMB | 1996 | 43.1811 | 935.529939 |
| Zimbabwe | ZWE | 1996 | 49.36137 | 1317.50986 |
| Algeria | DZA | 1997 | 68.91471 | 3281.10214 |
| Angola | AGO | 1997 | 44.35515 | 2015.01392 |
| Benin | BEN | 1997 | 55.04559 | 654.542812 |
| Botswana | BWA | 1997 | 52.15941 | 4641.80548 |
| Burkina Faso | BFA | 1997 | 49.60588 | 403.216944 |
| Burundi | BDI | 1997 | 50.1188 | 232.506872 |
| Cabo Verde | CPV | 1997 | 67.63473 | 1624.70297 |
| Cameroon | CMR | 1997 | 49.51922 | 1111.55138 |
| Central African Republic | CAF | 1997 | 45.1408 | 415.787312 |
| Chad | TCD | 1997 | 47.53271 | 489.095261 |
| Comoros | COM | 1997 | 59.13559 | 761.462178 |
| Congo, Dem. Rep. | COD | 1997 | 49.02446 | 338.411808 |
| Congo, Rep. | COG | 1997 | 52.14402 | 2368.34013 |
| Cote d'Ivoire | CIV | 1997 | 48.07505 | 1382.62159 |
| Djibouti | DJI | 1997 | 57.0112 | 1133.83373 |
| Egypt, Arab Rep. | EGY | 1997 | 67.66407 | 1772.21045 |
| Equatorial Guinea | GNQ | 1997 | 51.52322 | 3364.3529 |
| Eritrea | ERI | 1997 | 53.53763 | 622.236646 |
| Ethiopia | ETH | 1997 | 50.31856 | 199.111303 |
| Gabon | GAB | 1997 | 60.038 | 11816.5376 |
| Gambia, The | GMB | 1997 | 54.73788 | 498.20252 |
| Ghana | GHA | 1997 | 57.16424 | 919.640195 |
| Guinea | GIN | 1997 | 51.57802 | 549.08279 |
| Guinea-Bissau | GNB | 1997 | 51.5479 | 732.466382 |
| Kenya | KEN | 1997 | 52.59505 | 851.183572 |
| Lesotho | LSO | 1997 | 53.44676 | 857.462748 |
| Liberia | LBR | 1997 | 51.63332 | 235.451341 |
| Libya | LBY | 1997 | 70.22751 | |
| Madagascar | MDG | 1997 | 56.23351 | 414.774254 |
| Malawi | MWI | 1997 | 46.43559 | 387.63064 |
| Mali | MLI | 1997 | 46.80498 | 528.268275 |
| Mauritania | MRT | 1997 | 59.66827 | 992.595531 |
| Mauritius | MUS | 1997 | 70.40488 | 4843.14425 |
| Morocco | MAR | 1997 | 67.45793 | 1853.01285 |
| Mozambique | MOZ | 1997 | 46.64932 | 226.303923 |
| Namibia | NAM | 1997 | 58.42641 | 3661.05152 |
| Niger | NER | 1997 | 47.95329 | 331.896505 |
| Nigeria | NGA | 1997 | 45.92129 | 1276.24082 |
| Rwanda | RWA | 1997 | 39.97837 | 327.244053 |
| Sao Tome and Principe | STP | 1997 | 62.8599 | |
| Senegal | SEN | 1997 | 57.29734 | 810.998708 |
| Seychelles | SYC | 1997 | 71.41463 | 9163.68507 |

| Country Name | Country Code | Year | Life Expectancy at Birth | GDP Per Capita |
|---|---|---|---|---|
| Sierra Leone | SLE | 1997 | 36.4262 | 302.658833 |
| Somalia | SOM | 1997 | 48.97644 | |
| South Africa | ZAF | 1997 | 59.62115 | 5803.95782 |
| Sudan | SDN | 1997 | 57.36449 | 953.554864 |
| Swaziland | SWZ | 1997 | 53.19122 | 2904.69558 |
| Tanzania | TZA | 1997 | 49.86361 | 470.722368 |
| Togo | TGO | 1997 | 53.9699 | 568.984188 |
| Tunisia | TUN | 1997 | 72.35268 | 2668.81055 |
| Uganda | UGA | 1997 | 44.83239 | 387.600619 |
| Zambia | ZMB | 1997 | 43.33659 | 943.855469 |
| Zimbabwe | ZWE | 1997 | 47.96459 | 1330.67629 |
| Algeria | DZA | 1998 | 69.35732 | 3397.4102 |
| Angola | AGO | 1998 | 45.15959 | 2094.47853 |
| Benin | BEN | 1998 | 55.05471 | 660.631781 |
| Botswana | BWA | 1998 | 50.76239 | 4585.73993 |
| Burkina Faso | BFA | 1998 | 49.80666 | 420.723454 |
| Burundi | BDI | 1998 | 50.69251 | 240.627598 |
| Cabo Verde | CPV | 1998 | 68.25915 | 1787.99912 |
| Cameroon | CMR | 1998 | 49.51373 | 1132.95203 |
| Central African Republic | CAF | 1998 | 44.64976 | 425.63968 |
| Chad | TCD | 1998 | 47.55929 | 505.162085 |
| Comoros | COM | 1998 | 59.27093 | 751.129339 |
| Congo, Dem. Rep. | COD | 1998 | 49.19244 | 325.413959 |
| Congo, Rep. | COG | 1998 | 51.72902 | 2387.5613 |
| Cote d'Ivoire | CIV | 1998 | 47.46402 | 1410.73839 |
| Djibouti | DJI | 1998 | 56.98773 | 1102.17798 |
| Egypt, Arab Rep. | EGY | 1998 | 68.0361 | 1810.16933 |
| Equatorial Guinea | GNQ | 1998 | 51.96461 | 4002.27095 |
| Eritrea | ERI | 1998 | 54.12666 | 620.917485 |
| Ethiopia | ETH | 1998 | 50.83178 | 186.661402 |
| Gabon | GAB | 1998 | 59.74895 | 11925.7831 |
| Gambia, The | GMB | 1998 | 55.15683 | 501.082406 |
| Ghana | GHA | 1998 | 57.02393 | 940.035344 |
| Guinea | GIN | 1998 | 51.42246 | 558.028555 |
| Guinea-Bissau | GNB | 1998 | 51.80702 | 517.782951 |
| Kenya | KEN | 1998 | 52.10776 | 855.099649 |
| Lesotho | LSO | 1998 | 51.61559 | 860.737309 |
| Liberia | LBR | 1998 | 52.07076 | 283.431706 |
| Libya | LBY | 1998 | 70.3418 | |
| Madagascar | MDG | 1998 | 57.02044 | 417.666676 |
| Malawi | MWI | 1998 | 46.36871 | 390.582492 |
| Mali | MLI | 1998 | 47.08493 | 553.665074 |
| Mauritania | MRT | 1998 | 59.79002 | 989.103322 |
| Mauritius | MUS | 1998 | 70.60732 | 5083.42334 |
| Morocco | MAR | 1998 | 67.8198 | 1962.03424 |
| Mozambique | MOZ | 1998 | 47.22602 | 246.710099 |
| Namibia | NAM | 1998 | 57.44988 | 3673.8446 |

| Country Name | Country Code | Year | Life Expectancy at Birth | GDP Per Capita |
|---|---|---|---|---|
| Niger | NER | 1998 | 48.59968 | 353.417242 |
| Nigeria | NGA | 1998 | 45.99246 | 1278.65132 |
| Rwanda | RWA | 1998 | 43.55227 | 329.115107 |
| Sao Tome and Principe | STP | 1998 | 62.99746 | |
| Senegal | SEN | 1998 | 57.34912 | 838.605619 |
| Seychelles | SYC | 1998 | | 9741.3605 |
| Sierra Leone | SLE | 1998 | 37.0468 | 304.651371 |
| Somalia | SOM | 1998 | 49.76383 | |
| South Africa | ZAF | 1998 | 58.58544 | 5745.30237 |
| Sudan | SDN | 1998 | 57.71056 | 967.405135 |
| Swaziland | SWZ | 1998 | 51.50976 | 2916.38908 |
| Tanzania | TZA | 1998 | 50.26768 | 475.928709 |
| Togo | TGO | 1998 | 53.69 | 538.734044 |
| Tunisia | TUN | 1998 | 72.68354 | 2762.55429 |
| Uganda | UGA | 1998 | 45.40227 | 394.247295 |
| Zambia | ZMB | 1998 | 43.63602 | 913.412362 |
| Zimbabwe | ZWE | 1998 | 46.7021 | 1347.9718 |
| Algeria | DZA | 1999 | 69.81429 | 3457.13705 |
| Angola | AGO | 1999 | 46.07078 | 2101.94533 |
| Benin | BEN | 1999 | 55.13559 | 675.677482 |
| Botswana | BWA | 1999 | 49.66822 | 4939.59806 |
| Burkina Faso | BFA | 1999 | 50.06066 | 439.299726 |
| Burundi | BDI | 1999 | 51.1502 | 234.68485 |
| Cabo Verde | CPV | 1999 | 68.918 | 1946.8514 |
| Cameroon | CMR | 1999 | 49.6749 | 1152.35455 |
| Central African Republic | CAF | 1999 | 44.22946 | 431.472541 |
| Chad | TCD | 1999 | 47.56861 | 484.082559 |
| Comoros | COM | 1999 | 59.36568 | 746.092407 |
| Congo, Dem. Rep. | COD | 1999 | 49.51741 | 304.336648 |
| Congo, Rep. | COG | 1999 | 51.45315 | 2260.72982 |
| Cote d'Ivoire | CIV | 1999 | 46.99256 | 1396.99955 |
| Djibouti | DJI | 1999 | 56.98146 | 1094.8473 |
| Egypt, Arab Rep. | EGY | 1999 | 68.34368 | 1885.74314 |
| Equatorial Guinea | GNQ | 1999 | 52.38061 | 4831.07265 |
| Eritrea | ERI | 1999 | 54.69727 | 606.325513 |
| Ethiopia | ETH | 1999 | 51.36059 | 190.691548 |
| Gabon | GAB | 1999 | 59.47405 | 10593.2394 |
| Gambia, The | GMB | 1999 | 55.57041 | 517.775544 |
| Ghana | GHA | 1999 | 56.95371 | 957.967877 |
| Guinea | GIN | 1999 | 51.26454 | 569.227729 |
| Guinea-Bissau | GNB | 1999 | 52.03046 | 514.146652 |
| Kenya | KEN | 1999 | 51.80105 | 851.067757 |
| Lesotho | LSO | 1999 | 49.84112 | 855.848055 |
| Liberia | LBR | 1999 | 52.30117 | 321.904554 |
| Libya | LBY | 1999 | 70.45185 | 8782.82625 |
| Madagascar | MDG | 1999 | 57.77173 | 423.576141 |
| Malawi | MWI | 1999 | 46.35054 | 390.089367 |

| Country Name | Country Code | Year | Life Expectancy at Birth | GDP Per Capita |
|---|---|---|---|---|
| Mali | MLI | 1999 | 47.49739 | 569.704206 |
| Mauritania | MRT | 1999 | 59.8919 | 1033.13926 |
| Mauritius | MUS | 1999 | 70.96098 | 5150.24991 |
| Morocco | MAR | 1999 | 68.21427 | 1958.95379 |
| Mozambique | MOZ | 1999 | 47.76098 | 259.231825 |
| Namibia | NAM | 1999 | 56.4668 | 3700.59111 |
| Niger | NER | 1999 | 49.23254 | 338.847713 |
| Nigeria | NGA | 1999 | 46.10002 | 1253.04789 |
| Rwanda | RWA | 1999 | 46.36156 | 319.061172 |
| Sao Tome and Principe | STP | 1999 | 63.13702 | |
| Senegal | SEN | 1999 | 57.49468 | 870.793083 |
| Seychelles | SYC | 1999 | | 9730.69992 |
| Sierra Leone | SLE | 1999 | 37.81254 | 292.958493 |
| Somalia | SOM | 1999 | 50.40127 | |
| South Africa | ZAF | 1999 | 57.48271 | 5794.40652 |
| Sudan | SDN | 1999 | 58.06429 | 969.956951 |
| Swaziland | SWZ | 1999 | 49.88849 | 2946.11067 |
| Tanzania | TZA | 1999 | 50.79724 | 486.410931 |
| Togo | TGO | 1999 | 53.51505 | 535.322454 |
| Tunisia | TUN | 1999 | 72.98361 | 2897.98369 |
| Uganda | UGA | 1999 | 46.14868 | 412.798478 |
| Zambia | ZMB | 1999 | 44.0798 | 928.863582 |
| Zimbabwe | ZWE | 1999 | 45.63217 | 1317.96884 |
| Algeria | DZA | 2000 | 70.28568 | 3541.07204 |
| Angola | AGO | 2000 | 47.07676 | 2100.57238 |
| Benin | BEN | 2000 | 55.31076 | 694.243749 |
| Botswana | BWA | 2000 | 48.98259 | 4954.77429 |
| Burkina Faso | BFA | 2000 | 50.38285 | 434.76333 |
| Burundi | BDI | 2000 | 51.48793 | 228.247569 |
| Cabo Verde | CPV | 2000 | 69.5738 | 2179.98481 |
| Cameroon | CMR | 2000 | 49.99973 | 1163.43141 |
| Central African Republic | CAF | 2000 | 43.91429 | 411.938174 |
| Chad | TCD | 2000 | 47.57059 | 462.5286 |
| Comoros | COM | 2000 | 59.4389 | 806.429473 |
| Congo, Dem. Rep. | COD | 2000 | 50.00288 | 276.216683 |
| Congo, Rep. | COG | 2000 | 51.37734 | 2364.61292 |
| Cote d'Ivoire | CIV | 2000 | 46.69744 | 1336.42961 |
| Djibouti | DJI | 2000 | 57.01034 | 1072.61559 |
| Egypt, Arab Rep. | EGY | 2000 | 68.58832 | 1950.60698 |
| Equatorial Guinea | GNQ | 2000 | 52.76415 | 5484.30083 |
| Eritrea | ERI | 2000 | 55.26505 | 571.603231 |
| Ethiopia | ETH | 2000 | 51.93383 | 196.504962 |
| Gabon | GAB | 2000 | 59.2518 | 10137.5502 |
| Gambia, The | GMB | 2000 | 55.97802 | 530.101214 |
| Ghana | GHA | 2000 | 56.9851 | 969.223555 |
| Guinea | GIN | 2000 | 51.1738 | 573.223455 |
| Guinea-Bissau | GNB | 2000 | 52.22705 | 532.267639 |

| Country Name | Country Code | Year | Life Expectancy at Birth | GDP Per Capita |
|---|---|---|---|---|
| Kenya | KEN | 2000 | 51.74093 | 833.029813 |
| Lesotho | LSO | 2000 | 48.27851 | 880.371679 |
| Liberia | LBR | 2000 | 52.40761 | 392.490207 |
| Libya | LBY | 2000 | 70.57254 | 8967.24745 |
| Madagascar | MDG | 2000 | 58.4728 | 430.108996 |
| Malawi | MWI | 2000 | 46.43634 | 384.68017 |
| Mali | MLI | 2000 | 48.05234 | 553.578011 |
| Mauritania | MRT | 2000 | 59.98493 | 998.106968 |
| Mauritius | MUS | 2000 | 71.66341 | 5560.23465 |
| Morocco | MAR | 2000 | 68.65215 | 1972.30029 |
| Mozambique | MOZ | 2000 | 48.27007 | 256.53938 |
| Namibia | NAM | 2000 | 55.5421 | 3746.71312 |
| Niger | NER | 2000 | 49.8558 | 322.14989 |
| Nigeria | NGA | 2000 | 46.26444 | 1287.05926 |
| Rwanda | RWA | 2000 | 48.36061 | 327.096813 |
| Sao Tome and Principe | STP | 2000 | 63.29254 | 854.424169 |
| Senegal | SEN | 2000 | 57.75276 | 877.002253 |
| Seychelles | SYC | 2000 | | 9790.27077 |
| Sierra Leone | SLE | 2000 | 38.69015 | 303.789098 |
| Somalia | SOM | 2000 | 50.87827 | |
| South Africa | ZAF | 2000 | 56.36832 | 5945.99881 |
| Sudan | SDN | 2000 | 58.42424 | 1003.00205 |
| Swaziland | SWZ | 2000 | 48.44217 | 2953.2323 |
| Tanzania | TZA | 2000 | 51.45585 | 497.20418 |
| Togo | TGO | 2000 | 53.45971 | 515.669772 |
| Tunisia | TUN | 2000 | 73.25383 | 3004.61077 |
| Uganda | UGA | 2000 | 47.05117 | 412.19638 |
| Zambia | ZMB | 2000 | 44.67032 | 938.351157 |
| Zimbabwe | ZWE | 2000 | 44.81356 | 1261.16309 |
| Algeria | DZA | 2001 | 70.77202 | 3600.43725 |
| Angola | AGO | 2001 | 48.16263 | 2119.32593 |
| Benin | BEN | 2001 | 55.58917 | 709.469362 |
| Botswana | BWA | 2001 | 48.7832 | 4891.91484 |
| Burkina Faso | BFA | 2001 | 50.78861 | 450.452281 |
| Burundi | BDI | 2001 | 51.72876 | 227.428111 |
| Cabo Verde | CPV | 2001 | 70.18005 | 2185.25382 |
| Cameroon | CMR | 2001 | 50.46783 | 1183.43807 |
| Central African Republic | CAF | 2001 | 43.73359 | 421.659199 |
| Chad | TCD | 2001 | 47.58112 | 497.346803 |
| Comoros | COM | 2001 | 59.51015 | 805.155529 |
| Congo, Dem. Rep. | COD | 2001 | 50.62934 | 263.051269 |
| Congo, Rep. | COG | 2001 | 51.55654 | 2387.84864 |
| Cote d'Ivoire | CIV | 2001 | 46.59732 | 1310.28647 |
| Djibouti | DJI | 2001 | 57.08824 | 1071.98235 |
| Egypt, Arab Rep. | EGY | 2001 | 68.78302 | 1982.11163 |
| Equatorial Guinea | GNQ | 2001 | 53.11171 | 8603.95568 |
| Eritrea | ERI | 2001 | 55.85673 | 603.1051 |

| Country Name | Country Code | Year | Life Expectancy at Birth | GDP Per Capita |
|---|---|---|---|---|
| Ethiopia | ETH | 2001 | 52.5859 | 206.743143 |
| Gabon | GAB | 2001 | 59.1212 | 10098.6011 |
| Gambia, The | GMB | 2001 | 56.381 | 543.784995 |
| Ghana | GHA | 2001 | 57.13861 | 982.932667 |
| Guinea | GIN | 2001 | 51.22285 | 583.424778 |
| Guinea-Bissau | GNB | 2001 | 52.41156 | 533.498089 |
| Kenya | KEN | 2001 | 51.98785 | 841.22055 |
| Lesotho | LSO | 2001 | 47.07041 | 903.384777 |
| Liberia | LBR | 2001 | 52.52744 | 389.548438 |
| Libya | LBY | 2001 | 70.71678 | 8671.83645 |
| Madagascar | MDG | 2001 | 59.11361 | 442.135824 |
| Malawi | MWI | 2001 | 46.68434 | 355.550849 |
| Mali | MLI | 2001 | 48.74176 | 620.284784 |
| Mauritania | MRT | 2001 | 60.08015 | 988.470248 |
| Mauritius | MUS | 2001 | 71.76585 | 5658.44969 |
| Morocco | MAR | 2001 | 69.14029 | 2091.23452 |
| Mozambique | MOZ | 2001 | 48.78215 | 281.067691 |
| Namibia | NAM | 2001 | 54.73217 | 3723.5253 |
| Niger | NER | 2001 | 50.47798 | 332.755541 |
| Nigeria | NGA | 2001 | 46.50573 | 1310.50597 |
| Rwanda | RWA | 2001 | 49.73598 | 341.993367 |
| Sao Tome and Principe | STP | 2001 | 63.47951 | 862.903368 |
| Senegal | SEN | 2001 | 58.13205 | 894.511597 |
| Seychelles | SYC | 2001 | | 9559.55196 |
| Sierra Leone | SLE | 2001 | 39.64549 | 271.689644 |
| Somalia | SOM | 2001 | 51.2228 | |
| South Africa | ZAF | 2001 | 55.29466 | 6052.55932 |
| Sudan | SDN | 2001 | 58.79395 | 1038.58143 |
| Swaziland | SWZ | 2001 | 47.27054 | 2952.50837 |
| Tanzania | TZA | 2001 | 52.24012 | 512.96827 |
| Togo | TGO | 2001 | 53.52261 | 493.248301 |
| Tunisia | TUN | 2001 | 73.49961 | 3091.10277 |
| Uganda | UGA | 2001 | 48.08037 | 419.335784 |
| Zambia | ZMB | 2001 | 45.40998 | 961.499932 |
| Zimbabwe | ZWE | 2001 | 44.28759 | 1264.43062 |
| Algeria | DZA | 2002 | 71.27039 | 3754.51628 |
| Angola | AGO | 2002 | 49.30156 | 1906.08658 |
| Benin | BEN | 2002 | 55.94866 | 720.168277 |
| Botswana | BWA | 2002 | 49.04378 | 5115.89989 |
| Burkina Faso | BFA | 2002 | 51.28166 | 456.734135 |
| Burundi | BDI | 2002 | 51.9332 | 230.996154 |
| Cabo Verde | CPV | 2002 | 70.69876 | 2257.31667 |
| Cameroon | CMR | 2002 | 51.03176 | 1201.91208 |
| Central African Republic | CAF | 2002 | 43.69632 | 428.477229 |
| Chad | TCD | 2002 | 47.6151 | 519.27665 |
| Comoros | COM | 2002 | 59.59893 | 804.211318 |
| Congo, Dem. Rep. | COD | 2002 | 51.3468 | 262.972798 |

| Country Name | Country Code | Year | Life Expectancy at Birth | GDP Per Capita |
|---|---|---|---|---|
| Congo, Rep. | COG | 2002 | 51.99678 | 2430.28515 |
| Cote d'Ivoire | CIV | 2002 | 46.67254 | 1264.22231 |
| Djibouti | DJI | 2002 | 57.22056 | 1080.1369 |
| Egypt, Arab Rep. | EGY | 2002 | 68.94827 | 1990.99216 |
| Equatorial Guinea | GNQ | 2002 | 53.42924 | 9867.5621 |
| Eritrea | ERI | 2002 | 56.4931 | 601.034247 |
| Ethiopia | ETH | 2002 | 53.33868 | 203.905913 |
| Gabon | GAB | 2002 | 59.10559 | 9823.25199 |
| Gambia, The | GMB | 2002 | 56.78122 | 509.721395 |
| Ghana | GHA | 2002 | 57.39993 | 1001.23786 |
| Guinea | GIN | 2002 | 51.44454 | 602.395954 |
| Guinea-Bissau | GNB | 2002 | 52.602 | 517.619949 |
| Kenya | KEN | 2002 | 52.54276 | 823.091943 |
| Lesotho | LSO | 2002 | 46.26951 | 902.099835 |
| Liberia | LBR | 2002 | 52.79676 | 394.739885 |
| Libya | LBY | 2002 | 70.88554 | 8453.58472 |
| Madagascar | MDG | 2002 | 59.69917 | 374.489091 |
| Malawi | MWI | 2002 | 47.13034 | 352.028451 |
| Mali | MLI | 2002 | 49.52461 | 620.55831 |
| Mauritania | MRT | 2002 | 60.18954 | 966.472928 |
| Mauritius | MUS | 2002 | 71.96585 | 5738.05597 |
| Morocco | MAR | 2002 | 69.67015 | 2130.73392 |
| Mozambique | MOZ | 2002 | 49.32859 | 296.983486 |
| Namibia | NAM | 2002 | 54.07983 | 3845.05715 |
| Niger | NER | 2002 | 51.10954 | 330.548164 |
| Nigeria | NGA | 2002 | 46.82995 | 1326.24297 |
| Rwanda | RWA | 2002 | 50.91151 | 377.711879 |
| Sao Tome and Principe | STP | 2002 | 63.70493 | 863.494054 |
| Senegal | SEN | 2002 | 58.61222 | 877.648151 |
| Seychelles | SYC | 2002 | 72.95366 | 9384.15248 |
| Sierra Leone | SLE | 2002 | 40.6429 | 327.967423 |
| Somalia | SOM | 2002 | 51.50185 | |
| South Africa | ZAF | 2002 | 54.31495 | 6200.31658 |
| Sudan | SDN | 2002 | 59.17693 | 1074.6393 |
| Swaziland | SWZ | 2002 | 46.42112 | 3059.01387 |
| Tanzania | TZA | 2002 | 53.13015 | 534.696652 |
| Togo | TGO | 2002 | 53.67876 | 475.699197 |
| Tunisia | TUN | 2002 | 73.72139 | 3107.02064 |
| Uganda | UGA | 2002 | 49.19085 | 440.652174 |
| Zambia | ZMB | 2002 | 46.28622 | 978.053431 |
| Zimbabwe | ZWE | 2002 | 44.06063 | 1139.59007 |
| Algeria | DZA | 2003 | 71.77432 | 3974.17503 |
| Angola | AGO | 2003 | 50.46612 | 1936.59966 |
| Benin | BEN | 2003 | 56.3621 | 722.667195 |
| Botswana | BWA | 2003 | 49.71356 | 5280.21517 |
| Burkina Faso | BFA | 2003 | 51.85727 | 478.304352 |
| Burundi | BDI | 2003 | 52.15222 | 221.227482 |

| Country Name | Country Code | Year | Life Expectancy at Birth | GDP Per Capita |
|---|---|---|---|---|
| Cabo Verde | CPV | 2003 | 71.10793 | 2310.49442 |
| Cameroon | CMR | 2003 | 51.6441 | 1224.16103 |
| Central African Republic | CAF | 2003 | 43.80549 | 397.811327 |
| Chad | TCD | 2003 | 47.6909 | 573.334374 |
| Comoros | COM | 2003 | 59.7208 | 801.798756 |
| Congo, Dem. Rep. | COD | 2003 | 52.10678 | 269.243781 |
| Congo, Rep. | COG | 2003 | 52.68217 | 2383.35912 |
| Cote d'Ivoire | CIV | 2003 | 46.89424 | 1224.96834 |
| Djibouti | DJI | 2003 | 57.41122 | 1096.48923 |
| Egypt, Arab Rep. | EGY | 2003 | 69.10407 | 2015.898 |
| Equatorial Guinea | GNQ | 2003 | 53.72371 | 10788.0289 |
| Eritrea | ERI | 2003 | 57.18478 | 565.725054 |
| Ethiopia | ETH | 2003 | 54.19963 | 193.866915 |
| Gabon | GAB | 2003 | 59.21785 | 9788.87914 |
| Gambia, The | GMB | 2003 | 57.17863 | 527.504387 |
| Ghana | GHA | 2003 | 57.75015 | 1026.39836 |
| Guinea | GIN | 2003 | 51.85046 | 598.616262 |
| Guinea-Bissau | GNB | 2003 | 52.81217 | 509.656955 |
| Kenya | KEN | 2003 | 53.38451 | 824.470152 |
| Lesotho | LSO | 2003 | 45.89559 | 935.471224 |
| Liberia | LBR | 2003 | 53.3051 | 271.022142 |
| Libya | LBY | 2003 | 71.07485 | 9403.45365 |
| Madagascar | MDG | 2003 | 60.23551 | 398.901979 |
| Malawi | MWI | 2003 | 47.7912 | 362.371936 |
| Mali | MLI | 2003 | 50.3569 | 656.491888 |
| Mauritania | MRT | 2003 | 60.32107 | 995.194651 |
| Mauritius | MUS | 2003 | 72.1213 | 5905.00121 |
| Morocco | MAR | 2003 | 70.22973 | 2230.90475 |
| Mozambique | MOZ | 2003 | 49.92873 | 307.034073 |
| Namibia | NAM | 2003 | 53.62578 | 3958.87386 |
| Niger | NER | 2003 | 51.75898 | 335.66823 |
| Nigeria | NGA | 2003 | 47.23463 | 1426.90331 |
| Rwanda | RWA | 2003 | 52.20802 | 379.643977 |
| Sao Tome and Principe | STP | 2003 | 63.96973 | 898.652803 |
| Senegal | SEN | 2003 | 59.17183 | 912.250512 |
| Seychelles | SYC | 2003 | 71.02927 | 8932.19505 |
| Sierra Leone | SLE | 2003 | 41.64912 | 342.019024 |
| Somalia | SOM | 2003 | 51.7719 | |
| South Africa | ZAF | 2003 | 53.49044 | 6305.78791 |
| Sudan | SDN | 2003 | 59.57463 | 1125.7644 |
| Swaziland | SWZ | 2003 | 45.92402 | 3158.8261 |
| Tanzania | TZA | 2003 | 54.09834 | 555.496036 |
| Togo | TGO | 2003 | 53.90812 | 486.309191 |
| Tunisia | TUN | 2003 | 73.92315 | 3228.46383 |
| Uganda | UGA | 2003 | 50.33359 | 453.197793 |
| Zambia | ZMB | 2003 | 47.28207 | 1018.36197 |
| Zimbabwe | ZWE | 2003 | 44.13063 | 935.930158 |

| *Country Name* | *Country Code* | *Year* | *Life Expectancy at Birth* | *GDP Per Capita* |
|---|---|---|---|---|
| Algeria | DZA | 2004 | 72.27583 | 4091.14424 |
| Angola | AGO | 2004 | 51.63285 | 2071.90527 |
| Benin | BEN | 2004 | 56.81493 | 732.335423 |
| Botswana | BWA | 2004 | 50.74637 | 5349.00202 |
| Burkina Faso | BFA | 2004 | 52.50724 | 485.307404 |
| Burundi | BDI | 2004 | 52.4038 | 224.515553 |
| Cabo Verde | CPV | 2004 | 71.39854 | 2505.17251 |
| Cameroon | CMR | 2004 | 52.27388 | 1272.8512 |
| Central African Republic | CAF | 2004 | 44.05763 | 414.030231 |
| Chad | TCD | 2004 | 47.82241 | 737.987527 |
| Comoros | COM | 2004 | 59.88876 | 798.010572 |
| Congo, Dem. Rep. | COD | 2004 | 52.87927 | 278.476786 |
| Congo, Rep. | COG | 2004 | 53.58673 | 2395.81962 |
| Cote d'Ivoire | CIV | 2004 | 47.24459 | 1218.12035 |
| Djibouti | DJI | 2004 | 57.66363 | 1120.51907 |
| Egypt, Arab Rep. | EGY | 2004 | 69.26041 | 2059.37751 |
| Equatorial Guinea | GNQ | 2004 | 54.00202 | 14266.9279 |
| Eritrea | ERI | 2004 | 57.92485 | 556.03564 |
| Ethiopia | ETH | 2004 | 55.16122 | 214.044832 |
| Gabon | GAB | 2004 | 59.46378 | 9595.85149 |
| Gambia, The | GMB | 2004 | 57.57173 | 546.774803 |
| Ghana | GHA | 2004 | 58.17534 | 1056.00038 |
| Guinea | GIN | 2004 | 52.4339 | 600.980415 |
| Guinea-Bissau | GNB | 2004 | 53.05105 | 512.427534 |
| Kenya | KEN | 2004 | 54.47895 | 843.229371 |
| Lesotho | LSO | 2004 | 45.94846 | 943.61318 |
| Liberia | LBR | 2004 | 54.06415 | 272.855157 |
| Libya | LBY | 2004 | 71.2768 | 9670.08455 |
| Madagascar | MDG | 2004 | 60.72871 | 407.517462 |
| Malawi | MWI | 2004 | 48.67129 | 371.78737 |
| Mali | MLI | 2004 | 51.2081 | 645.922979 |
| Mauritania | MRT | 2004 | 60.48127 | 1022.75037 |
| Mauritius | MUS | 2004 | 72.27675 | 6205.2532 |
| Morocco | MAR | 2004 | 70.80856 | 2310.33845 |
| Mozambique | MOZ | 2004 | 50.58305 | 321.30288 |
| Namibia | NAM | 2004 | 53.41076 | 4394.41065 |
| Niger | NER | 2004 | 52.42778 | 323.969968 |
| Nigeria | NGA | 2004 | 47.71078 | 1860.06238 |
| Rwanda | RWA | 2004 | 53.69368 | 401.409684 |
| Sao Tome and Principe | STP | 2004 | 64.26795 | 911.005602 |
| Senegal | SEN | 2004 | 59.79729 | 940.686921 |
| Seychelles | SYC | 2004 | 72.60976 | 8709.78269 |
| Sierra Leone | SLE | 2004 | 42.6392 | 347.900129 |
| Somalia | SOM | 2004 | 52.0529 | |
| South Africa | ZAF | 2004 | 52.88032 | 6511.14013 |
| Sudan | SDN | 2004 | 59.98407 | 1137.56308 |
| Swaziland | SWZ | 2004 | 45.80341 | 3250.39922 |

| Country Name | Country Code | Year | Life Expectancy at Birth | GDP Per Capita |
|---|---|---|---|---|
| Tanzania | TZA | 2004 | 55.11705 | 581.772411 |
| Togo | TGO | 2004 | 54.2042 | 483.765465 |
| Tunisia | TUN | 2004 | 74.10688 | 3403.10523 |
| Uganda | UGA | 2004 | 51.46985 | 467.479965 |
| Zambia | ZMB | 2004 | 48.37946 | 1061.19773 |
| Zimbabwe | ZWE | 2004 | 44.50595 | 871.667105 |
| Algeria | DZA | 2005 | 72.76141 | 4273.31275 |
| Angola | AGO | 2005 | 52.78771 | 2364.19427 |
| Benin | BEN | 2005 | 57.28561 | 723.199959 |
| Botswana | BWA | 2005 | 52.07032 | 5512.81123 |
| Burkina Faso | BFA | 2005 | 53.21844 | 511.96759 |
| Burundi | BDI | 2005 | 52.70537 | 219.18655 |
| Cabo Verde | CPV | 2005 | 71.57559 | 2639.38264 |
| Cameroon | CMR | 2005 | 52.889 | 1264.1544 |
| Central African Republic | CAF | 2005 | 44.44283 | 410.414836 |
| Chad | TCD | 2005 | 48.02751 | 835.195542 |
| Comoros | COM | 2005 | 60.11078 | 801.33346 |
| Congo, Dem. Rep. | COD | 2005 | 53.63729 | 286.291577 |
| Congo, Rep. | COG | 2005 | 54.66551 | 2503.31205 |
| Cote d'Ivoire | CIV | 2005 | 47.69641 | 1216.20847 |
| Djibouti | DJI | 2005 | 57.98429 | 1137.58287 |
| Egypt, Arab Rep. | EGY | 2005 | 69.42434 | 2112.48797 |
| Equatorial Guinea | GNQ | 2005 | 54.27956 | 15941.647 |
| Eritrea | ERI | 2005 | 58.69778 | 554.488199 |
| Ethiopia | ETH | 2005 | 56.20893 | 232.7832 |
| Gabon | GAB | 2005 | 59.84256 | 9579.35612 |
| Gambia, The | GMB | 2005 | 57.95659 | 524.512768 |
| Ghana | GHA | 2005 | 58.65202 | 1089.46832 |
| Guinea | GIN | 2005 | 53.15693 | 606.874402 |
| Guinea-Bissau | GNB | 2005 | 53.3219 | 522.486155 |
| Kenya | KEN | 2005 | 55.78022 | 868.92282 |
| Lesotho | LSO | 2005 | 46.38702 | 968.399912 |
| Liberia | LBR | 2005 | 55.03107 | 279.796234 |
| Libya | LBY | 2005 | 71.471 | 10653.7844 |
| Madagascar | MDG | 2005 | 61.18729 | 413.867495 |
| Malawi | MWI | 2005 | 49.77156 | 373.232125 |
| Mali | MLI | 2005 | 52.04071 | 666.257623 |
| Mauritania | MRT | 2005 | 60.67359 | 1083.19527 |
| Mauritius | MUS | 2005 | 72.4322 | 6245.19696 |
| Morocco | MAR | 2005 | 71.39285 | 2358.44358 |
| Mozambique | MOZ | 2005 | 51.279 | 339.132244 |
| Namibia | NAM | 2005 | 53.4888 | 4454.63476 |
| Niger | NER | 2005 | 53.12241 | 326.33171 |
| Nigeria | NGA | 2005 | 48.23837 | 1875.02964 |
| Rwanda | RWA | 2005 | 55.36659 | 430.633605 |
| Sao Tome and Principe | STP | 2005 | 64.58356 | 952.679774 |
| Senegal | SEN | 2005 | 60.47532 | 967.49872 |

| Country Name | Country Code | Year | Life Expectancy at Birth | GDP Per Capita |
|---|---|---|---|---|
| Seychelles | SYC | 2005 | 72.13171 | 9450.27943 |
| Sierra Leone | SLE | 2005 | 43.60307 | 348.94474 |
| Somalia | SOM | 2005 | 52.35485 | |
| South Africa | ZAF | 2005 | 52.56317 | 6767.63258 |
| Sudan | SDN | 2005 | 60.40673 | 1189.96099 |
| Swaziland | SWZ | 2005 | 46.07483 | 3411.67334 |
| Tanzania | TZA | 2005 | 56.1539 | 610.822326 |
| Togo | TGO | 2005 | 54.5729 | 476.671548 |
| Tunisia | TUN | 2005 | 74.27217 | 3492.16594 |
| Uganda | UGA | 2005 | 52.5668 | 480.095353 |
| Zambia | ZMB | 2005 | 49.57493 | 1107.72817 |
| Zimbabwe | ZWE | 2005 | 45.21095 | 811.562953 |
| Algeria | DZA | 2006 | 73.21956 | 4282.32823 |
| Angola | AGO | 2006 | 53.92712 | 2754.41364 |
| Benin | BEN | 2006 | 57.74912 | 730.275256 |
| Botswana | BWA | 2006 | 53.59368 | 5883.89906 |
| Burkina Faso | BFA | 2006 | 53.97524 | 527.962349 |
| Burundi | BDI | 2006 | 53.06378 | 223.40359 |
| Cabo Verde | CPV | 2006 | 71.66005 | 2813.1854 |
| Cameroon | CMR | 2006 | 53.46788 | 1272.88267 |
| Central African Republic | CAF | 2006 | 44.94322 | 422.438682 |
| Chad | TCD | 2006 | 48.32207 | 812.0086 |
| Comoros | COM | 2006 | 60.39183 | 803.113048 |
| Congo, Dem. Rep. | COD | 2006 | 54.36334 | 291.971436 |
| Congo, Rep. | COG | 2006 | 55.86007 | 2573.50988 |
| Cote d'Ivoire | CIV | 2006 | 48.21883 | 1210.66821 |
| Djibouti | DJI | 2006 | 58.37768 | 1172.7889 |
| Egypt, Arab Rep. | EGY | 2006 | 69.59834 | 2217.39483 |
| Equatorial Guinea | GNQ | 2006 | 54.57022 | 16413.5404 |
| Eritrea | ERI | 2006 | 59.47593 | 535.929673 |
| Ethiopia | ETH | 2006 | 57.31883 | 251.056047 |
| Gabon | GAB | 2006 | 60.33988 | 9041.67368 |
| Gambia, The | GMB | 2006 | 58.32832 | 513.754354 |
| Ghana | GHA | 2006 | 59.15122 | 1129.23952 |
| Guinea | GIN | 2006 | 53.95624 | 609.330658 |
| Guinea-Bissau | GNB | 2006 | 53.62324 | 522.509422 |
| Kenya | KEN | 2006 | 57.22798 | 900.100565 |
| Lesotho | LSO | 2006 | 47.12468 | 1001.08707 |
| Liberia | LBR | 2006 | 56.11334 | 292.037742 |
| Libya | LBY | 2006 | 71.63107 | 11175.1299 |
| Madagascar | MDG | 2006 | 61.62388 | 422.141167 |
| Malawi | MWI | 2006 | 51.08 | 379.438608 |
| Mali | MLI | 2006 | 52.82127 | 674.740126 |
| Mauritania | MRT | 2006 | 60.89754 | 1251.63016 |
| Mauritius | MUS | 2006 | 72.4322 | 6746.88662 |
| Morocco | MAR | 2006 | 71.96785 | 2507.67466 |
| Mozambique | MOZ | 2006 | 51.99212 | 361.745038 |

| *Country Name* | *Country Code* | *Year* | *Life Expectancy at Birth* | *GDP Per Capita* |
|---|---|---|---|---|
| Namibia | NAM | 2006 | 53.90246 | 4715.10597 |
| Niger | NER | 2006 | 53.84683 | 332.710876 |
| Nigeria | NGA | 2006 | 48.79285 | 1976.70847 |
| Rwanda | RWA | 2006 | 57.15278 | 459.412163 |
| Sao Tome and Principe | STP | 2006 | 64.89605 | 1015.39539 |
| Senegal | SEN | 2006 | 61.19305 | 965.109503 |
| Seychelles | SYC | 2006 | 72.21707 | 10126.2905 |
| Sierra Leone | SLE | 2006 | 44.54507 | 356.244959 |
| Somalia | SOM | 2006 | 52.67678 | |
| South Africa | ZAF | 2006 | 52.60461 | 7053.9447 |
| Sudan | SDN | 2006 | 60.8421 | 1275.26203 |
| Swaziland | SWZ | 2006 | 46.72783 | 3568.85728 |
| Tanzania | TZA | 2006 | 57.1779 | 620.059709 |
| Togo | TGO | 2006 | 55.02312 | 482.859636 |
| Tunisia | TUN | 2006 | 74.41515 | 3641.5434 |
| Uganda | UGA | 2006 | 53.60395 | 513.75276 |
| Zambia | ZMB | 2006 | 50.87144 | 1163.30273 |
| Zimbabwe | ZWE | 2006 | 46.26705 | 772.472586 |
| Algeria | DZA | 2007 | 73.64271 | 4359.37575 |
| Angola | AGO | 2007 | 55.04751 | 3258.47528 |
| Benin | BEN | 2007 | 58.18898 | 752.215215 |
| Botswana | BWA | 2007 | 55.20961 | 6270.47408 |
| Burkina Faso | BFA | 2007 | 54.75566 | 541.268695 |
| Burundi | BDI | 2007 | 53.46646 | 226.304442 |
| Cabo Verde | CPV | 2007 | 71.69141 | 3202.37926 |
| Cameroon | CMR | 2007 | 54.0079 | 1299.29093 |
| Central African Republic | CAF | 2007 | 45.52646 | 434.250473 |
| Chad | TCD | 2007 | 48.7011 | 811.016282 |
| Comoros | COM | 2007 | 60.71937 | 790.367477 |
| Congo, Dem. Rep. | COD | 2007 | 55.05393 | 300.291829 |
| Congo, Rep. | COG | 2007 | 57.09446 | 2447.51163 |
| Cote d'Ivoire | CIV | 2007 | 48.78029 | 1207.08719 |
| Djibouti | DJI | 2007 | 58.83188 | 1212.50931 |
| Egypt, Arab Rep. | EGY | 2007 | 69.77944 | 2333.46731 |
| Equatorial Guinea | GNQ | 2007 | 54.88298 | 18075.1768 |
| Eritrea | ERI | 2007 | 60.23012 | 532.231477 |
| Ethiopia | ETH | 2007 | 58.45002 | 272.391198 |
| Gabon | GAB | 2007 | 60.92212 | 9299.46399 |
| Gambia, The | GMB | 2007 | 58.68456 | 515.77195 |
| Ghana | GHA | 2007 | 59.64388 | 1147.8665 |
| Guinea | GIN | 2007 | 54.75751 | 635.168547 |
| Guinea-Bissau | GNB | 2007 | 53.9478 | 526.841286 |
| Kenya | KEN | 2007 | 58.73907 | 935.656508 |
| Lesotho | LSO | 2007 | 48.0232 | 1040.66757 |
| Liberia | LBR | 2007 | 57.18327 | 307.399619 |
| Libya | LBY | 2007 | 71.73866 | 11707.9854 |
| Madagascar | MDG | 2007 | 62.05154 | 435.717245 |

| Country Name | Country Code | Year | Life Expectancy at Birth | GDP Per Capita |
|---|---|---|---|---|
| Malawi | MWI | 2007 | 52.53927 | 403.494597 |
| Mali | MLI | 2007 | 53.53429 | 675.409209 |
| Mauritania | MRT | 2007 | 61.14661 | 1251.15438 |
| Mauritius | MUS | 2007 | 72.57073 | 7100.86182 |
| Morocco | MAR | 2007 | 72.52024 | 2566.2167 |
| Mozambique | MOZ | 2007 | 52.69551 | 377.383272 |
| Namibia | NAM | 2007 | 54.62463 | 4968.66403 |
| Niger | NER | 2007 | 54.59456 | 330.633212 |
| Nigeria | NGA | 2007 | 49.34627 | 2056.83859 |
| Rwanda | RWA | 2007 | 58.90234 | 482.139939 |
| Sao Tome and Principe | STP | 2007 | 65.18493 | 1024.17906 |
| Senegal | SEN | 2007 | 61.93317 | 985.749914 |
| Seychelles | SYC | 2007 | 73.19268 | 11124.6571 |
| Sierra Leone | SLE | 2007 | 45.48139 | 374.282875 |
| Somalia | SOM | 2007 | 53.00517 | |
| South Africa | ZAF | 2007 | 52.99702 | 7333.23986 |
| Sudan | SDN | 2007 | 61.2871 | 1385.41003 |
| Swaziland | SWZ | 2007 | 47.67998 | 3668.48073 |
| Tanzania | TZA | 2007 | 58.16983 | 651.903658 |
| Togo | TGO | 2007 | 55.55371 | 480.775908 |
| Tunisia | TUN | 2007 | 74.53541 | 3847.40697 |
| Uganda | UGA | 2007 | 54.58156 | 538.039369 |
| Zambia | ZMB | 2007 | 52.2541 | 1226.54055 |
| Zimbabwe | ZWE | 2007 | 47.63585 | 732.769983 |
| Algeria | DZA | 2008 | 74.02532 | 4390.49963 |
| Angola | AGO | 2008 | 56.13929 | 3578.87281 |
| Benin | BEN | 2008 | 58.59071 | 767.057379 |
| Botswana | BWA | 2008 | 56.81946 | 6552.77664 |
| Burkina Faso | BFA | 2008 | 55.53571 | 563.447065 |
| Burundi | BDI | 2008 | 53.90188 | 229.834701 |
| Cabo Verde | CPV | 2008 | 71.70668 | 3378.6462 |
| Cameroon | CMR | 2008 | 54.51063 | 1308.2355 |
| Central African Republic | CAF | 2008 | 46.16317 | 436.073716 |
| Chad | TCD | 2008 | 49.15368 | 808.889004 |
| Comoros | COM | 2008 | 61.07934 | 774.684921 |
| Congo, Dem. Rep. | COD | 2008 | 55.70602 | 308.652808 |
| Congo, Rep. | COG | 2008 | 58.3008 | 2496.50231 |
| Cote d'Ivoire | CIV | 2008 | 49.35146 | 1211.62384 |
| Djibouti | DJI | 2008 | 59.32841 | 1261.73998 |
| Egypt, Arab Rep. | EGY | 2008 | 69.9631 | 2456.73143 |
| Equatorial Guinea | GNQ | 2008 | 55.22188 | 20333.9404 |
| Eritrea | ERI | 2008 | 60.93771 | 471.166625 |
| Ethiopia | ETH | 2008 | 59.56112 | 293.853313 |
| Gabon | GAB | 2008 | 61.5528 | 8715.45672 |
| Gambia, The | GMB | 2008 | 59.02295 | 528.371603 |
| Ghana | GHA | 2008 | 60.10602 | 1220.71327 |
| Guinea | GIN | 2008 | 55.50159 | 646.968779 |

| Country Name | Country Code | Year | Life Expectancy at Birth | GDP Per Capita |
|---|---|---|---|---|
| Guinea-Bissau | GNB | 2008 | 54.28668 | 530.930642 |
| Kenya | KEN | 2008 | 60.22856 | 912.376719 |
| Lesotho | LSO | 2008 | 48.95744 | 1101.00442 |
| Liberia | LBR | 2008 | 58.14171 | 315.876086 |
| Libya | LBY | 2008 | 71.78695 | 11856.0205 |
| Madagascar | MDG | 2008 | 62.48032 | 453.636564 |
| Malawi | MWI | 2008 | 54.08012 | 421.226145 |
| Mali | MLI | 2008 | 54.17432 | 684.494418 |
| Mauritania | MRT | 2008 | 61.41022 | 1229.45439 |
| Mauritius | MUS | 2008 | 72.57073 | 7456.36925 |
| Morocco | MAR | 2008 | 73.03812 | 2686.2283 |
| Mozambique | MOZ | 2008 | 53.36678 | 391.710147 |
| Namibia | NAM | 2008 | 55.60134 | 5036.2547 |
| Niger | NER | 2008 | 55.35312 | 349.00468 |
| Nigeria | NGA | 2008 | 49.87756 | 2128.66663 |
| Rwanda | RWA | 2008 | 60.4938 | 521.54528 |
| Sao Tome and Principe | STP | 2008 | 65.43571 | 1082.71488 |
| Senegal | SEN | 2008 | 62.67502 | 994.380234 |
| Seychelles | SYC | 2008 | 73.16341 | 10645.0867 |
| Sierra Leone | SLE | 2008 | 46.41517 | 384.898031 |
| Somalia | SOM | 2008 | 53.33154 | |
| South Africa | ZAF | 2008 | 53.70407 | 7464.37166 |
| Sudan | SDN | 2008 | 61.7342 | 1455.31837 |
| Swaziland | SWZ | 2008 | 48.8351 | 3633.31559 |
| Tanzania | TZA | 2008 | 59.11812 | 666.81324 |
| Togo | TGO | 2008 | 56.15007 | 478.361776 |
| Tunisia | TUN | 2008 | 74.63698 | 3968.35256 |
| Uganda | UGA | 2008 | 55.49546 | 565.067858 |
| Zambia | ZMB | 2008 | 53.68846 | 1285.86453 |
| Zimbabwe | ZWE | 2008 | 49.24944 | 593.127247 |
| Algeria | DZA | 2009 | 74.36785 | 4386.0389 |
| Angola | AGO | 2009 | 57.181 | 3536.7983 |
| Benin | BEN | 2009 | 58.9468 | 763.105014 |
| Botswana | BWA | 2009 | 58.35466 | 5948.85325 |
| Burkina Faso | BFA | 2009 | 56.29488 | 562.841935 |
| Burundi | BDI | 2009 | 54.36202 | 230.053171 |
| Cabo Verde | CPV | 2009 | 71.72839 | 3300.55099 |
| Cameroon | CMR | 2009 | 54.97263 | 1300.84144 |
| Central African Republic | CAF | 2009 | 46.83493 | 437.601384 |
| Chad | TCD | 2009 | 49.66337 | 815.968047 |
| Comoros | COM | 2009 | 61.46024 | 770.994711 |
| Congo, Dem. Rep. | COD | 2009 | 56.31261 | 307.109163 |
| Congo, Rep. | COG | 2009 | 59.43215 | 2595.7485 |
| Cote d'Ivoire | CIV | 2009 | 49.91137 | 1223.51062 |
| Djibouti | DJI | 2009 | 59.84885 | 1303.21679 |
| Egypt, Arab Rep. | EGY | 2009 | 70.15078 | 2524.43244 |
| Equatorial Guinea | GNQ | 2009 | 55.58498 | 19684.697 |

| Country Name | Country Code | Year | Life Expectancy at Birth | GDP Per Capita |
|---|---|---|---|---|
| Eritrea | ERI | 2009 | 61.58712 | 480.608925 |
| Ethiopia | ETH | 2009 | 60.6222 | 311.367744 |
| Gabon | GAB | 2009 | 62.20502 | 8449.93976 |
| Gambia, The | GMB | 2009 | 59.34351 | 544.958565 |
| Ghana | GHA | 2009 | 60.52363 | 1247.46274 |
| Guinea | GIN | 2009 | 56.16356 | 622.938229 |
| Guinea-Bissau | GNB | 2009 | 54.6382 | 535.280987 |
| Kenya | KEN | 2009 | 61.63163 | 917.043827 |
| Lesotho | LSO | 2009 | 49.8538 | 1113.98481 |
| Liberia | LBR | 2009 | 58.95163 | 319.655736 |
| Libya | LBY | 2009 | 71.78051 | 11631.719 |
| Madagascar | MDG | 2009 | 62.91524 | 423.305741 |
| Malawi | MWI | 2009 | 55.64271 | 442.557285 |
| Mali | MLI | 2009 | 54.73629 | 693.546068 |
| Mauritania | MRT | 2009 | 61.68183 | 1182.37837 |
| Mauritius | MUS | 2009 | 72.88244 | 7683.12492 |
| Morocco | MAR | 2009 | 73.51346 | 2765.85615 |
| Mozambique | MOZ | 2009 | 54.00051 | 404.59502 |
| Namibia | NAM | 2009 | 56.77773 | 4978.68 |
| Niger | NER | 2009 | 56.11005 | 333.690293 |
| Nigeria | NGA | 2009 | 50.37573 | 2216.49939 |
| Rwanda | RWA | 2009 | 61.88834 | 539.378799 |
| Sao Tome and Principe | STP | 2009 | 65.64293 | 1083.66427 |
| Senegal | SEN | 2009 | 63.39863 | 990.320872 |
| Seychelles | SYC | 2009 | 73.03415 | 10486.1899 |
| Sierra Leone | SLE | 2009 | 47.33327 | 393.545483 |
| Somalia | SOM | 2009 | 53.65839 | |
| South Africa | ZAF | 2009 | 54.68346 | 7247.44939 |
| Sudan | SDN | 2009 | 62.17578 | 1464.2546 |
| Swaziland | SWZ | 2009 | 50.11861 | 3622.112 |
| Tanzania | TZA | 2009 | 60.01044 | 680.80613 |
| Togo | TGO | 2009 | 56.79068 | 481.960278 |
| Tunisia | TUN | 2009 | 74.72529 | 4044.62969 |
| Uganda | UGA | 2009 | 56.33224 | 583.097021 |
| Zambia | ZMB | 2009 | 55.13159 | 1365.40234 |
| Zimbabwe | ZWE | 2009 | 51.0289 | 652.288733 |
| Algeria | DZA | 2010 | 74.66978 | 4463.39467 |
| Angola | AGO | 2010 | 58.14112 | 3529.05348 |
| Benin | BEN | 2010 | 59.25927 | 757.695907 |
| Botswana | BWA | 2010 | 59.78093 | 6346.1562 |
| Burkina Faso | BFA | 2010 | 57.01468 | 575.446453 |
| Burundi | BDI | 2010 | 54.837 | 231.194326 |
| Cabo Verde | CPV | 2010 | 71.77454 | 3312.82598 |
| Cameroon | CMR | 2010 | 55.40115 | 1309.12221 |
| Central African Republic | CAF | 2010 | 47.53271 | 446.443449 |
| Chad | TCD | 2010 | 50.20634 | 896.569734 |
| Comoros | COM | 2010 | 61.84707 | 769.174288 |

| *Country Name* | *Country Code* | *Year* | *Life Expectancy at Birth* | *GDP Per Capita* |
|---|---|---|---|---|
| Congo, Dem. Rep. | COD | 2010 | 56.87017 | 318.075752 |
| Congo, Rep. | COG | 2010 | 60.45261 | 2737.34233 |
| Cote d'Ivoire | CIV | 2010 | 50.45071 | 1219.7491 |
| Djibouti | DJI | 2010 | 60.36673 | 1325.99072 |
| Egypt, Arab Rep. | EGY | 2010 | 70.34141 | 2602.47955 |
| Equatorial Guinea | GNQ | 2010 | 55.95895 | 17136.4457 |
| Eritrea | ERI | 2010 | 62.17585 | 482.14909 |
| Ethiopia | ETH | 2010 | 61.60185 | 341.309909 |
| Gabon | GAB | 2010 | 62.85654 | 8754.11392 |
| Gambia, The | GMB | 2010 | 59.64573 | 562.482516 |
| Ghana | GHA | 2010 | 60.89373 | 1312.60756 |
| Guinea | GIN | 2010 | 56.74324 | 635.671485 |
| Guinea-Bissau | GNB | 2010 | 55.00054 | 546.721669 |
| Kenya | KEN | 2010 | 62.88815 | 967.340077 |
| Lesotho | LSO | 2010 | 50.66122 | 1169.26784 |
| Liberia | LBR | 2010 | 59.60551 | 327.42051 |
| Libya | LBY | 2010 | 71.73698 | 12120.5622 |
| Madagascar | MDG | 2010 | 63.3578 | 412.730934 |
| Malawi | MWI | 2010 | 57.15624 | 458.868174 |
| Mali | MLI | 2010 | 55.22976 | 708.370763 |
| Mauritania | MRT | 2010 | 61.95137 | 1203.38366 |
| Mauritius | MUS | 2010 | 72.96732 | 8000.37643 |
| Morocco | MAR | 2010 | 73.94107 | 2834.20472 |
| Mozambique | MOZ | 2010 | 54.60176 | 419.225815 |
| Namibia | NAM | 2010 | 58.07461 | 5191.58308 |
| Niger | NER | 2010 | 56.84541 | 348.151511 |
| Nigeria | NGA | 2010 | 50.83727 | 2327.32067 |
| Rwanda | RWA | 2010 | 63.06556 | 563.491049 |
| Sao Tome and Principe | STP | 2010 | 65.80861 | 1129.75496 |
| Senegal | SEN | 2010 | 64.08363 | 1002.52994 |
| Seychelles | SYC | 2010 | 73.19756 | 10804.6845 |
| Sierra Leone | SLE | 2010 | 48.212 | 405.128402 |
| Somalia | SOM | 2010 | 53.9912 | |
| South Africa | ZAF | 2010 | 55.86961 | 7361.75585 |
| Sudan | SDN | 2010 | 62.60076 | 1476.47809 |
| Swaziland | SWZ | 2010 | 51.4482 | 3690.23923 |
| Tanzania | TZA | 2010 | 60.85568 | 701.60455 |
| Togo | TGO | 2010 | 57.44251 | 487.923891 |
| Tunisia | TUN | 2010 | 74.81127 | 4140.15177 |
| Uganda | UGA | 2010 | 57.07763 | 595.206173 |
| Zambia | ZMB | 2010 | 56.52449 | 1463.21357 |
| Zimbabwe | ZWE | 2010 | 52.8778 | 719.979517 |
| Algeria | DZA | 2011 | 74.93756 | 4504.9201 |
| Angola | AGO | 2011 | 58.99124 | 3538.71569 |
| Benin | BEN | 2011 | 59.53661 | 758.577521 |
| Botswana | BWA | 2011 | 61.0981 | 6610.33192 |
| Burkina Faso | BFA | 2011 | 57.68112 | 595.393248 |

| Country Name | Country Code | Year | Life Expectancy at Birth | GDP Per Capita |
|---|---|---|---|---|
| Burundi | BDI | 2011 | 55.31441 | 233.518126 |
| Cabo Verde | CPV | 2011 | 71.85417 | 3405.78186 |
| Cameroon | CMR | 2011 | 55.80893 | 1326.64601 |
| Central African Republic | CAF | 2011 | 48.25698 | 458.332773 |
| Chad | TCD | 2011 | 50.75224 | 867.999063 |
| Comoros | COM | 2011 | 62.2248 | 770.322758 |
| Congo, Dem. Rep. | COD | 2011 | 57.38117 | 328.750569 |
| Congo, Rep. | COG | 2011 | 61.35024 | 2751.91068 |
| Cote d'Ivoire | CIV | 2011 | 50.97234 | 1138.66496 |
| Djibouti | DJI | 2011 | 60.85459 | 1361.56856 |
| Egypt, Arab Rep. | EGY | 2011 | 70.5349 | 2593.5969 |
| Equatorial Guinea | GNQ | 2011 | 56.32602 | 17461.5519 |
| Eritrea | ERI | 2011 | 62.71193 | 514.179598 |
| Ethiopia | ETH | 2011 | 62.47663 | 369.58442 |
| Gabon | GAB | 2011 | 63.48868 | 9060.66199 |
| Gambia, The | GMB | 2011 | 59.93056 | 521.611531 |
| Ghana | GHA | 2011 | 61.22078 | 1460.64566 |
| Guinea | GIN | 2011 | 57.26066 | 655.923443 |
| Guinea-Bissau | GNB | 2011 | 55.37366 | 576.013039 |
| Kenya | KEN | 2011 | 63.96059 | 998.998391 |
| Lesotho | LSO | 2011 | 51.3612 | 1235.66278 |
| Liberia | LBR | 2011 | 60.1288 | 343.6464 |
| Libya | LBY | 2011 | 71.68334 | 4578.53181 |
| Madagascar | MDG | 2011 | 63.80546 | 407.327282 |
| Malawi | MWI | 2011 | 58.55737 | 466.963342 |
| Mali | MLI | 2011 | 55.67463 | 709.39938 |
| Mauritania | MRT | 2011 | 62.20976 | 1223.3446 |
| Mauritius | MUS | 2011 | 73.26683 | 8313.27125 |
| Morocco | MAR | 2011 | 74.32024 | 2942.03882 |
| Mozambique | MOZ | 2011 | 55.18759 | 436.143182 |
| Namibia | NAM | 2011 | 59.40393 | 5351.36975 |
| Niger | NER | 2011 | 57.53629 | 342.859308 |
| Nigeria | NGA | 2011 | 51.26968 | 2376.63877 |
| Rwanda | RWA | 2011 | 64.03159 | 591.821409 |
| Sao Tome and Principe | STP | 2011 | 65.9408 | 1152.89978 |
| Senegal | SEN | 2011 | 64.71332 | 990.680473 |
| Seychelles | SYC | 2011 | 72.72439 | 11967.3623 |
| Sierra Leone | SLE | 2011 | 49.02427 | 414.791671 |
| Somalia | SOM | 2011 | 54.33549 | |
| South Africa | ZAF | 2011 | 57.18107 | 7493.30312 |
| Sudan | SDN | 2011 | 62.99702 | 1592.9644 |
| Swaziland | SWZ | 2011 | 52.75373 | 3704.14066 |
| Tanzania | TZA | 2011 | 61.67444 | 733.670799 |
| Togo | TGO | 2011 | 58.06861 | 498.242898 |
| Tunisia | TUN | 2011 | 74.90668 | 4014.91679 |
| Uganda | UGA | 2011 | 57.722 | 629.240447 |
| Zambia | ZMB | 2011 | 57.80861 | 1499.72831 |

| *Country Name* | *Country Code* | *Year* | *Life Expectancy at Birth* | *GDP Per Capita* |
|---|---|---|---|---|
| Zimbabwe | ZWE | 2011 | 54.6972 | 813.83401 |
| Algeria | DZA | 2012 | 75.1812 | 4564.43502 |
| Angola | AGO | 2012 | 59.71844 | 3591.02744 |
| Benin | BEN | 2012 | 59.79785 | 773.137026 |
| Botswana | BWA | 2012 | 62.34724 | 6779.3939 |
| Burkina Faso | BFA | 2012 | 58.29583 | 615.097084 |
| Burundi | BDI | 2012 | 55.78288 | 235.705288 |
| Cabo Verde | CPV | 2012 | 71.96283 | 3403.03108 |
| Cameroon | CMR | 2012 | 56.21768 | 1349.95171 |
| Central African Republic | CAF | 2012 | 49.01215 | 475.667387 |
| Chad | TCD | 2012 | 51.27476 | 914.118651 |
| Comoros | COM | 2012 | 62.58146 | 774.470989 |
| Congo, Dem. Rep. | COD | 2012 | 57.85807 | 340.714023 |
| Congo, Rep. | COG | 2012 | 62.14907 | 2782.11188 |
| Cote d'Ivoire | CIV | 2012 | 51.49017 | 1229.7782 |
| Djibouti | DJI | 2012 | 61.29546 | 1402.79944 |
| Egypt, Arab Rep. | EGY | 2012 | 70.7282 | 2593.22647 |
| Equatorial Guinea | GNQ | 2012 | 56.66834 | 18106.3367 |
| Eritrea | ERI | 2012 | 63.21293 | |
| Ethiopia | ETH | 2012 | 63.24859 | 391.131795 |
| Gabon | GAB | 2012 | 64.09534 | 9212.29127 |
| Gambia, The | GMB | 2012 | 60.20139 | 533.776842 |
| Ghana | GHA | 2012 | 61.52432 | 1558.45662 |
| Guinea | GIN | 2012 | 57.76112 | 679.556106 |
| Guinea-Bissau | GNB | 2012 | 55.75778 | 551.637377 |
| Kenya | KEN | 2012 | 64.85993 | 1016.8277 |
| Lesotho | LSO | 2012 | 51.98656 | 1293.63341 |
| Liberia | LBR | 2012 | 60.58954 | 361.232507 |
| Libya | LBY | 2012 | 71.65007 | |
| Madagascar | MDG | 2012 | 64.24912 | 408.342126 |
| Malawi | MWI | 2012 | 59.81473 | 461.887342 |
| Mali | MLI | 2012 | 56.10244 | 683.001597 |
| Mauritania | MRT | 2012 | 62.45095 | 1256.20197 |
| Mauritius | MUS | 2012 | 73.86341 | 8580.08565 |
| Morocco | MAR | 2012 | 74.66066 | 2987.31592 |
| Mozambique | MOZ | 2012 | 55.77654 | 454.106824 |
| Namibia | NAM | 2012 | 60.68471 | 5502.25887 |
| Niger | NER | 2012 | 58.17024 | 368.942844 |
| Nigeria | NGA | 2012 | 51.69049 | 2412.86078 |
| Rwanda | RWA | 2012 | 64.83546 | 627.852382 |
| Sao Tome and Principe | STP | 2012 | 66.05654 | 1162.5374 |
| Senegal | SEN | 2012 | 65.28559 | 1003.99153 |
| Seychelles | SYC | 2012 | 74.22683 | 12633.8883 |
| Sierra Leone | SLE | 2012 | 49.75359 | 466.861199 |
| Somalia | SOM | 2012 | 54.69576 | |
| South Africa | ZAF | 2012 | 58.52041 | 7545.78322 |
| Sudan | SDN | 2012 | 63.36005 | 1797.10607 |

| Country Name | Country Code | Year | Life Expectancy at Birth | GDP Per Capita |
|---|---|---|---|---|
| Swaziland | SWZ | 2012 | 53.99044 | 3807.74132 |
| Tanzania | TZA | 2012 | 62.48729 | 747.664453 |
| Togo | TGO | 2012 | 58.64456 | 508.540042 |
| Tunisia | TUN | 2012 | 75.0189 | 4127.40078 |
| Uganda | UGA | 2012 | 58.27483 | 631.555118 |
| Zambia | ZMB | 2012 | 58.94749 | 1565.90033 |
| Zimbabwe | ZWE | 2012 | 56.40771 | 913.53063 |
| Algeria | DZA | 2013 | 75.41217 | 4596.21963 |
| Angola | AGO | 2013 | 60.32176 | 3702.59918 |
| Benin | BEN | 2013 | 60.05651 | 805.944941 |
| Botswana | BWA | 2013 | 63.55066 | 7409.42116 |
| Burkina Faso | BFA | 2013 | 58.86037 | 631.612184 |
| Burundi | BDI | 2013 | 56.23451 | 239.331065 |
| Cabo Verde | CPV | 2013 | 72.09654 | 3389.94 |
| Cameroon | CMR | 2013 | 56.64198 | 1385.23544 |
| Central African Republic | CAF | 2013 | 49.79566 | 300.479582 |
| Chad | TCD | 2013 | 51.75451 | 934.702546 |
| Comoros | COM | 2013 | 62.90907 | 782.516902 |
| Congo, Dem. Rep. | COD | 2013 | 58.31239 | 357.570338 |
| Congo, Rep. | COG | 2013 | 62.8701 | 2806.34743 |
| Cote d'Ivoire | CIV | 2013 | 52.01605 | 1305.70923 |
| Djibouti | DJI | 2013 | 61.67737 | 1447.47222 |
| Egypt, Arab Rep. | EGY | 2013 | 70.92024 | 2591.05945 |
| Equatorial Guinea | GNQ | 2013 | 56.978 | 16634.7677 |
| Eritrea | ERI | 2013 | 63.6949 | |
| Ethiopia | ETH | 2013 | 63.92417 | 421.384136 |
| Gabon | GAB | 2013 | 64.67088 | 9408.0062 |
| Gambia, The | GMB | 2013 | 60.46217 | 542.131869 |
| Ghana | GHA | 2013 | 61.82032 | 1633.49404 |
| Guinea | GIN | 2013 | 58.27961 | 690.666992 |
| Guinea-Bissau | GNB | 2013 | 56.14966 | 554.911608 |
| Kenya | KEN | 2013 | 65.60307 | 1048.26921 |
| Lesotho | LSO | 2013 | 52.56502 | 1300.40615 |
| Liberia | LBR | 2013 | 61.04117 | 383.07944 |
| Libya | LBY | 2013 | 71.6591 | |
| Madagascar | MDG | 2013 | 64.68176 | 406.374993 |
| Malawi | MWI | 2013 | 60.90644 | 471.840466 |
| Mali | MLI | 2013 | 56.53612 | 678.756281 |
| Mauritania | MRT | 2013 | 62.67195 | 1293.55549 |
| Mauritius | MUS | 2013 | 74.01707 | 8848.88703 |
| Morocco | MAR | 2013 | 74.97015 | 3077.31501 |
| Mozambique | MOZ | 2013 | 56.37961 | 472.590637 |
| Namibia | NAM | 2013 | 61.84544 | 5679.27865 |
| Niger | NER | 2013 | 58.7388 | 373.736875 |
| Nigeria | NGA | 2013 | 52.11271 | 2475.94806 |
| Rwanda | RWA | 2013 | 65.52271 | 640.947437 |
| Sao Tome and Principe | STP | 2013 | 66.17134 | 1191.43677 |

| Country Name | Country Code | Year | Life Expectancy at Birth | GDP Per Capita |
|---|---|---|---|---|
| Senegal | SEN | 2013 | 65.80073 | 1008.02404 |
| Seychelles | SYC | 2013 | 73.11951 | 13153.0387 |
| Sierra Leone | SLE | 2013 | 50.39254 | 550.875982 |
| Somalia | SOM | 2013 | 55.07249 | |
| South Africa | ZAF | 2013 | 59.80007 | 7616.77912 |
| Sudan | SDN | 2013 | 63.68578 | 1832.31378 |
| Swaziland | SWZ | 2013 | 55.11929 | 3977.97643 |
| Tanzania | TZA | 2013 | 63.30561 | 777.403631 |
| Togo | TGO | 2013 | 59.15046 | 514.944966 |
| Tunisia | TUN | 2013 | 75.15429 | 4196.75249 |
| Uganda | UGA | 2013 | 58.74902 | 632.486138 |
| Zambia | ZMB | 2013 | 59.9202 | 1595.91504 |
| Zimbabwe | ZWE | 2013 | 57.94051 | 942.038655 |
| Algeria | DZA | 2014 | 75.63502 | 4675.88502 |
| Angola | AGO | 2014 | 60.80673 | 3747.56836 |
| Benin | BEN | 2014 | 60.31812 | 833.662487 |
| Botswana | BWA | 2014 | 64.69439 | 7574.2821 |
| Burkina Faso | BFA | 2014 | 59.37529 | 639.709551 |
| Burundi | BDI | 2014 | 56.66332 | 243.101912 |
| Cabo Verde | CPV | 2014 | 72.25432 | 3369.64271 |
| Cameroon | CMR | 2014 | 57.0878 | 1428.21567 |
| Central African Republic | CAF | 2014 | 50.59105 | 302.546369 |
| Chad | TCD | 2014 | 52.18107 | 967.102777 |
| Comoros | COM | 2014 | 63.20215 | 779.839822 |
| Congo, Dem. Rep. | COD | 2014 | 58.74861 | 378.79141 |
| Congo, Rep. | COG | 2014 | 63.51532 | 2922.97318 |
| Cote d'Ivoire | CIV | 2014 | 52.54707 | 1384.91035 |
| Djibouti | DJI | 2014 | 61.99432 | 1508.29166 |
| Egypt, Arab Rep. | EGY | 2014 | 71.10956 | 2608.3752 |
| Equatorial Guinea | GNQ | 2014 | 57.25554 | 16028.2495 |
| Eritrea | ERI | 2014 | 64.16339 | |
| Ethiopia | ETH | 2014 | 64.5069 | 452.778236 |
| Gabon | GAB | 2014 | 65.20302 | 9508.14829 |
| Gambia, The | GMB | 2014 | 60.71385 | 530.317659 |
| Ghana | GHA | 2014 | 62.11378 | 1659.77614 |
| Guinea | GIN | 2014 | 58.8249 | 699.964084 |
| Guinea-Bissau | GNB | 2014 | 56.54822 | 545.89852 |
| Kenya | KEN | 2014 | 66.19415 | 1075.63876 |
| Lesotho | LSO | 2014 | 53.09322 | 1323.23773 |
| Liberia | LBR | 2014 | 61.50124 | 376.588857 |
| Libya | LBY | 2014 | 71.71939 | |
| Madagascar | MDG | 2014 | 65.10132 | 408.661033 |
| Malawi | MWI | 2014 | 61.81661 | 484.368625 |
| Mali | MLI | 2014 | 56.98671 | 705.788473 |
| Mauritania | MRT | 2014 | 62.87024 | 1326.15865 |
| Mauritius | MUS | 2014 | 74.19439 | 9163.63335 |
| Morocco | MAR | 2014 | 75.25515 | 3110.20901 |

| Country Name | Country Code | Year | Life Expectancy at Birth | GDP Per Capita |
|---|---|---|---|---|
| Mozambique | MOZ | 2014 | 56.99434 | 493.252236 |
| Namibia | NAM | 2014 | 62.83893 | 5901.24289 |
| Niger | NER | 2014 | 59.24051 | 386.7258 |
| Nigeria | NGA | 2014 | 52.54134 | 2563.09212 |
| Rwanda | RWA | 2014 | 66.11334 | 672.748919 |
| Sao Tome and Principe | STP | 2014 | 66.29071 | 1240.9981 |
| Senegal | SEN | 2014 | 66.25783 | 1018.39275 |
| Seychelles | SYC | 2014 | 73.22927 | 13379.5906 |
| Sierra Leone | SLE | 2014 | 50.94261 | 563.174505 |
| Somalia | SOM | 2014 | 55.46568 | |
| South Africa | ZAF | 2014 | 60.95478 | 7626.81018 |
| Sudan | SDN | 2014 | 63.97473 | 1837.13836 |
| Swaziland | SWZ | 2014 | 56.10146 | 3980.77445 |
| Tanzania | TZA | 2014 | 64.11849 | 806.150078 |
| Togo | TGO | 2014 | 59.57634 | 531.156102 |
| Tunisia | TUN | 2014 | 75.31434 | 4265.14557 |
| Uganda | UGA | 2014 | 59.1558 | 642.877314 |
| Zambia | ZMB | 2014 | 60.71534 | 1620.82329 |
| Zimbabwe | ZWE | 2014 | 59.24432 | 939.780273 |
| Algeria | DZA | 2015 | 75.85529 | 4759.59524 |
| Angola | AGO | 2015 | 61.18934 | 3730.16906 |
| Benin | BEN | 2015 | 60.58468 | 827.845967 |
| Botswana | BWA | 2015 | 65.7511 | 7308.61151 |
| Burkina Faso | BFA | 2015 | 59.84466 | 645.369843 |
| Burundi | BDI | 2015 | 57.06934 | 226.528058 |
| Cabo Verde | CPV | 2015 | 72.43517 | 3364.17997 |
| Cameroon | CMR | 2015 | 57.55751 | 1469.63774 |
| Central African Republic | CAF | 2015 | 51.37785 | 314.926517 |
| Chad | TCD | 2015 | 52.55395 | 953.591407 |
| Comoros | COM | 2015 | 63.46068 | 769.477378 |
| Congo, Dem. Rep. | COD | 2015 | 59.17322 | 391.718545 |
| Congo, Rep. | COG | 2015 | 64.09073 | 2925.52775 |
| Cote d'Ivoire | CIV | 2015 | 53.07824 | 1469.73018 |
| Djibouti | DJI | 2015 | 62.24983 | 1579.92434 |
| Egypt, Arab Rep. | EGY | 2015 | 71.29566 | 2665.35161 |
| Equatorial Guinea | GNQ | 2015 | 57.50839 | 14010.9428 |
| Eritrea | ERI | 2015 | 64.62439 | |
| Ethiopia | ETH | 2015 | 65.00829 | 487.290011 |
| Gabon | GAB | 2015 | 65.68441 | 9598.30367 |
| Gambia, The | GMB | 2015 | 60.95744 | 536.41292 |
| Ghana | GHA | 2015 | 62.40724 | 1685.98612 |
| Guinea | GIN | 2015 | 59.39895 | 707.366223 |
| Guinea-Bissau | GNB | 2015 | 56.95039 | 564.722084 |
| Kenya | KEN | 2015 | 66.64566 | 1107.91806 |
| Lesotho | LSO | 2015 | 53.5701 | 1338.53537 |
| Liberia | LBR | 2015 | 61.98022 | 367.475978 |
| Libya | LBY | 2015 | 71.83039 | |

| Country Name | Country Code | Year | Life Expectancy at Birth | GDP Per Capita |
|---|---|---|---|---|
| Madagascar | MDG | 2015 | 65.50783 | 410.194159 |
| Malawi | MWI | 2015 | 62.54337 | 483.628811 |
| Mali | MLI | 2015 | 57.45771 | 726.248067 |
| Mauritania | MRT | 2015 | 63.04637 | 1306.64963 |
| Mauritius | MUS | 2015 | 74.35317 | 9468.9407 |
| Morocco | MAR | 2015 | 75.52015 | 3204.75361 |
| Mozambique | MOZ | 2015 | 57.60927 | 510.79208 |
| Namibia | NAM | 2015 | 63.63644 | 6114.05563 |
| Niger | NER | 2015 | 59.68188 | 386.903644 |
| Nigeria | NGA | 2015 | 52.97793 | 2562.52222 |
| Rwanda | RWA | 2015 | 66.62088 | 714.543175 |
| Sao Tome and Principe | STP | 2015 | 66.41666 | 1260.32203 |
| Senegal | SEN | 2015 | 66.66144 | 1052.95882 |
| Seychelles | SYC | 2015 | 73.22927 | 13542.2281 |
| Sierra Leone | SLE | 2015 | 51.41285 | 437.996902 |
| Somalia | SOM | 2015 | 55.87285 | |
| South Africa | ZAF | 2015 | 61.9341 | 7604.35669 |
| Sudan | SDN | 2015 | 64.22941 | 1881.89526 |
| Swaziland | SWZ | 2015 | 56.91237 | 3923.88968 |
| Tanzania | TZA | 2015 | 64.90332 | 835.970946 |
| Togo | TGO | 2015 | 59.92371 | 544.898506 |
| Tunisia | TUN | 2015 | 75.49705 | 4264.51604 |
| Uganda | UGA | 2015 | 59.50876 | 654.136505 |
| Zambia | ZMB | 2015 | 61.33959 | 1618.45767 |
| Zimbabwe | ZWE | 2015 | 60.27934 | 933.503264 |

## EDUCATION, POPULATION DENSITY, MINOR WAR, CIVIL WAR, AND CONFLICT DATA ACROSS ALL THE 54 REGIONS OF AFRICA

| Country Name | Year | Education | Population Density | Minor War | Civil War | Conflict |
|---|---|---|---|---|---|---|
| Algeria | 1960 | 0.871 | 11000.95 | 1 | 1 | 1 |
| Angola | 1960 | 0.975 | 11272.88 | 1 | 0 | 1 |
| Benin | 1960 | 1.027 | 11612.86 | 0 | 0 | 0 |
| Botswana | 1960 | 1.079 | 11963.09 | 0 | 0 | 0 |
| Burkina Faso | 1960 | 1.315 | 12339.14 | 0 | 0 | 0 |
| Burundi | 1960 | 1.433 | 12760.5 | 0 | 0 | 0 |
| Cabo Verde | 1960 | 1.492 | 13146.27 | 0 | 0 | 0 |
| Cameroon | 1960 | 1.5215 | 13528.3 | 0 | 0 | 0 |
| Central African Republic | 1960 | 1.551 | 13931.85 | 0 | 0 | 0 |
| Chad | 1960 | 1.8875 | 14335.39 | 0 | 0 | 0 |
| Comoros | 1960 | 2.05575 | 14760.79 | 0 | 0 | 0 |
| Congo, Dem. Rep. | 1960 | 2.139875 | 15197.72 | 0 | 0 | 0 |
| Congo, Rep. | 1960 | 2.181938 | 15653.2 | 0 | 0 | 0 |

| Country Name | Year | Education | Population Density | Minor War | Civil War | Conflict |
|---|---|---|---|---|---|---|
| Cote d'Ivoire | 1960 | 2.224 | 16140.25 | 0 | 0 | 0 |
| Djibouti | 1960 | 2.64 | 16634.62 | 0 | 0 | 0 |
| Egypt, Arab Rep. | 1960 | 2.848 | 17152.8 | 0 | 0 | 0 |
| Equatorial Guinea | 1960 | 2.952 | 17685.77 | 0 | 0 | 0 |
| Eritrea | 1960 | 3.004 | 18229.93 | 0 | 0 | 0 |
| Ethiopia | 1960 | 3.056 | 18806.06 | 0 | 0 | 0 |
| Gabon | 1960 | 3.6165 | 19407.04 | 0 | 0 | 0 |
| Gambia, The | 1960 | 3.89675 | 20033.75 | 0 | 0 | 0 |
| Ghana | 1960 | 4.036875 | 20680.98 | 0 | 0 | 0 |
| Guinea | 1960 | 4.106938 | 21340.55 | 0 | 0 | 0 |
| Guinea-Bissau | 1960 | 4.177 | 22008.45 | 0 | 0 | 0 |
| Kenya | 1960 | 4.72 | 22642.54 | 0 | 0 | 0 |
| Lesotho | 1960 | 4.9915 | 23254.96 | 0 | 0 | 0 |
| Liberia | 1960 | 5.12725 | 23880.77 | 0 | 0 | 0 |
| Libya | 1960 | 5.195125 | 24496.31 | 0 | 0 | 0 |
| Madagascar | 1960 | 5.263 | 25089.03 | 0 | 0 | 0 |
| Malawi | 1960 | 5.764 | 25687.08 | 1 | 0 | 1 |
| Mali | 1960 | 6.0145 | 26298.45 | 1 | 0 | 1 |
| Mauritania | 1960 | 6.13975 | 26916.44 | 0 | 1 | 1 |
| Mauritius | 1960 | 6.202375 | 27521.48 | 0 | 1 | 1 |
| Morocco | 1960 | 6.265 | 28089.15 | 0 | 1 | 1 |
| Mozambique | 1960 | 6.649 | 28604.04 | 0 | 1 | 1 |
| Namibia | 1960 | 6.841 | 29083.56 | 0 | 1 | 1 |
| Niger | 1960 | 6.937 | 29535.58 | 0 | 1 | 1 |
| Nigeria | 1960 | 6.985 | 29979.82 | 0 | 1 | 1 |
| Rwanda | 1960 | 7.033 | 30429.23 | 0 | 1 | 1 |
| Sao Tome and Principe | 1960 | 7.374 | 30874.31 | 0 | 1 | 1 |
| Senegal | 1960 | 7.5445 | 31312.48 | 1 | 1 | 1 |
| Seychelles | 1960 | 7.62975 | 31740.9 | 1 | 1 | 1 |
| Sierra Leone | 1960 | 7.672375 | 32157.67 | 1 | 1 | 1 |
| Somalia | 1960 | 7.715 | 32560.74 | 1 | 1 | 1 |
| South Africa | 1960 | 8.0055 | 32959.25 | 1 | 1 | 1 |
| Sudan | 1960 | 8.15075 | 33362.74 | 1 | 1 | 1 |
| Swaziland | 1960 | 8.223375 | 33770 | 1 | 1 | 1 |
| Tanzania | 1960 | 8.296 | 34178 | 1 | 1 | 1 |
| Togo | 1960 | | | | | |
| Tunisia | 1960 | | 4826.015 | 0 | 1 | 1 |
| Uganda | 1960 | | 4919.586 | 1 | 1 | 1 |
| Zambia | 1960 | | 5026.044 | 1 | 1 | 1 |
| Zimbabwe | 1960 | | 5134.818 | 1 | 1 | 1 |
| Algeria | 1961 | | 5201.25 | 1 | 1 | 1 |
| Angola | 1961 | | 5247.469 | 1 | 1 | 1 |
| Benin | 1961 | | 5350.384 | 1 | 1 | 1 |
| Botswana | 1961 | | 5471.641 | 1 | 1 | 1 |
| Burkina Faso | 1961 | | 5605.626 | 1 | 1 | 1 |
| Burundi | 1961 | | 5752.957 | 1 | 1 | 1 |
| Cabo Verde | 1961 | | 5895.212 | 1 | 1 | 1 |
| Cameroon | 1961 | | 6026.363 | 1 | 1 | 1 |

| *Country Name* | *Year* | *Education* | *Population Density* | *Minor War* | *Civil War* | *Conflict* |
|---|---|---|---|---|---|---|
| Central African Republic | 1961 | | 5987.492 | 1 | 1 | 1 |
| Chad | 1961 | | 5885.455 | 0 | 1 | 1 |
| Comoros | 1961 | | 5943.466 | 0 | 1 | 1 |
| Congo, Dem. Rep. | 1961 | | 6163.714 | 0 | 1 | 1 |
| Congo, Rep. | 1961 | | 6287.18 | 0 | 1 | 1 |
| Cote d'Ivoire | 1961 | | 6452.546 | 0 | 1 | 1 |
| Djibouti | 1961 | | 6743.08 | 0 | 1 | 1 |
| Egypt, Arab Rep. | 1961 | | 6879.574 | 0 | 1 | 1 |
| Equatorial Guinea | 1961 | | 7018.526 | 0 | 1 | 1 |
| Eritrea | 1961 | | 7240.535 | 0 | 1 | 1 |
| Ethiopia | 1961 | | 7442.448 | 0 | 1 | 1 |
| Gabon | 1961 | | 7584.709 | 0 | 1 | 1 |
| Gambia, The | 1961 | | 7748.632 | 0 | 1 | 1 |
| Ghana | 1961 | | 7878.396 | 0 | 1 | 1 |
| Guinea | 1961 | | 8023.39 | 0 | 1 | 1 |
| Guinea-Bissau | 1961 | | 8153.844 | 0 | 1 | 1 |
| Kenya | 1961 | | 8296.606 | 0 | 1 | 1 |
| Lesotho | 1961 | | 8496.81 | 0 | 1 | 1 |
| Liberia | 1961 | | 8741.838 | 0 | 1 | 1 |
| Libya | 1961 | | 8966.258 | 0 | 1 | 1 |
| Madagascar | 1961 | | 9172.28 | 0 | 1 | 1 |
| Malawi | 1961 | | 9419.124 | 0 | 1 | 1 |
| Mali | 1961 | | 9650.607 | 0 | 1 | 1 |
| Mauritania | 1961 | | 9855.579 | 0 | 1 | 1 |
| Mauritius | 1961 | | 10039.17 | 0 | 1 | 1 |
| Morocco | 1961 | | 10215.44 | 0 | 1 | 1 |
| Mozambique | 1961 | | 10377.27 | 0 | 1 | 1 |
| Namibia | 1961 | | 10538.39 | 0 | 1 | 1 |
| Niger | 1961 | | 10760.51 | 0 | 1 | 1 |
| Nigeria | 1961 | | 11057.09 | 1 | 0 | 0 |
| Rwanda | 1961 | | 11391.13 | 1 | 0 | 0 |
| Sao Tome and Principe | 1961 | | 11706.95 | 1 | 0 | 0 |
| Senegal | 1961 | | 11992.81 | 1 | 0 | 0 |
| Seychelles | 1961 | | 12263.6 | 1 | 0 | 0 |
| Sierra Leone | 1961 | | 12531 | 1 | 0 | 0 |
| Somalia | 1961 | | 12799 | 1 | 0 | 0 |
| South Africa | 1961 | 0.706 | 2151.895 | 0 | 0 | 0 |
| Sudan | 1961 | 0.736 | 2202.775 | 0 | 0 | 0 |
| Swaziland | 1961 | 0.751 | 2255.76 | 0 | 0 | 0 |
| Tanzania | 1961 | 0.766 | 2310.714 | 0 | 0 | 0 |
| Togo | 1961 | 0.805 | 2367.951 | 0 | 0 | 0 |
| Tunisia | 1961 | 0.8245 | 2427.334 | 0 | 0 | 0 |
| Uganda | 1961 | 0.83425 | 2488.957 | 0 | 0 | 0 |
| Zambia | 1961 | 0.839125 | 2553.162 | 0 | 0 | 0 |
| Zimbabwe | 1961 | 0.844 | 2619.809 | 0 | 0 | 0 |
| Algeria | 1962 | 0.8925 | 2689.271 | 0 | 0 | 0 |
| Angola | 1962 | 0.91675 | 2761.407 | 0 | 0 | 0 |
| Benin | 1962 | 0.928875 | 2836.325 | 0 | 0 | 0 |

| Country Name | Year | Education | Population Density | Minor War | Civil War | Conflict |
|---|---|---|---|---|---|---|
| Botswana | 1962 | 0.934938 | 2914.439 | 0 | 0 | 0 |
| Burkina Faso | 1962 | 0.941 | 2995.605 | 0 | 0 | 0 |
| Burundi | 1962 | 1.079 | 3080.268 | 0 | 0 | 0 |
| Cabo Verde | 1962 | 1.148 | 3168.267 | 0 | 0 | 0 |
| Cameroon | 1962 | 1.1825 | 3259.76 | 0 | 0 | 0 |
| Central African Republic | 1962 | 1.19975 | 3354.798 | 0 | 0 | 0 |
| Chad | 1962 | 1.217 | 3458.062 | 0 | 0 | 0 |
| Comoros | 1962 | 1.471 | 3564.85 | 0 | 0 | 0 |
| Congo, Dem. Rep. | 1962 | 1.598 | 3675.13 | 0 | 0 | 0 |
| Congo, Rep. | 1962 | 1.6615 | 3789.035 | 0 | 0 | 0 |
| Cote d'Ivoire | 1962 | 1.69325 | 3907.047 | 0 | 0 | 0 |
| Djibouti | 1962 | 1.725 | 4030.484 | 0 | 0 | 0 |
| Egypt, Arab Rep. | 1962 | 1.928 | 4157.854 | 0 | 0 | 0 |
| Equatorial Guinea | 1962 | 2.0295 | 4287.908 | 0 | 0 | 0 |
| Eritrea | 1962 | 2.08025 | 4422.114 | 0 | 0 | 0 |
| Ethiopia | 1962 | 2.105625 | 4561.161 | 0 | 0 | 0 |
| Gabon | 1962 | 2.131 | 4705.442 | 0 | 0 | 0 |
| Gambia, The | 1962 | 2.3685 | 4855.063 | 0 | 0 | 0 |
| Ghana | 1962 | 2.48725 | 5010.143 | 0 | 0 | 0 |
| Guinea | 1962 | 2.546625 | 5250.36 | 0 | 0 | 0 |
| Guinea-Bissau | 1962 | 2.576313 | 5488.151 | 0 | 0 | 0 |
| Kenya | 1962 | 2.606 | 5646.826 | 0 | 0 | 0 |
| Lesotho | 1962 | 2.8585 | 5820.226 | 0 | 0 | 0 |
| Liberia | 1962 | 2.98475 | 6006.23 | 0 | 0 | 0 |
| Libya | 1962 | 3.047875 | 6202.318 | 0 | 0 | 0 |
| Madagascar | 1962 | 3.079438 | 6406.766 | 0 | 0 | 0 |
| Malawi | 1962 | 3.111 | 6619.12 | 0 | 0 | 0 |
| Mali | 1962 | 3.3615 | 6839.006 | 0 | 0 | 0 |
| Mauritania | 1962 | 3.48675 | 7064.487 | 0 | 0 | 0 |
| Mauritius | 1962 | 3.549375 | 7293.71 | 0 | 0 | 0 |
| Morocco | 1962 | 3.580688 | 7526.831 | 0 | 0 | 0 |
| Mozambique | 1962 | 3.612 | 7777.709 | 0 | 0 | 0 |
| Namibia | 1962 | 3.9145 | 8031.708 | 0 | 0 | 0 |
| Niger | 1962 | 4.06575 | 8278.158 | 0 | 0 | 0 |
| Nigeria | 1962 | 4.141375 | 8533 | 0 | 0 | 0 |
| Rwanda | 1962 | 4.217 | 8792 | 0 | 0 | 0 |
| Sao Tome and Principe | 1962 | 1.316 | 512.764 | 0 | 0 | 0 |
| Senegal | 1962 | 1.425 | 521.237 | 0 | 0 | 0 |
| Seychelles | 1962 | 1.4795 | 529.966 | 0 | 0 | 0 |
| Sierra Leone | 1962 | 1.534 | 538.1 | 0 | 0 | 0 |
| Somalia | 1962 | 1.839 | 545.965 | 0 | 0 | 0 |
| South Africa | 1962 | 1.9915 | 553.541 | 0 | 0 | 0 |
| Sudan | 1962 | 2.06775 | 561.941 | 0 | 0 | 0 |
| Swaziland | 1962 | 2.105875 | 571.874 | 0 | 0 | 0 |
| Tanzania | 1962 | 2.144 | 583.999 | 0 | 0 | 0 |
| Togo | 1962 | 2.3625 | 599.647 | 0 | 0 | 0 |
| Tunisia | 1962 | 2.47175 | 619.351 | 0 | 0 | 0 |
| Uganda | 1962 | 2.526375 | 643.076 | 0 | 0 | 0 |

| Country Name | Year | Education | Population Density | Minor War | Civil War | Conflict |
|---|---|---|---|---|---|---|
| Zambia | 1962 | 2.553688 | 671.769 | 0 | 0 | 0 |
| Zimbabwe | 1962 | 2.581 | 704.591 | 0 | 0 | 0 |
| Algeria | 1963 | 2.85 | 741.273 | 0 | 0 | 0 |
| Angola | 1963 | 2.9845 | 781.472 | 0 | 0 | 0 |
| Benin | 1963 | 3.05175 | 822.247 | 0 | 0 | 0 |
| Botswana | 1963 | 3.085375 | 862.602 | 0 | 0 | 0 |
| Burkina Faso | 1963 | 3.119 | 900.476 | 0 | 0 | 0 |
| Burundi | 1963 | 4.176 | 934.438 | 0 | 0 | 0 |
| Cabo Verde | 1963 | 4.7045 | 970.651 | 0 | 0 | 0 |
| Cameroon | 1963 | 4.96875 | 1007.017 | 0 | 0 | 0 |
| Central African Republic | 1963 | 5.100875 | 1043.396 | 0 | 0 | 0 |
| Chad | 1963 | 5.233 | 1079.692 | 0 | 0 | 0 |
| Comoros | 1963 | 6.0295 | 1115.756 | 0 | 0 | 0 |
| Congo, Dem. Rep. | 1963 | 6.42775 | 1152.012 | 0 | 0 | 0 |
| Congo, Rep. | 1963 | 6.626875 | 1188.941 | 0 | 0 | 0 |
| Cote d'Ivoire | 1963 | 6.726438 | 1226.517 | 0 | 0 | 0 |
| Djibouti | 1963 | 6.826 | 1264.612 | 0 | 0 | 0 |
| Egypt, Arab Rep. | 1963 | 7.513 | 1303.104 | 0 | 0 | 0 |
| Equatorial Guinea | 1963 | 7.8565 | 1344.726 | 0 | 0 | 0 |
| Eritrea | 1963 | 8.02825 | 1389.35 | 0 | 0 | 0 |
| Ethiopia | 1963 | 8.114125 | 1433.688 | 0 | 0 | 0 |
| Gabon | 1963 | 8.2 | 1477.591 | 0 | 0 | 0 |
| Gambia, The | 1963 | 8.498 | 1520.912 | 0 | 0 | 0 |
| Ghana | 1963 | 8.647 | 1563.19 | 0 | 0 | 0 |
| Guinea | 1963 | 8.7215 | 1604.007 | 0 | 0 | 0 |
| Guinea-Bissau | 1963 | 8.75875 | 1642.943 | 0 | 0 | 0 |
| Kenya | 1963 | 8.796 | 1679.68 | 0 | 0 | 0 |
| Lesotho | 1963 | 9.019 | 1714.009 | 0 | 0 | 0 |
| Liberia | 1963 | 9.1305 | 1746.177 | 0 | 0 | 0 |
| Libya | 1963 | 9.18625 | 1777.092 | 0 | 0 | 0 |
| Madagascar | 1963 | 9.214125 | 1807.832 | 0 | 0 | 0 |
| Malawi | 1963 | 9.242 | 1840.116 | 0 | 0 | 0 |
| Mali | 1963 | 9.4025 | 1875.778 | 0 | 0 | 0 |
| Mauritania | 1963 | 9.48275 | 1913.422 | 0 | 0 | 0 |
| Mauritius | 1963 | 9.522875 | 1952 | 0 | 0 | 0 |
| Morocco | 1963 | 9.563 | 1991 | 0 | 0 | 0 |
| Mozambique | 1963 | | 4919.632 | 0 | 0 | 0 |
| Namibia | 1963 | | 4952.695 | 0 | 0 | 0 |
| Niger | 1963 | | 4989.961 | 0 | 0 | 0 |
| Nigeria | 1963 | | 5031.519 | 0 | 0 | 0 |
| Rwanda | 1963 | | 5077.473 | 0 | 0 | 0 |
| Sao Tome and Principe | 1963 | | 5127.935 | 0 | 0 | 0 |
| Senegal | 1963 | | 5183.033 | 0 | 0 | 0 |
| Seychelles | 1963 | | 5242.904 | 0 | 0 | 0 |
| Sierra Leone | 1963 | | 5303.777 | 0 | 0 | 0 |
| Somalia | 1963 | | 5366.018 | 0 | 0 | 0 |
| South Africa | 1963 | | 5433.886 | 0 | 0 | 0 |
| Sudan | 1963 | | 5507.594 | 0 | 0 | 0 |

| Country Name | Year | Education | Population Density | Minor War | Civil War | Conflict |
|---|---|---|---|---|---|---|
| Swaziland | 1963 | | 5587.373 | 0 | 0 | 0 |
| Tanzania | 1963 | | 5673.472 | 0 | 0 | 0 |
| Togo | 1963 | | 5764.606 | 0 | 0 | 0 |
| Tunisia | 1963 | | 5891.063 | 0 | 0 | 0 |
| Uganda | 1963 | | 6025.544 | 0 | 0 | 0 |
| Zambia | 1963 | | 6168.269 | 0 | 0 | 0 |
| Zimbabwe | 1963 | | 6318.189 | 0 | 0 | 0 |
| Algeria | 1964 | | 6474.37 | 0 | 0 | 0 |
| Angola | 1964 | | 6637.227 | 0 | 0 | 0 |
| Benin | 1964 | | 6807.281 | 0 | 0 | 0 |
| Botswana | 1964 | | 6985.039 | 0 | 0 | 0 |
| Burkina Faso | 1964 | | 7170.932 | 1 | 0 | 1 |
| Burundi | 1964 | | 7371.099 | 0 | 0 | 0 |
| Cabo Verde | 1964 | | 7591.809 | 1 | 0 | 1 |
| Cameroon | 1964 | | 7833.491 | 0 | 0 | 0 |
| Central African Republic | 1964 | | 8091.541 | 0 | 0 | 0 |
| Chad | 1964 | | 8361.039 | 0 | 0 | 0 |
| Comoros | 1964 | | 8642.245 | 0 | 0 | 0 |
| Congo, Dem. Rep. | 1964 | | 8934.969 | 0 | 0 | 0 |
| Congo, Rep. | 1964 | | 9237.704 | 0 | 0 | 0 |
| Cote d'Ivoire | 1964 | | 9570.647 | 0 | 0 | 0 |
| Djibouti | 1964 | | 9902.779 | 0 | 0 | 0 |
| Egypt, Arab Rep. | 1964 | | 10220.18 | 0 | 0 | 0 |
| Equatorial Guinea | 1964 | | 10542.57 | 0 | 0 | 0 |
| Eritrea | 1964 | | 10872.71 | 0 | 0 | 0 |
| Ethiopia | 1964 | | 11225.31 | 0 | 0 | 0 |
| Gabon | 1964 | | 11587.75 | 0 | 0 | 0 |
| Gambia, The | 1964 | | 12039.36 | 0 | 0 | 0 |
| Ghana | 1964 | | 12584.96 | 0 | 0 | 0 |
| Guinea | 1964 | | 13065.39 | 0 | 0 | 0 |
| Guinea-Bissau | 1964 | | 13478.09 | 0 | 0 | 0 |
| Kenya | 1964 | | 13903.89 | 0 | 0 | 0 |
| Lesotho | 1964 | | 14343.53 | 0 | 0 | 0 |
| Liberia | 1964 | | 14797.17 | 0 | 0 | 0 |
| Libya | 1964 | | 15265 | 0 | 0 | 0 |
| Madagascar | 1964 | | 15746 | 0 | 0 | 0 |
| Malawi | 1964 | 0.644 | 2961.915 | 0 | 0 | 0 |
| Mali | 1964 | 0.7165 | 3008.458 | 0 | 0 | 0 |
| Mauritania | 1964 | 0.75275 | 3088.827 | 0 | 0 | 0 |
| Mauritius | 1964 | 0.789 | 3170.653 | 1 | 0 | 1 |
| Morocco | 1964 | 0.9075 | 3253.61 | 0 | 0 | 0 |
| Mozambique | 1964 | 0.96675 | 3330.989 | 0 | 0 | 0 |
| Namibia | 1964 | 0.996375 | 3400.775 | 0 | 0 | 0 |
| Niger | 1964 | 1.011188 | 3460.144 | 0 | 0 | 0 |
| Nigeria | 1964 | 1.026 | 3521.913 | 0 | 0 | 0 |
| Rwanda | 1964 | 1.136 | 3596.811 | 0 | 0 | 0 |
| Sao Tome and Principe | 1964 | 1.191 | 3529.983 | 0 | 0 | 0 |
| Senegal | 1964 | 1.2185 | 3540.066 | 0 | 0 | 0 |

| Country Name | Year | Education | Population Density | Minor War | Civil War | Conflict |
|---|---|---|---|---|---|---|
| Seychelles | 1964 | 1.23225 | 3594.958 | 0 | 0 | 0 |
| Sierra Leone | 1964 | 1.246 | 3676.308 | 0 | 0 | 0 |
| Somalia | 1964 | 1.329 | 3749.077 | 0 | 0 | 0 |
| South Africa | 1964 | 1.3705 | 3834.415 | 0 | 0 | 0 |
| Sudan | 1964 | 1.39125 | 3929.974 | 0 | 0 | 0 |
| Swaziland | 1964 | 1.401625 | 4119.789 | 0 | 0 | 0 |
| Tanzania | 1964 | 1.412 | 4299.555 | 0 | 0 | 0 |
| Togo | 1964 | 1.457 | 4480.338 | 0 | 0 | 0 |
| Tunisia | 1964 | 1.4795 | 4580.41 | 0 | 0 | 0 |
| Uganda | 1964 | 1.49075 | 4692.262 | 0 | 0 | 0 |
| Zambia | 1964 | 1.496375 | 4802.889 | 0 | 0 | 0 |
| Zimbabwe | 1964 | 1.502 | 4906.862 | 0 | 0 | 0 |
| Algeria | 1965 | 1.616 | 5002.688 | 0 | 0 | 0 |
| Angola | 1965 | 1.673 | 5126.023 | 0 | 0 | 0 |
| Benin | 1965 | 1.7015 | 5257.314 | 0 | 0 | 0 |
| Botswana | 1965 | 1.71575 | 5379.124 | 0 | 0 | 0 |
| Burkina Faso | 1965 | 1.73 | 5505.113 | 0 | 0 | 0 |
| Burundi | 1965 | 1.9425 | 5674 | 1 | 0 | 1 |
| Cabo Verde | 1965 | 2.04875 | 5856 | 1 | 0 | 1 |
| Cameroon | 1965 | 2.101875 | 5685 | 1 | 0 | 1 |
| Central African Republic | 1965 | 2.128438 | 5750 | 1 | 0 | 1 |
| Chad | 1965 | 2.155 | 6165 | 1 | 0 | 1 |
| Comoros | 1965 | 2.3445 | 6204 | 1 | 0 | 1 |
| Congo, Dem. Rep. | 1965 | 2.43925 | 6244 | 1 | 1 | 1 |
| Congo, Rep. | 1965 | 2.486625 | 6417 | 1 | 1 | 2 |
| Cote d'Ivoire | 1965 | 2.510313 | 6631 | 1 | 1 | 1 |
| Djibouti | 1965 | 2.534 | 6823 | 0 | 1 | 1 |
| Egypt, Arab Rep. | 1965 | 2.6975 | 7043 | 0 | 1 | 1 |
| Equatorial Guinea | 1965 | 2.77925 | 7287 | 0 | 1 | 1 |
| Eritrea | 1965 | 2.820125 | 7553 | 1 | 1 | 1 |
| Ethiopia | 1965 | 2.840563 | 7859 | 1 | 1 | 1 |
| Gabon | 1965 | 2.861 | 8162 | 1 | 1 | 1 |
| Gambia, The | 1965 | 3.067 | 8465 | 1 | 1 | 1 |
| Ghana | 1965 | 3.17 | 8783 | 1 | 1 | 1 |
| Guinea | 1965 | 3.2215 | 9139 | 1 | 1 | 1 |
| Guinea-Bissau | 1965 | 3.273 | 9511 | 1 | 1 | 1 |
| Kenya | 1965 | 0.527 | 1523.478 | 0 | 0 | 0 |
| Lesotho | 1965 | 0.576 | 1553.368 | 0 | 0 | 0 |
| Liberia | 1965 | 0.6005 | 1584.615 | 0 | 0 | 0 |
| Libya | 1965 | 0.625 | 1627.54 | 0 | 0 | 0 |
| Madagascar | 1965 | 0.7325 | 1685.107 | 0 | 0 | 0 |
| Malawi | 1965 | 0.78625 | 1733.638 | 0 | 0 | 0 |
| Mali | 1965 | 0.813125 | 1763.062 | 0 | 0 | 0 |
| Mauritania | 1965 | 0.826563 | 1794.675 | 0 | 0 | 0 |
| Mauritius | 1965 | 0.84 | 1839.245 | 0 | 0 | 0 |
| Morocco | 1965 | 0.994 | 1883.905 | 0 | 0 | 0 |
| Mozambique | 1965 | 1.071 | 1927.26 | 0 | 0 | 0 |
| Namibia | 1965 | 1.1095 | 1965.058 | 0 | 0 | 0 |

| Country Name | Year | Education | Population Density | Minor War | Civil War | Conflict |
|---|---|---|---|---|---|---|
| Niger | 1965 | 1.12875 | 2006.137 | 0 | 0 | 0 |
| Nigeria | 1965 | 1.148 | 2057.734 | 0 | 0 | 0 |
| Rwanda | 1965 | 1.3965 | 2111.993 | 0 | 0 | 0 |
| Sao Tome and Principe | 1965 | 1.52075 | 2167.513 | 0 | 0 | 0 |
| Senegal | 1965 | 1.582875 | 2224.645 | 0 | 0 | 0 |
| Seychelles | 1965 | 1.613938 | 2285.053 | 0 | 0 | 0 |
| Sierra Leone | 1965 | 1.645 | 2348.575 | 0 | 0 | 0 |
| Somalia | 1965 | 1.851 | 2412.522 | 0 | 0 | 0 |
| South Africa | 1965 | 1.954 | 2477.275 | 0 | 0 | 0 |
| Sudan | 1965 | 2.0055 | 2542.882 | 0 | 0 | 0 |
| Swaziland | 1965 | 2.03125 | 2628.466 | 0 | 0 | 0 |
| Tanzania | 1965 | 2.057 | 2713.438 | 0 | 0 | 0 |
| Togo | 1965 | 2.3595 | 2775.133 | 0 | 0 | 0 |
| Tunisia | 1965 | 2.51075 | 2841.087 | 0 | 0 | 0 |
| Uganda | 1965 | 2.586375 | 2917.596 | 0 | 0 | 0 |
| Zambia | 1965 | 2.624188 | 3000.18 | 0 | 0 | 0 |
| Zimbabwe | 1965 | 2.662 | 3085.222 | 0 | 0 | 0 |
| Algeria | 1966 | 2.817 | 3174.955 | 0 | 0 | 0 |
| Angola | 1966 | 2.8945 | 3267.335 | 0 | 0 | 0 |
| Benin | 1966 | 2.93325 | 3367.951 | 0 | 0 | 0 |
| Botswana | 1966 | 2.952625 | 3466.753 | 0 | 0 | 0 |
| Burkina Faso | 1966 | 2.972 | 3544.495 | 0 | 0 | 0 |
| Burundi | 1966 | 3.118 | 3619.335 | 1 | 0 | 1 |
| Cabo Verde | 1966 | 3.191 | 3700.422 | 1 | 0 | 1 |
| Cameroon | 1966 | 3.2275 | 3783.066 | 0 | 0 | 0 |
| Central African Republic | 1966 | 3.24575 | 3863.414 | 0 | 0 | 0 |
| Chad | 1966 | 3.264 | 3980 | 0 | 0 | 0 |
| Comoros | 1966 | 3.378 | 4054 | 1 | 0 | 1 |
| Congo, Dem. Rep. | 1966 | 3.435 | 4128 | 1 | 0 | 1 |
| Congo, Rep. | 1966 | 3.4635 | 4215 | 0 | 0 | 0 |
| Cote d'Ivoire | 1966 | 3.47775 | 4289 | 0 | 0 | 0 |
| Djibouti | 1966 | 3.492 | 4363 | 0 | 0 | 0 |
| Egypt, Arab Rep. | 1966 | 3.5555 | 4449 | 1 | 0 | 1 |
| Equatorial Guinea | 1966 | 3.58725 | 4544 | 0 | 0 | 0 |
| Eritrea | 1966 | 3.603125 | 4641 | 0 | 0 | 0 |
| Ethiopia | 1966 | 3.619 | 4742 | 0 | 0 | 0 |
| Gabon | 1966 | 1.084 | 5793.633 | 0 | 0 | 0 |
| Gambia, The | 1966 | 1.258 | 5892.378 | 0 | 0 | 0 |
| Ghana | 1966 | 1.345 | 5995.682 | 0 | 0 | 0 |
| Guinea | 1966 | 1.432 | 6103.788 | 0 | 0 | 0 |
| Guinea-Bissau | 1966 | 1.622 | 6216.951 | 0 | 0 | 0 |
| Kenya | 1966 | 1.717 | 6335.506 | 0 | 0 | 0 |
| Lesotho | 1966 | 1.7645 | 6459.744 | 0 | 0 | 0 |
| Liberia | 1966 | 1.78825 | 6590.041 | 0 | 0 | 0 |
| Libya | 1966 | 1.812 | 6726.733 | 0 | 0 | 0 |
| Madagascar | 1966 | 2.111 | 6870.244 | 0 | 0 | 0 |
| Malawi | 1966 | 2.2605 | 7021.028 | 0 | 0 | 0 |
| Mali | 1966 | 2.33525 | 7179.499 | 0 | 0 | 0 |

| Country Name | Year | Education | Population Density | Minor War | Civil War | Conflict |
|---|---|---|---|---|---|---|
| Mauritania | 1966 | 2.372625 | 7346.174 | 0 | 0 | 0 |
| Mauritius | 1966 | 2.41 | 7521.53 | 0 | 0 | 0 |
| Morocco | 1966 | 2.7185 | 7721.125 | 0 | 0 | 0 |
| Mozambique | 1966 | 2.87275 | 7962.216 | 0 | 0 | 0 |
| Namibia | 1966 | 2.949875 | 8212.692 | 0 | 0 | 0 |
| Niger | 1966 | 2.988438 | 8461.756 | 0 | 0 | 0 |
| Nigeria | 1966 | 3.027 | 8762.486 | 0 | 0 | 0 |
| Rwanda | 1966 | 3.3475 | 9047.915 | 0 | 0 | 0 |
| Sao Tome and Principe | 1966 | 3.50775 | 9282.553 | 0 | 0 | 0 |
| Senegal | 1966 | 3.587875 | 9562.721 | 0 | 0 | 0 |
| Seychelles | 1966 | 3.627938 | 9867.132 | 1 | 1 | 1 |
| Sierra Leone | 1966 | 3.668 | 10191.37 | 0 | 0 | 0 |
| Somalia | 1966 | 4.0025 | 10530.15 | 0 | 0 | 0 |
| South Africa | 1966 | 4.16975 | 10867.1 | 0 | 0 | 0 |
| Sudan | 1966 | 4.253375 | 11200.98 | 0 | 0 | 0 |
| Swaziland | 1966 | 4.295188 | 11540.12 | 0 | 0 | 0 |
| Tanzania | 1966 | 4.337 | 11884.5 | 0 | 0 | 0 |
| Togo | 1966 | 4.6505 | 12230.3 | 0 | 0 | 0 |
| Tunisia | 1966 | 4.80725 | 12574.75 | 0 | 0 | 0 |
| Uganda | 1966 | 4.885625 | 12920.47 | 0 | 0 | 0 |
| Zambia | 1966 | 4.924813 | 13264.17 | 0 | 0 | 0 |
| Zimbabwe | 1966 | 4.964 | 13603.16 | 0 | 0 | 0 |
| Algeria | 1967 | 5.1955 | 13944.74 | 1 | 0 | 1 |
| Angola | 1967 | 5.31125 | 14290.13 | 0 | 0 | 0 |
| Benin | 1967 | 5.369125 | 14637.98 | 0 | 0 | 0 |
| Botswana | 1967 | 5.398063 | 14988.5 | 0 | 0 | 0 |
| Burkina Faso | 1967 | 5.427 | 15343.04 | 0 | 0 | 0 |
| Burundi | 1967 | 5.5885 | 15706.86 | 0 | 0 | 0 |
| Cabo Verde | 1967 | 5.66925 | 16094.44 | 0 | 0 | 0 |
| Cameroon | 1967 | 5.709625 | 16489.01 | 0 | 0 | 0 |
| Central African Republic | 1967 | 5.729813 | 16872.75 | 0 | 0 | 0 |
| Chad | 1967 | 5.75 | 17261.47 | 0 | 0 | 0 |
| Comoros | 1967 | 5.909 | 17657.86 | 0 | 0 | 0 |
| Congo, Dem. Rep. | 1967 | 5.9885 | 18060.38 | 0 | 0 | 0 |
| Congo, Rep. | 1967 | 6.02825 | 18468 | 0 | 0 | 0 |
| Cote d'Ivoire | 1967 | 6.068 | 18879 | 0 | 0 | 0 |
| Djibouti | 1967 | | 209.878 | 0 | 0 | 0 |
| Egypt, Arab Rep. | 1967 | | 216.919 | 0 | 0 | 0 |
| Equatorial Guinea | 1967 | | 224.264 | 0 | 0 | 0 |
| Eritrea | 1967 | | 231.719 | 0 | 0 | 0 |
| Ethiopia | 1967 | | 239.23 | 0 | 0 | 0 |
| Gabon | 1967 | | 246.787 | 0 | 0 | 0 |
| Gambia, The | 1967 | | 254.303 | 0 | 0 | 0 |
| Ghana | 1967 | | 261.602 | 0 | 0 | 0 |
| Guinea | 1967 | | 268.867 | 0 | 0 | 0 |
| Guinea-Bissau | 1967 | | 273.381 | 0 | 0 | 0 |
| Kenya | 1967 | | 275.392 | 0 | 0 | 0 |
| Lesotho | 1967 | | 277.218 | 0 | 0 | 0 |

| Country Name | Year | Education | Population Density | Minor War | Civil War | Conflict |
|---|---|---|---|---|---|---|
| Liberia | 1967 | | 278.617 | 0 | 0 | 0 |
| Libya | 1967 | | 280.259 | 0 | 0 | 0 |
| Madagascar | 1967 | | 282.516 | 0 | 0 | 0 |
| Malawi | 1967 | | 285.691 | 0 | 0 | 0 |
| Mali | 1967 | | 288.855 | 0 | 0 | 0 |
| Mauritania | 1967 | | 292.276 | 0 | 0 | 0 |
| Mauritius | 1967 | | 296.042 | 0 | 0 | 0 |
| Morocco | 1967 | | 299.978 | 0 | 0 | 0 |
| Mozambique | 1967 | | 304.196 | 0 | 0 | 0 |
| Namibia | 1967 | | 308.737 | 0 | 0 | 0 |
| Niger | 1967 | | 313.61 | 0 | 0 | 0 |
| Nigeria | 1967 | | 318.802 | 0 | 0 | 0 |
| Rwanda | 1967 | | 324.292 | 0 | 0 | 0 |
| Sao Tome and Principe | 1967 | | 330.057 | 0 | 0 | 0 |
| Senegal | 1967 | | 336.065 | 0 | 0 | 0 |
| Seychelles | 1967 | | 342.27 | 0 | 0 | 0 |
| Sierra Leone | 1967 | | 348.617 | 0 | 0 | 0 |
| Somalia | 1967 | | 347 | 0 | 0 | 0 |
| South Africa | 1967 | | 356 | 0 | 0 | 0 |
| Sudan | 1967 | | 366 | 0 | 0 | 0 |
| Swaziland | 1967 | | 376 | 0 | 0 | 0 |
| Tanzania | 1967 | | 385 | 0 | 0 | 0 |
| Togo | 1967 | | 395 | 0 | 0 | 0 |
| Tunisia | 1967 | | 404 | 0 | 0 | 0 |
| Uganda | 1967 | | 413 | 0 | 0 | 0 |
| Zambia | 1967 | | 422 | 0 | 0 | 0 |
| Zimbabwe | 1967 | | 430 | 0 | 0 | 0 |
| Algeria | 1968 | | 438 | 0 | 0 | 0 |
| Angola | 1968 | | 447 | 0 | 0 | 0 |
| Benin | 1968 | | 455 | 0 | 0 | 0 |
| Botswana | 1968 | | 463 | 0 | 0 | 0 |
| Burkina Faso | 1968 | | 471 | 0 | 0 | 0 |
| Burundi | 1968 | | 478 | 0 | 0 | 0 |
| Cabo Verde | 1968 | | 486 | 0 | 0 | 0 |
| Cameroon | 1968 | | 494 | 0 | 0 | 0 |
| Central African Republic | 1968 | | 501 | 0 | 0 | 0 |
| Chad | 1968 | | 3150.417 | 0 | 0 | 0 |
| Comoros | 1968 | | 3207.638 | 0 | 0 | 0 |
| Congo, Dem. Rep. | 1968 | | 3271.357 | 0 | 0 | 0 |
| Congo, Rep. | 1968 | | 3344.52 | 0 | 0 | 0 |
| Cote d'Ivoire | 1968 | | 3419.366 | 1 | 0 | 1 |
| Djibouti | 1968 | | 3495.635 | 1 | 0 | 1 |
| Egypt, Arab Rep. | 1968 | | 3572.229 | 1 | 0 | 1 |
| Equatorial Guinea | 1968 | | 3649.335 | 1 | 1 | 1 |
| Eritrea | 1968 | | 3727.238 | 1 | 1 | 1 |
| Ethiopia | 1968 | | 3806.002 | 1 | 1 | 1 |
| Gabon | 1968 | | 3886.643 | 1 | 1 | 1 |
| Gambia, The | 1968 | | 3969.803 | 0 | 1 | 0 |

| Country Name | Year | Education | Population Density | Minor War | Civil War | Conflict |
|---|---|---|---|---|---|---|
| Ghana | 1968 | | 4055.702 | 0 | 1 | 0 |
| Guinea | 1968 | | 4144.061 | 0 | 1 | 0 |
| Guinea-Bissau | 1968 | | 4234.743 | 1 | 1 | 1 |
| Kenya | 1968 | | 4327.777 | 1 | 1 | 1 |
| Lesotho | 1968 | | 4424.045 | 0 | 1 | 1 |
| Liberia | 1968 | | 4524.409 | 0 | 1 | 1 |
| Libya | 1968 | | 4522.391 | 0 | 1 | 0 |
| Madagascar | 1968 | | 4514.94 | 1 | 1 | 1 |
| Malawi | 1968 | | 4732.876 | 1 | 1 | 1 |
| Mali | 1968 | | 4971.162 | 1 | 1 | 1 |
| Mauritania | 1968 | | 5025.174 | 1 | 1 | 1 |
| Mauritius | 1968 | | 5066.042 | 1 | 1 | 1 |
| Morocco | 1968 | | 5214.2 | 1 | 1 | 1 |
| Mozambique | 1968 | | 5391.517 | 0 | 1 | 1 |
| Namibia | 1968 | | 5556.341 | 0 | 1 | 0 |
| Niger | 1968 | | 5714.913 | 1 | 1 | 1 |
| Nigeria | 1968 | | 5841.411 | 0 | 1 | 1 |
| Rwanda | 1968 | | 6028.221 | 1 | 1 | 1 |
| Sao Tome and Principe | 1968 | | 6263.272 | 1 | 1 | 1 |
| Senegal | 1968 | | 6379.099 | 1 | 1 | 1 |
| Seychelles | 1968 | | 6496.685 | 1 | 1 | 1 |
| Sierra Leone | 1968 | | 6769.686 | 1 | 1 | 1 |
| Somalia | 1968 | | 7051 | 1 | 1 | 2 |
| South Africa | 1968 | | 7261.713 | 1 | 1 | 1 |
| Sudan | 1968 | | 7479.317 | 1 | 1 | 1 |
| Swaziland | 1968 | | 7708.743 | 1 | 1 | 1 |
| Tanzania | 1968 | | 7942.675 | 1 | 1 | 1 |
| Togo | 1968 | | 8179.408 | 1 | 1 | 1 |
| Tunisia | 1968 | | 8436.193 | 1 | 1 | 1 |
| Uganda | 1968 | | 8745.74 | 0 | 1 | 0 |
| Zambia | 1968 | | 9097.655 | 0 | 1 | 0 |
| Zimbabwe | 1968 | | 9400.658 | 1 | 1 | 1 |
| Algeria | 1969 | | 9648.955 | 0 | 1 | 1 |
| Angola | 1969 | | 9885.661 | 1 | 1 | 1 |
| Benin | 1969 | | 10111 | 1 | 1 | 1 |
| Botswana | 1969 | | 10329 | 0 | 1 | 0 |
| Burkina Faso | 1969 | | 191.689 | 0 | 0 | 0 |
| Burundi | 1969 | | 196.348 | 0 | 0 | 0 |
| Cabo Verde | 1969 | | 201.208 | 0 | 0 | 0 |
| Cameroon | 1969 | | 206.279 | 0 | 0 | 0 |
| Central African Republic | 1969 | | 211.571 | 0 | 0 | 0 |
| Chad | 1969 | | 217.378 | 0 | 0 | 0 |
| Comoros | 1969 | | 223.443 | 0 | 0 | 0 |
| Congo, Dem. Rep. | 1969 | | 229.732 | 0 | 0 | 0 |
| Congo, Rep. | 1969 | | 236.252 | 0 | 0 | 0 |
| Cote d'Ivoire | 1969 | | 243.014 | 0 | 0 | 0 |
| Djibouti | 1969 | | 250.027 | 0 | 0 | 0 |
| Egypt, Arab Rep. | 1969 | | 257.303 | 0 | 0 | 0 |

| Country Name | Year | Education | Population Density | Minor War | Civil War | Conflict |
|---|---|---|---|---|---|---|
| Equatorial Guinea | 1969 | | 264.851 | 0 | 0 | 0 |
| Eritrea | 1969 | | 272.685 | 0 | 0 | 0 |
| Ethiopia | 1969 | | 280.815 | 0 | 0 | 0 |
| Gabon | 1969 | | 304.739 | 0 | 0 | 0 |
| Gambia, The | 1969 | | 313.97 | 0 | 0 | 0 |
| Ghana | 1969 | | 323.557 | 0 | 0 | 0 |
| Guinea | 1969 | | 333.514 | 0 | 0 | 0 |
| Guinea-Bissau | 1969 | | 340.879 | 0 | 0 | 0 |
| Kenya | 1969 | | 348.82 | 0 | 0 | 0 |
| Lesotho | 1969 | | 357.203 | 0 | 0 | 0 |
| Liberia | 1969 | | 366.026 | 0 | 0 | 0 |
| Libya | 1969 | | 375.3 | 0 | 0 | 0 |
| Madagascar | 1969 | | 385.045 | 0 | 0 | 0 |
| Malawi | 1969 | | 395.282 | 0 | 0 | 0 |
| Mali | 1969 | | 406.029 | 0 | 0 | 0 |
| Mauritania | 1969 | | 417.307 | 1 | 0 | 1 |
| Mauritius | 1969 | | 429.136 | 0 | 0 | 0 |
| Morocco | 1969 | | 441.535 | 0 | 0 | 0 |
| Mozambique | 1969 | | 454.525 | 0 | 0 | 0 |
| Namibia | 1969 | | 468.101 | 0 | 0 | 0 |
| Niger | 1969 | | 482.255 | 0 | 0 | 0 |
| Nigeria | 1969 | | 497.008 | 0 | 0 | 0 |
| Rwanda | 1969 | | 512.315 | 0 | 0 | 0 |
| Sao Tome and Principe | 1969 | | 528.122 | 1 | 0 | 1 |
| Senegal | 1969 | | 544.435 | 0 | 0 | 0 |
| Seychelles | 1969 | | 561.261 | 0 | 0 | 0 |
| Sierra Leone | 1969 | | 578.626 | 0 | 0 | 0 |
| Somalia | 1969 | | 596.457 | 0 | 0 | 0 |
| South Africa | 1969 | | 614.67 | 0 | 0 | 0 |
| Sudan | 1969 | | 633.272 | 0 | 0 | 0 |
| Swaziland | 1969 | | 652.26 | 0 | 0 | 0 |
| Tanzania | 1969 | | 671.638 | 0 | 0 | 0 |
| Togo | 1969 | | 691.37 | 0 | 0 | 0 |
| Tunisia | 1969 | | 711.417 | 0 | 0 | 0 |
| Uganda | 1969 | | 732 | 0 | 0 | 0 |
| Zambia | 1969 | | 752 | 0 | 0 | 0 |
| Zimbabwe | 1969 | 1.19 | 1047.924 | 0 | 0 | 0 |
| Algeria | 1970 | 1.4165 | 1072.198 | 0 | 0 | 0 |
| Angola | 1970 | 1.52975 | 1097.474 | 0 | 0 | 0 |
| Benin | 1970 | 1.643 | 1123.795 | 0 | 0 | 0 |
| Botswana | 1970 | 1.887 | 1151.207 | 0 | 0 | 0 |
| Burkina Faso | 1970 | 2.009 | 1179.76 | 0 | 0 | 0 |
| Burundi | 1970 | 2.07 | 1209.505 | 0 | 0 | 0 |
| Cabo Verde | 1970 | 2.1005 | 1240.372 | 0 | 0 | 0 |
| Cameroon | 1970 | 2.131 | 1272.408 | 0 | 0 | 0 |
| Central African Republic | 1970 | 2.6845 | 1305.794 | 0 | 0 | 0 |
| Chad | 1970 | 2.96125 | 1340.458 | 0 | 0 | 0 |
| Comoros | 1970 | 3.099625 | 1376.455 | 0 | 0 | 0 |

| *Country Name* | *Year* | *Education* | *Population Density* | *Minor War* | *Civil War* | *Conflict* |
|---|---|---|---|---|---|---|
| Congo, Dem. Rep. | 1970 | 3.168813 | 1414.408 | 0 | 0 | 0 |
| Congo, Rep. | 1970 | 3.238 | 1453.65 | 0 | 0 | 0 |
| Cote d'Ivoire | 1970 | 3.6955 | 1494.47 | 0 | 0 | 0 |
| Djibouti | 1970 | 3.92425 | 1536.889 | 0 | 0 | 0 |
| Egypt, Arab Rep. | 1970 | 4.038625 | 1580.962 | 0 | 0 | 0 |
| Equatorial Guinea | 1970 | 4.095813 | 1626.73 | 0 | 0 | 0 |
| Eritrea | 1970 | 4.153 | 1674.288 | 0 | 0 | 0 |
| Ethiopia | 1970 | 4.559 | 1723.743 | 0 | 0 | 0 |
| Gabon | 1970 | 4.762 | 1775.157 | 0 | 0 | 0 |
| Gambia, The | 1970 | 4.8635 | 1828.563 | 0 | 0 | 0 |
| Ghana | 1970 | 4.91425 | 1883.981 | 0 | 0 | 0 |
| Guinea | 1970 | 4.965 | 1941.765 | 0 | 0 | 0 |
| Guinea-Bissau | 1970 | 5.1955 | 2002.137 | 0 | 0 | 0 |
| Kenya | 1970 | 5.31075 | 2064.973 | 0 | 0 | 0 |
| Lesotho | 1970 | 5.368375 | 2130.061 | 0 | 0 | 0 |
| Liberia | 1970 | 5.397188 | 2197.165 | 0 | 0 | 0 |
| Libya | 1970 | 5.426 | 2266.001 | 0 | 0 | 0 |
| Madagascar | 1970 | 5.5865 | 2337.401 | 0 | 0 | 0 |
| Malawi | 1970 | 5.66675 | 2410.397 | 0 | 0 | 0 |
| Mali | 1970 | 5.706875 | 2488.937 | 1 | 0 | 1 |
| Mauritania | 1970 | 5.726938 | 2570.292 | 1 | 0 | 1 |
| Mauritius | 1970 | 5.747 | 2649.999 | 0 | 0 | 0 |
| Morocco | 1970 | 5.802 | 2731.246 | 0 | 0 | 0 |
| Mozambique | 1970 | 5.8295 | 2802.469 | 0 | 1 | 1 |
| Namibia | 1970 | 5.84325 | 2879.995 | 0 | 1 | 1 |
| Niger | 1970 | 5.850125 | 2972.317 | 0 | 1 | 0 |
| Nigeria | 1970 | 5.857 | 3103.941 | 0 | 1 | 0 |
| Rwanda | 1970 | 5.891 | 3239.986 | 0 | 1 | 0 |
| Sao Tome and Principe | 1970 | 5.908 | 3330.421 | 1 | 1 | 1 |
| Senegal | 1970 | 5.9165 | 3414.253 | 1 | 1 | 1 |
| Seychelles | 1970 | 5.92075 | 3503.742 | 1 | 1 | 1 |
| Sierra Leone | 1970 | 5.925 | 3604.002 | 0 | 0 | 0 |
| Somalia | 1970 | 5.983 | 3704.056 | 0 | 0 | 0 |
| South Africa | 1970 | 6.012 | 3802.332 | 0 | 0 | 0 |
| Sudan | 1970 | 6.0265 | 3905 | 0 | 0 | 0 |
| Swaziland | 1970 | 6.041 | 4013 | 0 | 0 | 0 |
| Tanzania | 1970 | 0.921 | 3842.85 | 0 | 0 | 0 |
| Togo | 1970 | 0.976 | 4001.575 | 0 | 0 | 0 |
| Tunisia | 1970 | 1.0035 | 4171.038 | 0 | 0 | 0 |
| Uganda | 1970 | 1.031 | 4356.37 | 0 | 0 | 0 |
| Zambia | 1970 | 1.1455 | 4563.607 | 0 | 0 | 0 |
| Zimbabwe | 1970 | 1.20275 | 4790.271 | 0 | 0 | 0 |
| Algeria | 1971 | 1.231375 | 5038.277 | 0 | 0 | 0 |
| Angola | 1971 | 1.245688 | 5299.106 | 0 | 0 | 0 |
| Benin | 1971 | 1.26 | 5579.014 | 0 | 0 | 0 |
| Botswana | 1971 | 1.466 | 5873.709 | 0 | 0 | 0 |
| Burkina Faso | 1971 | 1.569 | 6171.63 | 0 | 0 | 0 |
| Burundi | 1971 | 1.6205 | 6465.22 | 0 | 0 | 0 |

| Country Name | Year | Education | Population Density | Minor War | Civil War | Conflict |
|---|---|---|---|---|---|---|
| Cabo Verde | 1971 | 1.64625 | 6749.048 | 0 | 0 | 0 |
| Cameroon | 1971 | 1.672 | 7030.905 | 0 | 0 | 0 |
| Central African Republic | 1971 | 1.87 | 7334.543 | 0 | 0 | 0 |
| Chad | 1971 | 1.969 | 7642.397 | 0 | 0 | 0 |
| Comoros | 1971 | 2.0185 | 7954.372 | 0 | 0 | 0 |
| Congo, Dem. Rep. | 1971 | 2.04325 | 8270.975 | 0 | 0 | 0 |
| Congo, Rep. | 1971 | 2.068 | 8593.262 | 0 | 0 | 0 |
| Cote d'Ivoire | 1971 | 2.2185 | 8922.474 | 0 | 0 | 0 |
| Djibouti | 1971 | 2.29375 | 9259.826 | 0 | 0 | 0 |
| Egypt, Arab Rep. | 1971 | 2.331375 | 9606.456 | 0 | 0 | 0 |
| Equatorial Guinea | 1971 | 2.350188 | 9963.431 | 0 | 0 | 0 |
| Eritrea | 1971 | 2.369 | 10331.68 | 0 | 0 | 0 |
| Ethiopia | 1971 | 2.529 | 10712.06 | 0 | 0 | 0 |
| Gabon | 1971 | 2.609 | 11105.27 | 0 | 0 | 0 |
| Gambia, The | 1971 | 2.649 | 11511.74 | 0 | 0 | 0 |
| Ghana | 1971 | 2.669 | 11930.65 | 0 | 0 | 0 |
| Guinea | 1971 | 2.689 | 12490.88 | 0 | 0 | 0 |
| Guinea-Bissau | 1971 | 2.9935 | 13039.52 | 0 | 0 | 0 |
| Kenya | 1971 | 3.14575 | 13422.14 | 0 | 0 | 0 |
| Lesotho | 1971 | 3.221875 | 13860.57 | 0 | 0 | 0 |
| Liberia | 1971 | 3.259938 | 14379.92 | 0 | 0 | 0 |
| Libya | 1971 | 3.298 | 14845.8 | 0 | 0 | 0 |
| Madagascar | 1971 | 3.58 | 15281.45 | 0 | 0 | 0 |
| Malawi | 1971 | 3.721 | 15686.23 | 0 | 0 | 0 |
| Mali | 1971 | 3.7915 | 16045.36 | 0 | 0 | 0 |
| Mauritania | 1971 | 3.82675 | 16456.88 | 0 | 0 | 0 |
| Mauritius | 1971 | 3.862 | 16884.58 | 0 | 0 | 0 |
| Morocco | 1971 | 4.0355 | 17310.97 | 0 | 0 | 0 |
| Mozambique | 1971 | 4.12225 | 17687.65 | 1 | 0 | 1 |
| Namibia | 1971 | 4.165625 | 18068 | 1 | 0 | 1 |
| Niger | 1971 | 4.187313 | 18504.38 | 1 | 0 | 1 |
| Nigeria | 1971 | 4.209 | 18920.5 | 0 | 0 | 0 |
| Rwanda | 1971 | 4.355 | 19326.8 | 0 | 0 | 0 |
| Sao Tome and Principe | 1971 | 4.428 | 19746.95 | 0 | 0 | 0 |
| Senegal | 1971 | 4.4645 | 20180 | 0 | 0 | 0 |
| Seychelles | 1971 | 4.501 | 20617 | 0 | 0 | 0 |
| Sierra Leone | 1971 | 0.804 | 17486.43 | 1 | 0 | 1 |
| Somalia | 1971 | 0.8805 | 18027.17 | 0 | 0 | 0 |
| South Africa | 1971 | 0.91875 | 18432.65 | 0 | 1 | 1 |
| Sudan | 1971 | 0.957 | 18855.51 | 0 | 1 | 1 |
| Swaziland | 1971 | 1.0585 | 19343.38 | 0 | 0 | 0 |
| Tanzania | 1971 | 1.10925 | 19941.07 | 1 | 1 | 1 |
| Togo | 1971 | 1.134625 | 20570.63 | 0 | 0 | 0 |
| Tunisia | 1971 | 1.147313 | 21178.81 | 0 | 0 | 0 |
| Uganda | 1971 | 1.16 | 21780.96 | 0 | 0 | 0 |
| Zambia | 1971 | 1.3075 | 22385.56 | 0 | 0 | 0 |
| Zimbabwe | 1971 | 1.38125 | 23007.67 | 0 | 0 | 0 |
| Algeria | 1972 | 1.418125 | 23668.47 | 0 | 0 | 0 |

| Country Name | Year | Education | Population Density | Minor War | Civil War | Conflict |
|---|---|---|---|---|---|---|
| Angola | 1972 | 1.436563 | 24333.99 | 0 | 0 | 0 |
| Benin | 1972 | 1.455 | 25032.77 | 0 | 0 | 0 |
| Botswana | 1972 | 1.684 | 25741.48 | 0 | 0 | 0 |
| Burkina Faso | 1972 | 1.7985 | 26483.95 | 1 | 1 | 1 |
| Burundi | 1972 | 1.85575 | 27316.66 | 1 | 1 | 1 |
| Cabo Verde | 1972 | 1.884375 | 28203.77 | 0 | 0 | 0 |
| Cameroon | 1972 | 1.913 | 29012.55 | 0 | 0 | 0 |
| Central African Republic | 1972 | 2.2255 | 29808.02 | 0 | 0 | 0 |
| Chad | 1972 | 2.38175 | 30648.84 | 0 | 0 | 0 |
| Comoros | 1972 | 2.459875 | 31446.87 | 0 | 0 | 0 |
| Congo, Dem. Rep. | 1972 | 2.498938 | 32340.98 | 0 | 0 | 0 |
| Congo, Rep. | 1972 | 2.538 | 33344.22 | 0 | 0 | 0 |
| Cote d'Ivoire | 1972 | 2.785 | 34376.23 | 0 | 0 | 0 |
| Djibouti | 1972 | 2.9085 | 35482.16 | 0 | 0 | 0 |
| Egypt, Arab Rep. | 1972 | 2.97025 | 36628.16 | 0 | 0 | 0 |
| Equatorial Guinea | 1972 | 3.001125 | 37804.13 | 0 | 0 | 0 |
| Eritrea | 1972 | 3.032 | 39047.46 | 0 | 0 | 0 |
| Ethiopia | 1972 | 3.1345 | 40514 | 0 | 0 | 0 |
| Gabon | 1972 | 3.18575 | 41846 | 0 | 0 | 0 |
| Gambia, The | 1972 | 3.211375 | 43290 | 0 | 0 | 0 |
| Ghana | 1972 | 3.224188 | 44820 | 0 | 0 | 0 |
| Guinea | 1972 | 3.237 | 46705 | 0 | 0 | 0 |
| Guinea-Bissau | 1972 | 3.2995 | 47685 | 1 | 1 | 1 |
| Kenya | 1972 | 3.33075 | 48289 | 0 | 1 | 1 |
| Lesotho | 1972 | 3.346375 | 49349 | 0 | 1 | 1 |
| Liberia | 1972 | 3.354188 | 50890 | 0 | 1 | 1 |
| Libya | 1972 | 3.362 | 52445 | 0 | 1 | 1 |
| Madagascar | 1972 | 3.4125 | 54058 | 1 | 1 | 1 |
| Malawi | 1972 | 3.43775 | 55702 | 0 | 0 | 0 |
| Mali | 1972 | 3.450375 | 57303 | 0 | 0 | 0 |
| Mauritania | 1972 | 3.456688 | 58943 | 0 | 0 | 0 |
| Mauritius | 1972 | 3.463 | 60698 | 0 | 0 | 0 |
| Morocco | 1972 | 3.467 | 62522 | 1 | 1 | 1 |
| Mozambique | 1972 | 3.469 | 64355 | 1 | 1 | 1 |
| Namibia | 1972 | 3.47 | 66197 | 1 | 1 | 1 |
| Niger | 1972 | 3.471 | 69016 | 1 | 1 | 1 |
| Nigeria | 1972 | | 89.898 | 0 | 0 | 0 |
| Rwanda | 1972 | | 96.376 | 0 | 0 | 0 |
| Sao Tome and Principe | 1972 | | 103.354 | 0 | 0 | 0 |
| Senegal | 1972 | | 110.84 | 0 | 0 | 0 |
| Seychelles | 1972 | | 118.886 | 0 | 0 | 0 |
| Sierra Leone | 1972 | | 127.617 | 0 | 0 | 0 |
| Somalia | 1972 | | 137.047 | 0 | 0 | 0 |
| South Africa | 1972 | | 147.181 | 0 | 0 | 0 |
| Sudan | 1972 | | 158.034 | 0 | 0 | 0 |
| Swaziland | 1972 | | 168.6 | 0 | 0 | 0 |
| Tanzania | 1972 | | 178.848 | 0 | 0 | 0 |
| Togo | 1972 | | 188.75 | 0 | 0 | 0 |

| *Country Name* | *Year* | *Education* | *Population Density* | *Minor War* | *Civil War* | *Conflict* |
|---|---|---|---|---|---|---|
| Tunisia | 1972 | | 198.279 | 0 | 0 | 0 |
| Uganda | 1972 | | 207.959 | 0 | 0 | 0 |
| Zambia | 1972 | | 217.219 | 0 | 0 | 0 |
| Zimbabwe | 1972 | | 228.694 | 0 | 0 | 0 |
| Algeria | 1973 | | 247.883 | 0 | 0 | 0 |
| Angola | 1973 | | 263.409 | 0 | 0 | 0 |
| Benin | 1973 | | 279.149 | 0 | 0 | 0 |
| Botswana | 1973 | | 293.659 | 0 | 0 | 0 |
| Burkina Faso | 1973 | | 305.991 | 0 | 0 | 0 |
| Burundi | 1973 | | 316.123 | 0 | 0 | 0 |
| Cabo Verde | 1973 | | 289.431 | 0 | 0 | 0 |
| Cameroon | 1973 | | 296.544 | 0 | 0 | 0 |
| Central African Republic | 1973 | | 303.756 | 0 | 0 | 0 |
| Chad | 1973 | | 311.025 | 0 | 0 | 0 |
| Comoros | 1973 | | 326.58 | 0 | 0 | 0 |
| Congo, Dem. Rep. | 1973 | | 349.928 | 0 | 0 | 0 |
| Congo, Rep. | 1973 | | 366.088 | 0 | 0 | 0 |
| Cote d'Ivoire | 1973 | | 552 | 1 | 0 | 1 |
| Djibouti | 1973 | | 547 | 1 | 0 | 1 |
| Egypt, Arab Rep. | 1973 | | 534 | 1 | 0 | 1 |
| Equatorial Guinea | 1973 | | 547 | 1 | 0 | 1 |
| Eritrea | 1973 | | 553 | 0 | 0 | 0 |
| Ethiopia | 1973 | | 568 | 0 | 0 | 0 |
| Gabon | 1973 | | 592 | 0 | 0 | 0 |
| Gambia, The | 1973 | | 621 | 0 | 0 | 0 |
| Ghana | 1973 | | 426.507 | 1 | 0 | 1 |
| Guinea | 1973 | | | | | |
| Guinea-Bissau | 1973 | | 669 | 0 | 0 | 0 |
| Kenya | 1973 | | 693 | 0 | 0 | 0 |
| Lesotho | 1973 | | 716 | 0 | 0 | 0 |
| Liberia | 1973 | | 691 | 0 | 0 | 0 |
| Libya | 1973 | | 657 | 0 | 0 | 0 |
| Madagascar | 1973 | | 666 | 0 | 0 | 0 |
| Malawi | 1973 | | 679 | 0 | 0 | 0 |
| Mali | 1973 | | 694 | 0 | 0 | 0 |
| Mauritania | 1973 | | 804.94 | 1 | 0 | 1 |
| Mauritius | 1973 | | 819.501 | 0 | 0 | 0 |
| Morocco | 1973 | | | | | |
| Mozambique | 1973 | 0.808 | 28173.31 | 0 | 0 | 0 |
| Namibia | 1973 | 0.923 | 28820.67 | 0 | 0 | 0 |
| Niger | 1973 | 0.9805 | 29533.07 | 0 | 0 | 0 |
| Nigeria | 1973 | 1.038 | 30265.15 | 0 | 0 | 0 |
| Rwanda | 1973 | 1.1715 | 30986.38 | 0 | 0 | 0 |
| Sao Tome and Principe | 1973 | 1.23825 | 31681.19 | 0 | 1 | 1 |
| Senegal | 1973 | 1.271625 | 32337.88 | 0 | 0 | 0 |
| Seychelles | 1973 | 1.288313 | 32966.24 | 1 | 1 | 1 |
| Sierra Leone | 1973 | | | | | |
| Somalia | 1973 | 1.305 | 33574.03 | 1 | 1 | 1 |

| Country Name | Year | Education | Population Density | Minor War | Civil War | Conflict |
|---|---|---|---|---|---|---|
| South Africa | 1973 | 1.4945 | 34183.99 | 0 | 0 | 0 |
| Sudan | 1973 | 1.58925 | 34807.42 | 0 | 0 | 0 |
| Swaziland | 1973 | 1.636625 | 35480.41 | 0 | 1 | 1 |
| Tanzania | 1973 | 1.660313 | 36216.31 | 0 | 0 | 0 |
| Togo | 1973 | 1.684 | 36952.5 | 0 | 0 | 0 |
| Tunisia | 1973 | 2.1645 | 37736.99 | 0 | 0 | 0 |
| Uganda | 1973 | 2.40475 | 38783.86 | 0 | 0 | 0 |
| Zambia | 1973 | 2.524875 | 40020.46 | 0 | 0 | 0 |
| Zimbabwe | 1973 | 2.584938 | 41257.72 | 0 | 0 | 0 |
| Algeria | 1974 | | | | | |
| Angola | 1974 | 2.645 | 42634.22 | 0 | 0 | 0 |
| Benin | 1974 | 3.1955 | 44196.1 | 0 | 0 | 0 |
| Botswana | 1974 | 3.47075 | 45681.81 | 0 | 0 | 0 |
| Burkina Faso | 1974 | 3.608375 | 47093.03 | 0 | 0 | 0 |
| Burundi | 1974 | 3.677188 | 48550.16 | 0 | 0 | 0 |
| Cabo Verde | 1974 | 3.746 | 50052.38 | 0 | 0 | 0 |
| Cameroon | 1974 | 4.062 | 51593.43 | 0 | 0 | 0 |
| Central African Republic | 1974 | 4.22 | 52793.54 | 0 | 0 | 0 |
| Chad | 1974 | 4.299 | 54015.07 | 0 | 0 | 0 |
| Comoros | 1974 | 4.3385 | 55251.81 | 0 | 0 | 0 |
| Congo, Dem. Rep. | 1974 | | | | | |
| Congo, Rep. | 1974 | 4.378 | 56683.22 | 0 | 0 | 0 |
| Cote d'Ivoire | 1974 | 4.721 | 55862 | 0 | 0 | 0 |
| Djibouti | 1974 | 4.8925 | 56625 | 0 | 0 | 0 |
| Egypt, Arab Rep. | 1974 | 4.97825 | 57384 | 1 | 0 | 1 |
| Equatorial Guinea | 1974 | 5.021125 | 58157 | 1 | 0 | 1 |
| Eritrea | 1974 | 5.064 | 58945 | 1 | 0 | 1 |
| Ethiopia | 1974 | 5.487 | 59758 | 1 | 0 | 1 |
| Gabon | 1974 | 5.6985 | 61072 | 1 | 0 | 1 |
| Gambia, The | 1974 | 5.80425 | 62412 | 1 | 0 | 1 |
| Ghana | 1974 | 5.857125 | 63773 | 0 | 0 | 0 |
| Guinea | 1974 | | | | | |
| Guinea-Bissau | 1974 | 5.91 | 65159 | 0 | 0 | 0 |
| Kenya | 1974 | 6.251 | 66574 | 0 | 0 | 0 |
| Lesotho | 1974 | 6.4215 | 68023 | 0 | 0 | 0 |
| Liberia | 1974 | 6.50675 | 69502 | 0 | 0 | 0 |
| Libya | 1974 | 6.549375 | 71009 | 0 | 0 | 0 |
| Madagascar | 1974 | 6.592 | 72544 | 0 | 0 | 0 |
| Malawi | 1974 | 6.8345 | 74101 | 0 | 0 | 0 |
| Mali | 1974 | 6.95575 | 75677 | 0 | 0 | 0 |
| Mauritania | 1974 | 7.016375 | 77267 | 0 | 0 | 0 |
| Mauritius | 1974 | 7.077 | 78867 | 0 | 0 | 0 |
| Morocco | 1974 | | | | | |
| Mozambique | 1974 | | 249.22 | 0 | 0 | 0 |
| Namibia | 1974 | | 250.419 | 0 | 0 | 0 |
| Niger | 1974 | | 251.623 | 0 | 0 | 0 |
| Nigeria | 1974 | | 252.833 | 0 | 0 | 0 |
| Rwanda | 1974 | | 256.349 | 0 | 0 | 0 |

| Country Name | Year | Education | Population Density | Minor War | Civil War | Conflict |
|---|---|---|---|---|---|---|
| Sao Tome and Principe | 1974 | | 259.864 | 0 | 0 | 0 |
| Senegal | 1974 | | 263.377 | 0 | 0 | 0 |
| Seychelles | 1974 | | 266.898 | 0 | 0 | 0 |
| Sierra Leone | 1974 | | | | | |
| Somalia | 1974 | | 270.435 | 0 | 0 | 0 |
| South Africa | 1974 | | 273.999 | 0 | 0 | 0 |
| Sudan | 1974 | | 277.603 | 0 | 0 | 0 |
| Swaziland | 1974 | | 271.301 | 0 | 0 | 0 |
| Tanzania | 1974 | | 249.952 | 0 | 0 | 0 |
| Togo | 1974 | | 213.292 | 0 | 0 | 0 |
| Tunisia | 1974 | | 190.808 | 0 | 0 | 0 |
| Uganda | 1974 | | 192.675 | 0 | 0 | 0 |
| Zambia | 1974 | | 194.597 | 0 | 0 | 0 |
| Zimbabwe | 1974 | | 221.299 | 1 | 0 | 1 |
| Algeria | 1975 | | | | | |
| Angola | 1975 | | 256.009 | 0 | 0 | 0 |
| Benin | 1975 | | 271.778 | 0 | 0 | 0 |
| Botswana | 1975 | | 285.483 | 0 | 0 | 0 |
| Burkina Faso | 1975 | | 299.577 | 0 | 0 | 0 |
| Burundi | 1975 | | 314.637 | 0 | 0 | 0 |
| Cabo Verde | 1975 | | 325.194 | 0 | 0 | 0 |
| Cameroon | 1975 | | 333.651 | 0 | 0 | 0 |
| Central African Republic | 1975 | | 342.469 | 0 | 0 | 0 |
| Chad | 1975 | | 351.649 | 0 | 0 | 0 |
| Comoros | 1975 | | 361.192 | 0 | 0 | 0 |
| Congo, Dem. Rep. | 1975 | | | | | |
| Congo, Rep. | 1975 | | 371.1 | 0 | 0 | 0 |
| Cote d'Ivoire | 1975 | | 381.377 | 0 | 0 | 0 |
| Djibouti | 1975 | | 392.024 | 0 | 0 | 0 |
| Egypt, Arab Rep. | 1975 | | 403.044 | 0 | 0 | 0 |
| Equatorial Guinea | 1975 | | 414.443 | 0 | 0 | 0 |
| Eritrea | 1975 | | 426.231 | 0 | 0 | 0 |
| Ethiopia | 1975 | | 438.42 | 0 | 0 | 0 |
| Gabon | 1975 | | 451.026 | 0 | 0 | 0 |
| Gambia, The | 1975 | | 464.06 | 0 | 0 | 0 |
| Ghana | 1975 | | 477.538 | 0 | 0 | 0 |
| Guinea | 1975 | | | | | |
| Guinea-Bissau | 1975 | | 491.483 | 0 | 0 | 0 |
| Kenya | 1975 | | 505.919 | 0 | 0 | 0 |
| Lesotho | 1975 | | 520.764 | 0 | 0 | 0 |
| Liberia | 1975 | | 535.927 | 0 | 0 | 0 |
| Libya | 1975 | | 551.415 | 0 | 0 | 0 |
| Madagascar | 1975 | | 567.232 | 0 | 0 | 0 |
| Malawi | 1975 | | 583.355 | 0 | 0 | 0 |
| Mali | 1975 | | 599.763 | 0 | 0 | 0 |
| Mauritania | 1975 | | 616 | 0 | 0 | 0 |
| Mauritius | 1975 | | 633 | 0 | 0 | 0 |
| Morocco | 1975 | | | | | |

| *Country Name* | *Year* | *Education* | *Population Density* | *Minor War* | *Civil War* | *Conflict* |
|---|---|---|---|---|---|---|
| Mozambique | 1975 | | 25145.37 | 0 | 0 | 0 |
| Namibia | 1975 | | 25659.68 | 0 | 0 | 0 |
| Niger | 1975 | | 26192.36 | 1 | 0 | 1 |
| Nigeria | 1975 | | 26740.27 | 1 | 0 | 1 |
| Rwanda | 1975 | | 27307.8 | 1 | 0 | 1 |
| Sao Tome and Principe | 1975 | | 27860.3 | 1 | 0 | 1 |
| Senegal | 1975 | | 28451.26 | 1 | 0 | 1 |
| Seychelles | 1975 | | 28962.28 | 1 | 0 | 1 |
| Sierra Leone | 1975 | | 29468.5 | 1 | 0 | 1 |
| Somalia | 1975 | | | | | |
| South Africa | 1975 | | 30099.66 | 1 | 0 | 1 |
| Sudan | 1975 | | 30770.37 | 1 | 0 | 1 |
| Swaziland | 1975 | | 31445.18 | 1 | 0 | 1 |
| Tanzania | 1975 | | 32199.37 | 1 | 0 | 1 |
| Togo | 1975 | | 32975.87 | 0 | 1 | 1 |
| Tunisia | 1975 | | 33824.84 | 0 | 1 | 1 |
| Uganda | 1975 | | 34617.8 | 1 | 1 | 2 |
| Zambia | 1975 | | 35216.32 | 1 | 1 | 2 |
| Zimbabwe | 1975 | | 35664.27 | 1 | 1 | 2 |
| Algeria | 1976 | | | | | |
| Angola | 1976 | | 36036.46 | 0 | 1 | 1 |
| Benin | 1976 | | 37720.09 | 0 | 1 | 1 |
| Botswana | 1976 | | 39478.54 | 0 | 1 | 1 |
| Burkina Faso | 1976 | | 40673.92 | 0 | 1 | 1 |
| Burundi | 1976 | | 41649.83 | 0 | 1 | 1 |
| Cabo Verde | 1976 | | 42227.14 | 0 | 1 | 1 |
| Cameroon | 1976 | | 43046 | 1 | 1 | 2 |
| Central African Republic | 1976 | | 44323.43 | 0 | 1 | 1 |
| Chad | 1976 | | 45725.36 | 0 | 1 | 1 |
| Comoros | 1976 | | 47086.92 | 0 | 1 | 1 |
| Congo, Dem. Rep. | 1976 | | | | | |
| Congo, Rep. | 1976 | | 48397.41 | 0 | 1 | 1 |
| Cote d'Ivoire | 1976 | | 50090.52 | 0 | 1 | 1 |
| Djibouti | 1976 | | 51673.32 | 1 | 1 | 1 |
| Egypt, Arab Rep. | 1976 | | 52803.02 | 1 | 1 | 1 |
| Equatorial Guinea | 1976 | | 54034.25 | 1 | 1 | 1 |
| Eritrea | 1976 | | 55549.97 | 1 | 1 | 1 |
| Ethiopia | 1976 | | 57192.65 | 1 | 1 | 1 |
| Gabon | 1976 | | 58805.42 | 1 | 1 | 1 |
| Gambia, The | 1976 | | 60483.9 | 1 | 1 | 1 |
| Ghana | 1976 | | 62279.4 | 1 | 1 | 1 |
| Guinea | 1976 | | | | | |
| Guinea-Bissau | 1976 | | 64164.97 | 1 | 1 | 1 |
| Kenya | 1976 | | 66122.58 | 1 | 1 | 1 |
| Lesotho | 1976 | | 68187.27 | 1 | 1 | 1 |
| Liberia | 1976 | | 70366.07 | 1 | 1 | 1 |
| Libya | 1976 | | 72637.21 | 1 | 1 | 1 |
| Madagascar | 1976 | | 74980.29 | 1 | 1 | 1 |

| Country Name | Year | Education | Population Density | Minor War | Civil War | Conflict |
|---|---|---|---|---|---|---|
| Malawi | 1976 | | 77411.4 | 1 | 1 | 1 |
| Mali | 1976 | | 79935.8 | 1 | 1 | 1 |
| Mauritania | 1976 | | 82545 | 1 | 1 | 1 |
| Mauritius | 1976 | | 85237 | 1 | 1 | 1 |
| Morocco | 1976 | | | | | |
| Mozambique | 1976 | 1.01 | 455.661 | 0 | 0 | 0 |
| Namibia | 1976 | 1.21 | 461.357 | 0 | 0 | 0 |
| Niger | 1976 | 1.31 | 467.592 | 1 | 0 | 1 |
| Nigeria | 1976 | 1.41 | 474.386 | 0 | 0 | 0 |
| Rwanda | 1976 | 1.618 | 481.519 | 0 | 0 | 0 |
| Sao Tome and Principe | 1976 | 1.722 | 489.004 | 0 | 0 | 0 |
| Senegal | 1976 | 1.774 | 496.853 | 0 | 0 | 0 |
| Seychelles | 1976 | 1.8 | 503.763 | 0 | 0 | 0 |
| Sierra Leone | 1976 | | | | | |
| Somalia | 1976 | 1.826 | 514.579 | 0 | 0 | 0 |
| South Africa | 1976 | 2.2015 | 525.93 | 0 | 0 | 0 |
| Sudan | 1976 | 2.38925 | 538.009 | 0 | 0 | 0 |
| Swaziland | 1976 | 2.483125 | 560.658 | 0 | 0 | 0 |
| Tanzania | 1976 | 2.530063 | 597.135 | 0 | 0 | 0 |
| Togo | 1976 | 2.577 | 647.436 | 0 | 0 | 0 |
| Tunisia | 1976 | 2.955 | 687.762 | 0 | 0 | 0 |
| Uganda | 1976 | 3.144 | 706.489 | 0 | 0 | 0 |
| Zambia | 1976 | 3.2385 | 726.421 | 0 | 0 | 0 |
| Zimbabwe | 1976 | 3.28575 | 722.911 | 0 | 0 | 0 |
| Algeria | 1977 | | | | | |
| Angola | 1977 | 3.333 | 713.827 | 0 | 0 | 0 |
| Benin | 1977 | 3.82 | 730.836 | 0 | 0 | 0 |
| Botswana | 1977 | 4.0635 | 754.241 | 0 | 0 | 0 |
| Burkina Faso | 1977 | 4.18525 | 779.018 | 0 | 0 | 0 |
| Burundi | 1977 | 4.246125 | 805.26 | 0 | 0 | 0 |
| Cabo Verde | 1977 | 4.307 | 833.036 | 0 | 0 | 0 |
| Cameroon | 1977 | 4.7555 | 859.448 | 0 | 0 | 0 |
| Central African Republic | 1977 | 4.97975 | 880.916 | 0 | 0 | 0 |
| Chad | 1977 | 5.091875 | 899.743 | 0 | 0 | 0 |
| Comoros | 1977 | 5.147938 | 918.835 | 0 | 0 | 0 |
| Congo, Dem. Rep. | 1977 | 5.204 | 938.084 | 0 | 0 | 0 |
| Congo, Rep. | 1977 | | | | | |
| Cote d'Ivoire | 1977 | 5.712 | 960.425 | 0 | 0 | 0 |
| Djibouti | 1977 | 5.966 | 986.367 | 0 | 0 | 0 |
| Egypt, Arab Rep. | 1977 | 6.093 | 1013.159 | 0 | 0 | 0 |
| Equatorial Guinea | 1977 | 6.1565 | 1040.811 | 0 | 0 | 0 |
| Eritrea | 1977 | 6.22 | 1069.065 | 0 | 0 | 0 |
| Ethiopia | 1977 | 6.6045 | 1097.708 | 0 | 0 | 0 |
| Gabon | 1977 | 6.79675 | 1126.94 | 0 | 0 | 0 |
| Gambia, The | 1977 | 6.892875 | 1157.171 | 0 | 0 | 0 |
| Ghana | 1977 | 6.940938 | 1195.647 | 0 | 0 | 0 |
| Guinea | 1977 | | | | | |
| Guinea-Bissau | 1977 | 6.989 | 1236.429 | 0 | 0 | 0 |

| Country Name | Year | Education | Population Density | Minor War | Civil War | Conflict |
|---|---|---|---|---|---|---|
| Kenya | 1977 | 7.3205 | 1269.154 | 0 | 0 | 0 |
| Lesotho | 1977 | 7.48625 | 1300.423 | 0 | 0 | 0 |
| Liberia | 1977 | 7.569125 | 1332.623 | 0 | 0 | 0 |
| Libya | 1977 | 7.610563 | 1364.412 | 0 | 0 | 0 |
| Madagascar | 1977 | 7.652 | 1395.69 | 0 | 0 | 0 |
| Malawi | 1977 | 8.0015 | 1426.392 | 0 | 0 | 0 |
| Mali | 1977 | 8.17625 | 1456.451 | 0 | 0 | 0 |
| Mauritania | 1977 | 8.263625 | 1486 | 0 | 0 | 0 |
| Mauritius | 1977 | 8.351 | 1515 | 0 | 0 | 0 |
| Morocco | 1977 | | | | | |
| Mozambique | 1977 | 0.464 | 374.02 | 0 | 0 | 0 |
| Namibia | 1977 | 0.4915 | 386.04 | 0 | 0 | 0 |
| Niger | 1977 | 0.50525 | 398.783 | 0 | 0 | 0 |
| Nigeria | 1977 | 0.519 | 411.947 | 0 | 0 | 0 |
| Rwanda | 1977 | 0.546 | 425.546 | 0 | 0 | 0 |
| Sao Tome and Principe | 1977 | 0.5595 | 439.593 | 0 | 0 | 0 |
| Senegal | 1977 | 0.56625 | 454.105 | 0 | 0 | 0 |
| Seychelles | 1977 | 0.569625 | 469.095 | 0 | 0 | 0 |
| Sierra Leone | 1977 | 0.573 | 484.58 | 0 | 0 | 0 |
| Somalia | 1977 | | | | | |
| South Africa | 1977 | 0.6515 | 500.576 | 0 | 0 | 0 |
| Sudan | 1977 | 0.69075 | 517.101 | 0 | 0 | 0 |
| Swaziland | 1977 | 0.710375 | 534.171 | 0 | 0 | 0 |
| Tanzania | 1977 | 0.720188 | 551.804 | 0 | 0 | 0 |
| Togo | 1977 | 0.73 | 570.02 | 0 | 0 | 0 |
| Tunisia | 1977 | 0.8485 | 588.836 | 0 | 0 | 0 |
| Uganda | 1977 | 0.90775 | 608.274 | 0 | 0 | 0 |
| Zambia | 1977 | 0.937375 | 628.354 | 0 | 0 | 0 |
| Zimbabwe | 1977 | 0.952188 | 649.096 | 0 | 0 | 0 |
| Algeria | 1978 | | | | | |
| Angola | 1978 | 0.967 | 670.523 | 0 | 0 | 0 |
| Benin | 1978 | 1.12 | 692.658 | 1 | 0 | 1 |
| Botswana | 1978 | 1.1965 | 715.523 | 0 | 0 | 0 |
| Burkina Faso | 1978 | 1.23475 | 739.143 | 0 | 0 | 0 |
| Burundi | 1978 | 1.253875 | 763.854 | 0 | 0 | 0 |
| Cabo Verde | 1978 | 1.273 | 790.282 | 0 | 0 | 0 |
| Cameroon | 1978 | 1.54 | 818.467 | 0 | 0 | 0 |
| Central African Republic | 1978 | 1.6735 | 848.406 | 0 | 0 | 0 |
| Chad | 1978 | 1.74025 | 880.17 | 0 | 0 | 0 |
| Comoros | 1978 | 1.773625 | 913.762 | 0 | 0 | 0 |
| Congo, Dem. Rep. | 1978 | | | | | |
| Congo, Rep. | 1978 | 1.807 | 949.255 | 0 | 0 | 0 |
| Cote d'Ivoire | 1978 | 2.129 | 986.512 | 0 | 0 | 0 |
| Djibouti | 1978 | 2.29 | 1025.384 | 0 | 0 | 0 |
| Egypt, Arab Rep. | 1978 | 2.3705 | 1065.906 | 0 | 0 | 0 |
| Equatorial Guinea | 1978 | 2.41075 | 1107.563 | 0 | 0 | 0 |
| Eritrea | 1978 | 2.451 | 1149.787 | 0 | 0 | 0 |
| Ethiopia | 1978 | 2.5445 | 1192.548 | 0 | 0 | 0 |

| Country Name | Year | Education | Population Density | Minor War | Civil War | Conflict |
|---|---|---|---|---|---|---|
| Gabon | 1978 | 2.59125 | 1235.767 | 0 | 0 | 0 |
| Gambia, The | 1978 | 2.614625 | 1279.41 | 0 | 0 | 0 |
| Ghana | 1978 | 2.626313 | 1323.467 | 0 | 0 | 0 |
| Guinea | 1978 | | | | | |
| Guinea-Bissau | 1978 | 2.638 | 1367.884 | 0 | 0 | 0 |
| Kenya | 1978 | 2.8535 | 1393 | 0 | 0 | 0 |
| Lesotho | 1978 | 2.96125 | 1431 | 0 | 0 | 0 |
| Liberia | 1978 | 3.015125 | 1469 | 0 | 0 | 0 |
| Libya | 1978 | 3.042063 | 1508 | 0 | 0 | 0 |
| Madagascar | 1978 | 3.069 | 1548 | 0 | 0 | 0 |
| Malawi | 1978 | 3.29 | 1589 | 0 | 0 | 0 |
| Mali | 1978 | 3.4005 | 1630 | 0 | 0 | 0 |
| Mauritania | 1978 | 3.45575 | 1671 | 0 | 0 | 0 |
| Mauritius | 1978 | 3.511 | 1713 | 0 | 0 | 0 |
| Morocco | 1978 | | | | | |
| Mozambique | 1978 | 1.076 | 7355.248 | 0 | 0 | 0 |
| Namibia | 1978 | 0.9365 | 7563.839 | 0 | 0 | 0 |
| Niger | 1978 | 0.86675 | 7781.813 | 0 | 0 | 0 |
| Nigeria | 1978 | 0.797 | 8009.602 | 0 | 0 | 0 |
| Rwanda | 1978 | 2.188 | 8245.481 | 1 | 0 | 1 |
| Sao Tome and Principe | 1978 | 2.8835 | 8490.213 | 0 | 0 | 0 |
| Senegal | 1978 | 3.23125 | 8744.302 | 0 | 0 | 0 |
| Seychelles | 1978 | 3.405125 | 9009.048 | 0 | 0 | 0 |
| Sierra Leone | 1978 | | | | | |
| Somalia | 1978 | 3.579 | 8788.945 | 0 | 0 | 0 |
| South Africa | 1978 | 3.9625 | 9065.186 | 0 | 0 | 0 |
| Sudan | 1978 | 4.15425 | 9353.659 | 0 | 0 | 0 |
| Swaziland | 1978 | 4.250125 | 9649.467 | 0 | 0 | 0 |
| Tanzania | 1978 | 4.298063 | 9904.862 | 0 | 0 | 0 |
| Togo | 1978 | 4.346 | 10117.86 | 0 | 0 | 0 |
| Tunisia | 1978 | 4.673 | 10332.93 | 0 | 0 | 0 |
| Uganda | 1978 | 4.8365 | 10538.04 | 0 | 0 | 0 |
| Zambia | 1978 | 4.91825 | 10720.78 | 0 | 0 | 0 |
| Zimbabwe | 1978 | 4.959125 | 10878.8 | 0 | 0 | 0 |
| Algeria | 1979 | | | | | |
| Angola | 1979 | 5 | 11016.64 | 0 | 0 | 0 |
| Benin | 1979 | 5.288 | 11177.98 | 1 | 0 | 1 |
| Botswana | 1979 | 5.432 | 11402.29 | 0 | 0 | 0 |
| Burkina Faso | 1979 | 5.504 | 12152.3 | 1 | 0 | 1 |
| Burundi | 1979 | 5.54 | 12832.61 | 0 | 0 | 0 |
| Cabo Verde | 1979 | 5.576 | 13228.43 | 0 | 0 | 0 |
| Cameroon | 1979 | 5.754 | 13781.21 | 0 | 0 | 0 |
| Central African Republic | 1979 | 5.843 | 14174.7 | 0 | 0 | 0 |
| Chad | 1979 | 5.8875 | 14576.59 | 0 | 0 | 0 |
| Comoros | 1979 | 5.90975 | 14987.05 | 0 | 0 | 0 |
| Congo, Dem. Rep. | 1979 | | | | | |
| Congo, Rep. | 1979 | 5.932 | 15413.8 | 0 | 0 | 0 |
| Cote d'Ivoire | 1979 | 6.0075 | 15848 | 0 | 0 | 0 |

| Country Name | Year | Education | Population Density | Minor War | Civil War | Conflict |
|---|---|---|---|---|---|---|
| Djibouti | 1979 | 6.04525 | 16293 | 0 | 0 | 0 |
| Egypt, Arab Rep. | 1979 | 6.064125 | 16805 | 0 | 0 | 0 |
| Equatorial Guinea | 1979 | 6.073563 | 17302 | 0 | 0 | 0 |
| Eritrea | 1979 | 6.083 | 17704 | 0 | 0 | 0 |
| Ethiopia | 1979 | 6.326 | 18085 | 0 | 0 | 0 |
| Gabon | 1979 | 6.4475 | 18474 | 0 | 0 | 0 |
| Gambia, The | 1979 | 6.50825 | 18888 | 0 | 0 | 0 |
| Ghana | 1979 | 6.538625 | 19314 | 0 | 0 | 0 |
| Guinea | 1979 | | | | | |
| Guinea-Bissau | 1979 | 6.569 | 19752 | 1 | 0 | 1 |
| Kenya | 1979 | 6.669 | 20196 | 1 | 0 | 1 |
| Lesotho | 1979 | 6.719 | 20661 | 0 | 0 | 0 |
| Liberia | 1979 | 6.744 | 21137 | 0 | 0 | 0 |
| Libya | 1979 | 6.7565 | 21601 | 0 | 0 | 0 |
| Madagascar | 1979 | 6.769 | 22062 | 0 | 0 | 0 |
| Malawi | 1979 | 6.9535 | 22524 | 0 | 0 | 0 |
| Mali | 1979 | 7.04575 | 22981 | 0 | 0 | 0 |
| Mauritania | 1979 | 7.091875 | 23435 | 0 | 0 | 0 |
| Mauritius | 1979 | 7.138 | 23888 | 0 | 0 | 0 |
| Morocco | 1979 | | | | | |
| Mozambique | 1979 | | 3136.138 | 0 | 0 | 0 |
| Namibia | 1979 | | 3193.668 | 0 | 0 | 0 |
| Niger | 1979 | | 3252.861 | 0 | 0 | 0 |
| Nigeria | 1979 | | 3313.707 | 0 | 0 | 0 |
| Rwanda | 1979 | | 3376.211 | 0 | 0 | 0 |
| Sao Tome and Principe | 1979 | | 3440.361 | 0 | 0 | 0 |
| Senegal | 1979 | | 3506.216 | 0 | 0 | 0 |
| Seychelles | 1979 | | 3573.863 | 0 | 0 | 0 |
| Sierra Leone | 1979 | | | | | |
| Somalia | 1979 | | 3643.361 | 0 | 0 | 0 |
| South Africa | 1979 | | 3714.679 | 0 | 0 | 0 |
| Sudan | 1979 | | 3787.796 | 0 | 0 | 0 |
| Swaziland | 1979 | | 3862.799 | 0 | 0 | 0 |
| Tanzania | 1979 | | 3939.774 | 0 | 0 | 0 |
| Togo | 1979 | | 4018.826 | 0 | 0 | 0 |
| Tunisia | 1979 | | 4100.005 | 0 | 0 | 0 |
| Uganda | 1979 | | 4183.359 | 0 | 0 | 0 |
| Zambia | 1979 | | 4268.975 | 0 | 0 | 0 |
| Zimbabwe | 1979 | | 4356.939 | 0 | 0 | 0 |
| Algeria | 1980 | | | | | |
| Angola | 1980 | | 4447.369 | 0 | 0 | 0 |
| Benin | 1980 | | 4540.361 | 0 | 0 | 0 |
| Botswana | 1980 | | 4636.011 | 0 | 0 | 0 |
| Burkina Faso | 1980 | | 4734.4 | 0 | 0 | 0 |
| Burundi | 1980 | | 4953.578 | 0 | 0 | 0 |
| Cabo Verde | 1980 | | 5226.741 | 0 | 0 | 0 |
| Cameroon | 1980 | | 5394.334 | 0 | 0 | 0 |
| Central African Republic | 1980 | | 5528.408 | 0 | 0 | 0 |

| Country Name | Year | Education | Population Density | Minor War | Civil War | Conflict |
|---|---|---|---|---|---|---|
| Chad | 1980 | | 5666.825 | 0 | 0 | 0 |
| Comoros | 1980 | | 5809.689 | 0 | 0 | 0 |
| Congo, Dem. Rep. | 1980 | | | | | |
| Congo, Rep. | 1980 | | 6118.452 | 0 | 0 | 0 |
| Cote d'Ivoire | 1980 | | 6552.474 | 0 | 0 | 0 |
| Djibouti | 1980 | | 6800.519 | 0 | 0 | 0 |
| Egypt, Arab Rep. | 1980 | | 6989.107 | 0 | 0 | 0 |
| Equatorial Guinea | 1980 | | 7209.485 | 0 | 0 | 0 |
| Eritrea | 1980 | | 7445.695 | 0 | 0 | 0 |
| Ethiopia | 1980 | | 7701.569 | 0 | 0 | 0 |
| Gabon | 1980 | | 7791.058 | 0 | 0 | 0 |
| Gambia, The | 1980 | | 7906.607 | 0 | 0 | 0 |
| Ghana | 1980 | | 8154.403 | 0 | 0 | 0 |
| Guinea | 1980 | | | | | |
| Guinea-Bissau | 1980 | | 8350.413 | 1 | 0 | 1 |
| Kenya | 1980 | | 8416.924 | 1 | 0 | 1 |
| Lesotho | 1980 | | 8520.304 | 0 | 0 | 0 |
| Liberia | 1980 | | 8755.538 | 0 | 0 | 0 |
| Libya | 1980 | | 8971.979 | 0 | 0 | 0 |
| Madagascar | 1980 | | 9153.73 | 0 | 0 | 0 |
| Malawi | 1980 | | 9345.729 | 0 | 0 | 0 |
| Mali | 1980 | | 9569.216 | 0 | 0 | 0 |
| Mauritania | 1980 | | 9807 | 0 | 0 | 0 |
| Mauritius | 1980 | | 10058 | 0 | 0 | 0 |
| Morocco | 1980 | | | | | |
| Mozambique | 1980 | | 627.82 | 0 | 0 | 0 |
| Namibia | 1980 | | 633.939 | 1 | 0 | 1 |
| Niger | 1980 | | 610.284 | 1 | 0 | 1 |
| Nigeria | 1980 | | 603.78 | 1 | 1 | 1 |
| Rwanda | 1980 | | 598.111 | 1 | 1 | 1 |
| Sao Tome and Principe | 1980 | | 601.287 | 1 | 1 | 1 |
| Senegal | 1980 | | 611.16 | 1 | 1 | 1 |
| Seychelles | 1980 | | 615.749 | 1 | 1 | 1 |
| Sierra Leone | 1980 | | | | | |
| Somalia | 1980 | | 620.02 | 1 | 1 | 1 |
| South Africa | 1980 | | 623.282 | 1 | 1 | 1 |
| Sudan | 1980 | | 625.361 | 1 | 1 | 1 |
| Swaziland | 1980 | | 633.266 | 1 | 1 | 1 |
| Tanzania | 1980 | | 640.043 | 0 | 0 | 0 |
| Togo | 1980 | | 680.919 | 0 | 0 | 0 |
| Tunisia | 1980 | | 732.707 | 0 | 0 | 0 |
| Uganda | 1980 | | 745.228 | 0 | 0 | 0 |
| Zambia | 1980 | | 758.113 | 0 | 0 | 0 |
| Zimbabwe | 1980 | | 771.376 | 0 | 0 | 0 |
| Algeria | 1981 | | | | | |
| Angola | 1981 | | 788.898 | 0 | 0 | 0 |
| Benin | 1981 | | 807.056 | 0 | 0 | 0 |
| Botswana | 1981 | | 825.767 | 0 | 0 | 0 |

| *Country Name* | *Year* | *Education* | *Population Density* | *Minor War* | *Civil War* | *Conflict* |
|---|---|---|---|---|---|---|
| Burkina Faso | 1981 | | 845.006 | 0 | 0 | 0 |
| Burundi | 1981 | | 864.775 | 0 | 0 | 0 |
| Cabo Verde | 1981 | | 885.063 | 0 | 0 | 0 |
| Cameroon | 1981 | | 905.93 | 0 | 0 | 0 |
| Central African Republic | 1981 | | 927.409 | 0 | 0 | 0 |
| Chad | 1981 | | 949.542 | 0 | 0 | 0 |
| Comoros | 1981 | | 972.389 | 0 | 0 | 0 |
| Congo, Dem. Rep. | 1981 | | | | | |
| Congo, Rep. | 1981 | | 995.989 | 0 | 0 | 0 |
| Cote d'Ivoire | 1981 | | 1020.216 | 0 | 0 | 0 |
| Djibouti | 1981 | | 1051.003 | 0 | 0 | 0 |
| Egypt, Arab Rep. | 1981 | | 1084.455 | 0 | 0 | 0 |
| Equatorial Guinea | 1981 | | 1116.514 | 0 | 0 | 0 |
| Eritrea | 1981 | | 1143.328 | 0 | 0 | 0 |
| Ethiopia | 1981 | | 1166.256 | 0 | 0 | 0 |
| Gabon | 1981 | | 1194.113 | 0 | 0 | 0 |
| Gambia, The | 1981 | | 1222.239 | 1 | 1 | 1 |
| Ghana | 1981 | | 1250.409 | 1 | 1 | 1 |
| Guinea | 1981 | | | | | |
| Guinea-Bissau | 1981 | | 1278.859 | 0 | 0 | 0 |
| Kenya | 1981 | | 1306.455 | 0 | 0 | 0 |
| Lesotho | 1981 | | 1333.12 | 0 | 0 | 0 |
| Liberia | 1981 | | 1359.917 | 0 | 0 | 0 |
| Libya | 1981 | | 1386.926 | 0 | 0 | 0 |
| Madagascar | 1981 | | 1414.159 | 0 | 0 | 0 |
| Malawi | 1981 | | 1442.747 | 0 | 0 | 0 |
| Mali | 1981 | | 1472.78 | 0 | 0 | 0 |
| Mauritania | 1981 | | 1503 | 0 | 0 | 0 |
| Mauritius | 1981 | | 1534 | 0 | 0 | 0 |
| Morocco | 1981 | | | | | |
| Mozambique | 1981 | 1.523 | 8678.557 | 0 | 0 | 0 |
| Namibia | 1981 | 1.6145 | 8957.178 | 0 | 0 | 0 |
| Niger | 1981 | 1.66025 | 9247.518 | 0 | 0 | 0 |
| Nigeria | 1981 | 1.706 | 9549.179 | 0 | 0 | 0 |
| Rwanda | 1981 | 1.94 | 9863.639 | 0 | 0 | 0 |
| Sao Tome and Principe | 1981 | 2.057 | 10191.51 | 0 | 0 | 0 |
| Senegal | 1981 | 2.1155 | 10532.39 | 0 | 0 | 0 |
| Seychelles | 1981 | 2.14475 | 10887.93 | 0 | 0 | 0 |
| Sierra Leone | 1981 | 2.174 | 11247.18 | 0 | 0 | 0 |
| Somalia | 1981 | | | | | |
| South Africa | 1981 | 2.522 | 11633.03 | 0 | 0 | 0 |
| Sudan | 1981 | 2.696 | 12044.79 | 0 | 0 | 0 |
| Swaziland | 1981 | 2.783 | 12482.05 | 0 | 0 | 0 |
| Tanzania | 1981 | 2.8265 | 12944.29 | 0 | 0 | 0 |
| Togo | 1981 | 2.87 | 13433.41 | 0 | 0 | 0 |
| Tunisia | 1981 | 3.3285 | 13951.44 | 0 | 0 | 0 |
| Uganda | 1981 | 3.55775 | 14500.4 | 0 | 0 | 0 |

| *Country Name* | *Year* | *Education* | *Population Density* | *Minor War* | *Civil War* | *Conflict* |
|---|---|---|---|---|---|---|
| Zambia | 1981 | 3.672375 | 15079.69 | 0 | 0 | 0 |
| Zimbabwe | 1981 | 3.729688 | 15690.25 | 0 | 0 | 0 |
| Algeria | 1982 | | | | | |
| Angola | 1982 | 3.787 | 16330.54 | 0 | 0 | 0 |
| Benin | 1982 | 4.263 | 16987.23 | 0 | 0 | 0 |
| Botswana | 1982 | 4.501 | 17659.97 | 1 | 0 | 1 |
| Burkina Faso | 1982 | 4.62 | 18347.99 | 0 | 0 | 0 |
| Burundi | 1982 | 4.6795 | 19050.21 | 0 | 0 | 0 |
| Cabo Verde | 1982 | 4.739 | 19761.49 | 0 | 0 | 0 |
| Cameroon | 1982 | 5.1675 | 20477.12 | 0 | 0 | 0 |
| Central African Republic | 1982 | 5.38175 | 21195.78 | 0 | 0 | 0 |
| Chad | 1982 | 5.488875 | 21915.87 | 0 | 0 | 0 |
| Comoros | 1982 | 5.542438 | 22634.77 | 0 | 0 | 0 |
| Congo, Dem. Rep. | 1982 | | | | | |
| Congo, Rep. | 1982 | 5.596 | 23354.48 | 0 | 0 | 0 |
| Cote d'Ivoire | 1982 | 5.8795 | 24121.43 | 0 | 0 | 0 |
| Djibouti | 1982 | 6.02125 | 25018.97 | 0 | 0 | 0 |
| Egypt, Arab Rep. | 1982 | 6.092125 | 25817.55 | 0 | 0 | 0 |
| Equatorial Guinea | 1982 | 6.127563 | 26454.52 | 0 | 0 | 0 |
| Eritrea | 1982 | 6.163 | 27123.91 | 0 | 0 | 0 |
| Ethiopia | 1982 | 6.3935 | 27790.29 | 0 | 0 | 0 |
| Gabon | 1982 | 6.50875 | 28458.61 | 0 | 0 | 0 |
| Gambia, The | 1982 | 6.566375 | 29122.89 | 1 | 0 | 1 |
| Ghana | 1982 | 6.595188 | 29795.5 | 0 | 0 | 0 |
| Guinea | 1982 | 6.624 | 30507.98 | 0 | 0 | 0 |
| Guinea-Bissau | 1982 | | | | | |
| Kenya | 1982 | 6.8625 | 31298.7 | 0 | 0 | 0 |
| Lesotho | 1982 | 6.98175 | 32155.32 | 0 | 0 | 0 |
| Liberia | 1982 | 7.041375 | 33041.79 | 0 | 0 | 0 |
| Libya | 1982 | 7.071188 | 33967.09 | 0 | 0 | 0 |
| Madagascar | 1982 | 7.101 | 34911.78 | 0 | 0 | 0 |
| Malawi | 1982 | 7.203 | 35890.65 | 0 | 0 | 0 |
| Mali | 1982 | 7.254 | 36913.72 | 0 | 0 | 0 |
| Mauritania | 1982 | 7.2795 | 37954 | 0 | 0 | 0 |
| Mauritius | 1982 | 7.305 | 39003 | 0 | 0 | 0 |
| Morocco | 1982 | | | | | |
| Mozambique | 1982 | 2.954 | 893.143 | 0 | 0 | 0 |
| Namibia | 1982 | 3.0945 | 912.006 | 0 | 0 | 0 |
| Niger | 1982 | 3.16475 | 931.826 | 0 | 0 | 0 |
| Nigeria | 1982 | 3.235 | 952.459 | 0 | 0 | 0 |
| Rwanda | 1982 | 3.377 | 973.983 | 0 | 0 | 0 |
| Sao Tome and Principe | 1982 | 3.448 | 996.38 | 0 | 0 | 0 |
| Senegal | 1982 | 3.4835 | 1019.394 | 0 | 0 | 0 |
| Seychelles | 1982 | 3.50125 | 1043.044 | 0 | 0 | 0 |
| Sierra Leone | 1982 | | | | | |
| Somalia | 1982 | 3.519 | 1067.136 | 0 | 0 | 0 |
| South Africa | 1982 | 3.684 | 1091.675 | 0 | 0 | 0 |

| *Country Name* | *Year* | *Education* | *Population Density* | *Minor War* | *Civil War* | *Conflict* |
|---|---|---|---|---|---|---|
| Sudan | 1982 | 3.7665 | 1116.779 | 0 | 0 | 0 |
| Swaziland | 1982 | 3.80775 | 1142.46 | 0 | 0 | 0 |
| Tanzania | 1982 | 3.828375 | 1168.731 | 0 | 0 | 0 |
| Togo | 1982 | 3.849 | 1195.487 | 0 | 0 | 0 |
| Tunisia | 1982 | 4.0355 | 1222.874 | 0 | 0 | 0 |
| Uganda | 1982 | 4.12875 | 1251.669 | 0 | 0 | 0 |
| Zambia | 1982 | 4.175375 | 1281.575 | 0 | 0 | 0 |
| Zimbabwe | 1982 | 4.198688 | 1312.582 | 0 | 0 | 0 |
| Algeria | 1983 | | | | | |
| Angola | 1983 | 4.222 | 1344.719 | 0 | 0 | 0 |
| Benin | 1983 | 4.327 | 1377.963 | 0 | 0 | 0 |
| Botswana | 1983 | 4.3795 | 1412.338 | 0 | 0 | 0 |
| Burkina Faso | 1983 | 4.40575 | 1447.79 | 0 | 0 | 0 |
| Burundi | 1983 | 4.418875 | 1484.3 | 0 | 0 | 0 |
| Cabo Verde | 1983 | 4.432 | 1521.78 | 0 | 0 | 0 |
| Cameroon | 1983 | 4.5575 | 1560.198 | 0 | 0 | 0 |
| Central African Republic | 1983 | 4.62025 | 1599.409 | 0 | 0 | 0 |
| Chad | 1983 | 4.651625 | 1639.388 | 0 | 0 | 0 |
| Comoros | 1983 | 4.667313 | 1680.026 | 0 | 0 | 0 |
| Congo, Dem. Rep. | 1983 | | | | | |
| Congo, Rep. | 1983 | 4.683 | 1721.26 | 0 | 0 | 0 |
| Cote d'Ivoire | 1983 | 4.8745 | 1732 | 0 | 0 | 0 |
| Djibouti | 1983 | 4.97025 | 1762 | 0 | 0 | 0 |
| Egypt, Arab Rep. | 1983 | 5.018125 | 1791 | 0 | 0 | 0 |
| Equatorial Guinea | 1983 | 5.042063 | 1819 | 0 | 0 | 0 |
| Eritrea | 1983 | 5.066 | 1848 | 0 | 0 | 0 |
| Ethiopia | 1983 | 5.2745 | 1869 | 0 | 0 | 0 |
| Gabon | 1983 | 5.37875 | 1884 | 0 | 0 | 0 |
| Gambia, The | 1983 | 5.430875 | 1897 | 1 | 0 | 1 |
| Ghana | 1983 | 5.456938 | 1908 | 0 | 0 | 0 |
| Guinea | 1983 | | | | | |
| Guinea-Bissau | 1983 | 5.483 | 1916 | 0 | 0 | 0 |
| Kenya | 1983 | 5.763 | 1922 | 0 | 0 | 0 |
| Lesotho | 1983 | 5.903 | 1926 | 0 | 0 | 0 |
| Liberia | 1983 | 5.973 | 1926 | 0 | 0 | 0 |
| Libya | 1983 | 6.008 | 1925 | 0 | 0 | 0 |
| Madagascar | 1983 | 6.043 | 1922 | 0 | 0 | 0 |
| Malawi | 1983 | 6.3355 | 1919 | 0 | 0 | 0 |
| Mali | 1983 | 6.48175 | 1917 | 0 | 0 | 0 |
| Mauritania | 1983 | 6.554875 | 1915 | 0 | 0 | 0 |
| Mauritius | 1983 | 6.628 | 1910 | 0 | 0 | 0 |
| Morocco | 1983 | | | | | |
| Mozambique | 1983 | 0.726 | 1112.796 | 0 | 0 | 0 |
| Namibia | 1983 | 0.822 | 1143.525 | 0 | 0 | 0 |
| Niger | 1983 | 0.87 | 1175.491 | 0 | 0 | 0 |
| Nigeria | 1983 | 0.918 | 1208.749 | 0 | 0 | 0 |
| Rwanda | 1983 | 1.0275 | 1243.371 | 0 | 0 | 0 |

| Country Name | Year | Education | Population Density | Minor War | Civil War | Conflict |
|---|---|---|---|---|---|---|
| Sao Tome and Principe | 1983 | 1.08225 | 1279.406 | 0 | 0 | 0 |
| Senegal | 1983 | 1.109625 | 1316.907 | 0 | 0 | 0 |
| Seychelles | 1983 | 1.123313 | 1355.941 | 0 | 0 | 0 |
| Sierra Leone | 1983 | | | | | |
| Somalia | 1983 | 1.137 | 1396.565 | 0 | 0 | 0 |
| South Africa | 1983 | 1.3975 | 1438.78 | 0 | 0 | 0 |
| Sudan | 1983 | 1.52775 | 1482.628 | 0 | 0 | 0 |
| Swaziland | 1983 | 1.592875 | 1528.162 | 0 | 0 | 0 |
| Tanzania | 1983 | 1.625438 | 1575.442 | 0 | 0 | 0 |
| Togo | 1983 | 1.658 | 1616.234 | 0 | 0 | 0 |
| Tunisia | 1983 | 1.8975 | 1658.886 | 0 | 0 | 0 |
| Uganda | 1983 | 2.01725 | 1703.381 | 0 | 0 | 0 |
| Zambia | 1983 | 2.077125 | 1749.771 | 0 | 0 | 0 |
| Zimbabwe | 1983 | 2.107063 | 1798.208 | 0 | 0 | 0 |
| Algeria | 1984 | | | | | |
| Angola | 1984 | 2.137 | 1848.799 | 1 | 0 | 1 |
| Benin | 1984 | 2.364 | 1901.617 | 0 | 0 | 0 |
| Botswana | 1984 | 2.4775 | 1956.765 | 0 | 0 | 0 |
| Burkina Faso | 1984 | 2.53425 | 2014.325 | 0 | 0 | 0 |
| Burundi | 1984 | 2.562625 | 2074.345 | 0 | 0 | 0 |
| Cabo Verde | 1984 | 2.591 | 2136.87 | 0 | 0 | 0 |
| Cameroon | 1984 | 2.7485 | 2201.96 | 0 | 0 | 0 |
| Central African Republic | 1984 | 2.82725 | 2269.658 | 0 | 0 | 0 |
| Chad | 1984 | 2.866625 | 2339.986 | 0 | 0 | 0 |
| Comoros | 1984 | 2.886313 | 2412.781 | 1 | 1 | 1 |
| Congo, Dem. Rep. | 1984 | | | | | |
| Congo, Rep. | 1984 | 2.906 | 2117.239 | 0 | 1 | 1 |
| Cote d'Ivoire | 1984 | 2.9565 | 1817.358 | 1 | 1 | 1 |
| Djibouti | 1984 | 2.98175 | 1913.344 | 0 | 1 | 1 |
| Egypt, Arab Rep. | 1984 | 2.994375 | 1989.814 | 1 | 1 | 1 |
| Equatorial Guinea | 1984 | 3.000688 | 1974.381 | 1 | 1 | 1 |
| Eritrea | 1984 | 3.007 | 1975.252 | 1 | 1 | 1 |
| Ethiopia | 1984 | 3.2205 | 2025.646 | 0 | 0 | 0 |
| Gabon | 1984 | 3.32725 | 2201.269 | 0 | 0 | 0 |
| Gambia, The | 1984 | 3.380625 | 2455.863 | 0 | 0 | 0 |
| Ghana | 1984 | 3.407313 | 2598.615 | 0 | 0 | 0 |
| Guinea | 1984 | | | | | |
| Guinea-Bissau | 1984 | 3.434 | 2601 | 1 | 1 | 1 |
| Kenya | 1984 | 3.841 | 2680 | 1 | 1 | 1 |
| Lesotho | 1984 | 4.0445 | 2753 | 1 | 1 | 1 |
| Liberia | 1984 | 4.14625 | 2770 | 1 | 1 | 2 |
| Libya | 1984 | 4.197125 | 2796 | 0 | 0 | 0 |
| Madagascar | 1984 | 4.248 | 2930 | 0 | 0 | 0 |
| Malawi | 1984 | 4.8385 | 3108 | 0 | 0 | 0 |
| Mali | 1984 | 5.13375 | 3270 | 0 | 0 | 0 |
| Mauritania | 1984 | 5.281375 | 3440 | 0 | 0 | 0 |
| Mauritius | 1984 | 5.429 | 3583 | 0 | 0 | 0 |

| Country Name | Year | Education | Population Density | Minor War | Civil War | Conflict |
|---|---|---|---|---|---|---|
| Morocco | 1984 | | | | | |
| Mozambique | 1984 | 0.673 | 1441.863 | 0 | 0 | 0 |
| Namibia | 1984 | 0.8355 | 1498.607 | 0 | 0 | 0 |
| Niger | 1984 | 0.91675 | 1560.361 | 0 | 0 | 0 |
| Nigeria | 1984 | 0.998 | 1623.77 | 0 | 0 | 0 |
| Rwanda | 1984 | 1.254 | 1693.925 | 0 | 0 | 0 |
| Sao Tome and Principe | 1984 | 1.382 | 1759.224 | 0 | 0 | 0 |
| Senegal | 1984 | 1.446 | 1833.726 | 0 | 0 | 0 |
| Seychelles | 1984 | 1.478 | 1922.974 | 0 | 0 | 0 |
| Sierra Leone | 1984 | | | | | |
| Somalia | 1984 | 1.51 | 1999.162 | 0 | 0 | 0 |
| South Africa | 1984 | 1.852 | 2077.381 | 0 | 0 | 0 |
| Sudan | 1984 | 2.023 | 2183.877 | 0 | 0 | 0 |
| Swaziland | 1984 | 2.1085 | 2312.369 | 0 | 0 | 0 |
| Tanzania | 1984 | 2.15125 | 2451.375 | 0 | 0 | 0 |
| Togo | 1984 | 2.194 | 2569.606 | 0 | 0 | 0 |
| Tunisia | 1984 | 2.729 | 2666.16 | 0 | 0 | 0 |
| Uganda | 1984 | 2.9965 | 2721.783 | 0 | 0 | 0 |
| Zambia | 1984 | 3.13025 | 2796.747 | 0 | 0 | 0 |
| Zimbabwe | 1984 | 3.197125 | 2928.575 | 0 | 0 | 0 |
| Algeria | 1985 | | | | | |
| Angola | 1985 | 3.264 | 3065.365 | 0 | 0 | 0 |
| Benin | 1985 | 3.7085 | 3204.071 | 0 | 0 | 0 |
| Botswana | 1985 | 3.93075 | 3344.074 | 0 | 0 | 0 |
| Burkina Faso | 1985 | 4.041875 | 3484.531 | 0 | 0 | 0 |
| Burundi | 1985 | 4.097438 | 3624.92 | 0 | 0 | 0 |
| Cabo Verde | 1985 | 4.153 | 3675.422 | 0 | 0 | 0 |
| Cameroon | 1985 | 4.605 | 3699.538 | 0 | 0 | 0 |
| Central African Republic | 1985 | 4.831 | 3799.845 | 0 | 0 | 0 |
| Chad | 1985 | 4.944 | 3913.314 | 0 | 0 | 0 |
| Comoros | 1985 | 5.0005 | 4026.847 | 0 | 0 | 0 |
| Congo, Dem. Rep. | 1985 | | | | | |
| Congo, Rep. | 1985 | 5.057 | 4139.825 | 0 | 0 | 0 |
| Cote d'Ivoire | 1985 | 5.386 | 4252.354 | 0 | 0 | 0 |
| Djibouti | 1985 | 5.5505 | 4364.501 | 0 | 0 | 0 |
| Egypt, Arab Rep. | 1985 | 5.63275 | 4475.679 | 0 | 0 | 0 |
| Equatorial Guinea | 1985 | 5.673875 | 4585.017 | 0 | 0 | 0 |
| Eritrea | 1985 | 5.715 | 4654.252 | 0 | 0 | 0 |
| Ethiopia | 1985 | 6.1185 | 4686.329 | 0 | 0 | 0 |
| Gabon | 1985 | 6.32025 | 4759.67 | 0 | 0 | 0 |
| Gambia, The | 1985 | 6.421125 | 4874.638 | 0 | 0 | 0 |
| Ghana | 1985 | 6.471563 | 4993.414 | 0 | 0 | 0 |
| Guinea | 1985 | | | | | |
| Guinea-Bissau | 1985 | 6.522 | 5115.45 | 0 | 0 | 0 |
| Kenya | 1985 | 6.882 | 5240.599 | 0 | 0 | 0 |
| Lesotho | 1985 | 7.062 | 5368.585 | 0 | 0 | 0 |
| Liberia | 1985 | 7.152 | 5499.074 | 0 | 0 | 0 |

| *Country Name* | *Year* | *Education* | *Population Density* | *Minor War* | *Civil War* | *Conflict* |
|---|---|---|---|---|---|---|
| Libya | 1985 | 7.197 | 5631.585 | 0 | 0 | 0 |
| Madagascar | 1985 | 7.242 | 5765.563 | 0 | 0 | 0 |
| Malawi | 1985 | 7.5465 | 5900.754 | 0 | 0 | 0 |
| Mali | 1985 | 7.69875 | 6036.914 | 0 | 0 | 0 |
| Mauritania | 1985 | 7.774875 | 6187 | 0 | 0 | 0 |
| Mauritius | 1985 | 7.851 | 6324 | 0 | 0 | 0 |
| Morocco | 1985 | | | | | |
| Mozambique | 1985 | | 5703.324 | 0 | 0 | 0 |
| Namibia | 1985 | | 5821.158 | 0 | 0 | 0 |
| Niger | 1985 | | 5943.744 | 0 | 0 | 0 |
| Nigeria | 1985 | | 6070.004 | 0 | 0 | 0 |
| Rwanda | 1985 | | 6200 | 0 | 0 | 0 |
| Sao Tome and Principe | 1985 | | 6334.556 | 0 | 0 | 0 |
| Senegal | 1985 | | 6473.179 | 0 | 0 | 0 |
| Seychelles | 1985 | | 6615.873 | 0 | 0 | 0 |
| Sierra Leone | 1985 | | | | | |
| Somalia | 1985 | | 6765.644 | 0 | 0 | 0 |
| South Africa | 1985 | | 6920.494 | 1 | 0 | 1 |
| Sudan | 1985 | | 7082.43 | 0 | 0 | 0 |
| Swaziland | 1985 | | 7250.455 | 0 | 0 | 0 |
| Tanzania | 1985 | | 7423.573 | 0 | 0 | 0 |
| Togo | 1985 | | 7603.79 | 0 | 0 | 0 |
| Tunisia | 1985 | | 7807.4 | 0 | 0 | 0 |
| Uganda | 1985 | | 8011.695 | 0 | 0 | 0 |
| Zambia | 1985 | | 8224.285 | 0 | 0 | 0 |
| Zimbabwe | 1985 | | 8453.131 | 0 | 0 | 0 |
| Algeria | 1986 | | | | | |
| Angola | 1986 | | 8691.245 | 0 | 0 | 0 |
| Benin | 1986 | | 8938.764 | 0 | 0 | 0 |
| Botswana | 1986 | | 9195.873 | 0 | 0 | 0 |
| Burkina Faso | 1986 | | 9463.017 | 0 | 0 | 0 |
| Burundi | 1986 | | 9740.535 | 0 | 0 | 0 |
| Cabo Verde | 1986 | | 10028.63 | 0 | 0 | 0 |
| Cameroon | 1986 | | 10327.39 | 0 | 0 | 0 |
| Central African Republic | 1986 | | 10636.88 | 0 | 0 | 0 |
| Chad | 1986 | | 10957.34 | 0 | 0 | 0 |
| Comoros | 1986 | | 11289.16 | 0 | 0 | 0 |
| Congo, Dem. Rep. | 1986 | | | | | |
| Congo, Rep. | 1986 | | 11632.87 | 0 | 0 | 0 |
| Cote d'Ivoire | 1986 | | 11988.71 | 0 | 0 | 0 |
| Djibouti | 1986 | | 12356.68 | 0 | 0 | 0 |
| Egypt, Arab Rep. | 1986 | | 12736.61 | 0 | 0 | 0 |
| Equatorial Guinea | 1986 | | 13128.41 | 0 | 0 | 0 |
| Eritrea | 1986 | | 13532.36 | 0 | 0 | 0 |
| Ethiopia | 1986 | | 13948.48 | 0 | 0 | 0 |
| Gabon | 1986 | | 14376.6 | 0 | 0 | 0 |
| Gambia, The | 1986 | | 14816.58 | 0 | 0 | 0 |

| Country Name | Year | Education | Population Density | Minor War | Civil War | Conflict |
|---|---|---|---|---|---|---|
| Ghana | 1986 | | 15271.26 | 0 | 0 | 0 |
| Guinea | 1986 | | | | | |
| Guinea-Bissau | 1986 | | 15741.94 | 0 | 0 | 0 |
| Kenya | 1986 | | 16226.82 | 0 | 0 | 0 |
| Lesotho | 1986 | | 16725.89 | 0 | 0 | 0 |
| Liberia | 1986 | | 17239.52 | 0 | 0 | 0 |
| Libya | 1986 | | 17768.15 | 0 | 0 | 0 |
| Madagascar | 1986 | | 18312.16 | 0 | 0 | 0 |
| Malawi | 1986 | | 18872.16 | 0 | 0 | 0 |
| Mali | 1986 | | 19448.82 | 0 | 0 | 0 |
| Mauritania | 1986 | | 20043 | 0 | 0 | 0 |
| Mauritius | 1986 | | 20654 | 0 | 0 | 0 |
| Morocco | 1986 | | | | | |
| Mozambique | 1986 | 1.085 | 3628.608 | 0 | 0 | 0 |
| Namibia | 1986 | 1.147 | 3726.394 | 0 | 0 | 0 |
| Niger | 1986 | 1.178 | 3816.197 | 0 | 0 | 0 |
| Nigeria | 1986 | 1.209 | 3914.095 | 0 | 0 | 0 |
| Rwanda | 1986 | 1.3875 | 4023 | 0 | 0 | 0 |
| Sao Tome and Principe | 1986 | 1.47675 | 4151.575 | 0 | 0 | 0 |
| Senegal | 1986 | 1.521375 | 4272.708 | 0 | 0 | 0 |
| Seychelles | 1986 | 1.543688 | 4392.979 | 0 | 0 | 0 |
| Sierra Leone | 1986 | | | | | |
| Somalia | 1986 | 1.566 | 4508.062 | 0 | 0 | 0 |
| South Africa | 1986 | 1.715 | 4630.328 | 0 | 0 | 0 |
| Sudan | 1986 | 1.7895 | 4760.666 | 0 | 0 | 0 |
| Swaziland | 1986 | 1.82675 | 4900.549 | 0 | 0 | 0 |
| Tanzania | 1986 | 1.845375 | 5072.873 | 0 | 0 | 0 |
| Togo | 1986 | 1.864 | 5317.309 | 0 | 0 | 0 |
| Tunisia | 1986 | 2.0965 | 5530.771 | 0 | 0 | 0 |
| Uganda | 1986 | 2.21275 | 5702.228 | 0 | 0 | 0 |
| Zambia | 1986 | 2.270875 | 5880.328 | 0 | 0 | 0 |
| Zimbabwe | 1986 | 2.299938 | 6065.654 | 0 | 0 | 0 |
| Algeria | 1987 | | | | | |
| Angola | 1987 | 2.329 | 6258.512 | 0 | 0 | 0 |
| Benin | 1987 | 2.4905 | 6459.263 | 0 | 0 | 0 |
| Botswana | 1987 | 2.57125 | 6668.216 | 0 | 0 | 0 |
| Burkina Faso | 1987 | 2.611625 | 6883.756 | 0 | 0 | 0 |
| Burundi | 1987 | 2.631813 | 7104.46 | 0 | 0 | 0 |
| Cabo Verde | 1987 | 2.652 | 7330.508 | 0 | 0 | 0 |
| Cameroon | 1987 | 2.772 | 7608.484 | 0 | 0 | 0 |
| Central African Republic | 1987 | 2.832 | 8049.175 | 0 | 0 | 0 |
| Chad | 1987 | 2.862 | 8579.782 | 0 | 0 | 0 |
| Comoros | 1987 | 2.877 | 9082.018 | 0 | 0 | 0 |
| Congo, Dem. Rep. | 1987 | | | | | |
| Congo, Rep. | 1987 | 2.892 | 9536.25 | 0 | 0 | 0 |
| Cote d'Ivoire | 1987 | 2.977 | 9919.733 | 0 | 0 | 0 |
| Djibouti | 1987 | 3.0195 | 10294.08 | 0 | 0 | 0 |

| Country Name | Year | Education | Population Density | Minor War | Civil War | Conflict |
|---|---|---|---|---|---|---|
| Egypt, Arab Rep. | 1987 | 3.04075 | 10475.43 | 0 | 0 | 0 |
| Equatorial Guinea | 1987 | 3.051375 | 10296.32 | 0 | 0 | 0 |
| Eritrea | 1987 | 3.062 | 10223.55 | 0 | 0 | 0 |
| Ethiopia | 1987 | 3.2695 | 10458.52 | 0 | 0 | 0 |
| Gabon | 1987 | 3.37325 | 10735.43 | 0 | 0 | 0 |
| Gambia, The | 1987 | 3.425125 | 11010.64 | 0 | 0 | 0 |
| Ghana | 1987 | 3.451063 | 11285.57 | 0 | 0 | 0 |
| Guinea | 1987 | | | | | |
| Guinea-Bissau | 1987 | 3.477 | 11802 | 0 | 0 | 0 |
| Kenya | 1987 | 3.926 | 12129 | 0 | 0 | 0 |
| Lesotho | 1987 | 4.1505 | 12460 | 0 | 0 | 0 |
| Liberia | 1987 | 4.26275 | 12797 | 0 | 0 | 0 |
| Libya | 1987 | 4.318875 | 13140 | 0 | 0 | 0 |
| Madagascar | 1987 | 4.375 | 13492 | 0 | 0 | 0 |
| Malawi | 1987 | 4.5375 | 13856 | 0 | 0 | 0 |
| Mali | 1987 | 4.61875 | 14233 | 0 | 0 | 0 |
| Mauritania | 1987 | 4.659375 | 14624 | 0 | 0 | 0 |
| Mauritius | 1987 | 4.7 | 15029 | 0 | 0 | 0 |
| Morocco | 1987 | | | | | |
| Mozambique | 1987 | 0.191 | 4678.528 | 0 | 0 | 0 |
| Namibia | 1987 | 0.2135 | 4774.976 | 0 | 0 | 0 |
| Niger | 1987 | 0.22475 | 4874.607 | 0 | 0 | 0 |
| Nigeria | 1987 | 0.236 | 4977.536 | 0 | 0 | 0 |
| Rwanda | 1987 | 0.2625 | 5083.886 | 0 | 0 | 0 |
| Sao Tome and Principe | 1987 | 0.27575 | 5193.779 | 0 | 0 | 0 |
| Senegal | 1987 | 0.282375 | 5307.348 | 0 | 0 | 0 |
| Seychelles | 1987 | 0.285688 | 5424.728 | 0 | 0 | 0 |
| Sierra Leone | 1987 | | | | | |
| Somalia | 1987 | 0.289 | 5546.065 | 0 | 0 | 0 |
| South Africa | 1987 | 0.368 | 5671.505 | 0 | 0 | 0 |
| Sudan | 1987 | 0.4075 | 5801.204 | 0 | 0 | 0 |
| Swaziland | 1987 | 0.42725 | 5935.323 | 0 | 0 | 0 |
| Tanzania | 1987 | 0.437125 | 6074.032 | 0 | 0 | 0 |
| Togo | 1987 | 0.447 | 6217.503 | 0 | 0 | 0 |
| Tunisia | 1987 | 0.531 | 6365.926 | 0 | 0 | 0 |
| Uganda | 1987 | 0.573 | 6454.823 | 0 | 0 | 0 |
| Zambia | 1987 | 0.594 | 6550.2 | 0 | 0 | 0 |
| Zimbabwe | 1987 | 0.6045 | 6651.246 | 0 | 0 | 0 |
| Algeria | 1988 | | | | | |
| Angola | 1988 | 0.615 | 6758.153 | 0 | 0 | 0 |
| Benin | 1988 | 0.696 | 6871.186 | 0 | 0 | 0 |
| Botswana | 1988 | 0.7365 | 6988.555 | 0 | 0 | 0 |
| Burkina Faso | 1988 | 0.75675 | 7108.978 | 0 | 0 | 0 |
| Burundi | 1988 | 0.766875 | 7233.025 | 0 | 0 | 0 |
| Cabo Verde | 1988 | 0.777 | 7361.326 | 0 | 0 | 0 |
| Cameroon | 1988 | 0.839 | 7494.408 | 0 | 0 | 0 |
| Central African Republic | 1988 | 0.87 | 7632.679 | 0 | 0 | 0 |

| Country Name | Year | Education | Population Density | Minor War | Civil War | Conflict |
|---|---|---|---|---|---|---|
| Chad | 1988 | 0.8855 | 7777.037 | 0 | 0 | 0 |
| Comoros | 1988 | 0.89325 | 7927.759 | 0 | 0 | 0 |
| Congo, Dem. Rep. | 1988 | | | | | |
| Congo, Rep. | 1988 | 0.901 | 8084.632 | 1 | 0 | 1 |
| Cote d'Ivoire | 1988 | 0.9615 | 8248.008 | 0 | 0 | 0 |
| Djibouti | 1988 | 0.99175 | 8417.713 | 0 | 0 | 0 |
| Egypt, Arab Rep. | 1988 | 1.006875 | 8593.64 | 0 | 0 | 0 |
| Equatorial Guinea | 1988 | 1.014438 | 8776.266 | 1 | 0 | 1 |
| Eritrea | 1988 | 1.022 | 8966.35 | 0 | 0 | 0 |
| Ethiopia | 1988 | 1.1145 | 9165.475 | 0 | 0 | 0 |
| Gabon | 1988 | 1.16075 | 9372.774 | 0 | 0 | 0 |
| Gambia, The | 1988 | 1.183875 | 9588.701 | 0 | 0 | 0 |
| Ghana | 1988 | 1.195438 | 9813.715 | 0 | 0 | 0 |
| Guinea | 1988 | | | | | |
| Guinea-Bissau | 1988 | 1.207 | 10621 | 0 | 0 | 0 |
| Kenya | 1988 | 1.3755 | 10918 | 0 | 0 | 0 |
| Lesotho | 1988 | 1.45975 | 11220 | 0 | 0 | 0 |
| Liberia | 1988 | 1.501875 | 11523 | 0 | 0 | 0 |
| Libya | 1988 | 1.522938 | 11827 | 0 | 0 | 0 |
| Madagascar | 1988 | 1.544 | 12134 | 0 | 0 | 0 |
| Malawi | 1988 | 1.7885 | 12447 | 0 | 0 | 0 |
| Mali | 1988 | 1.91075 | 12769 | 1 | 0 | 1 |
| Mauritania | 1988 | 1.971875 | 13101 | 1 | 0 | 1 |
| Mauritius | 1988 | 2.033 | 13443 | 0 | 0 | 0 |
| Morocco | 1988 | | | | | |
| Mozambique | 1988 | 1.545 | 1146.757 | 0 | 0 | 0 |
| Namibia | 1988 | 1.577 | 1162.199 | 0 | 0 | 0 |
| Niger | 1988 | 1.593 | 1178.277 | 0 | 0 | 0 |
| Nigeria | 1988 | 1.609 | 1195.012 | 0 | 0 | 0 |
| Rwanda | 1988 | 1.6665 | 1212.426 | 0 | 0 | 0 |
| Sao Tome and Principe | 1988 | 1.69525 | 1230.542 | 0 | 0 | 0 |
| Senegal | 1988 | 1.709625 | 1249.383 | 0 | 0 | 0 |
| Seychelles | 1988 | 1.716813 | 1269 | 0 | 0 | 0 |
| Sierra Leone | 1988 | | | | | |
| Somalia | 1988 | 1.724 | 1289.42 | 0 | 0 | 0 |
| South Africa | 1988 | 1.786 | 1310.672 | 0 | 0 | 0 |
| Sudan | 1988 | 1.817 | 1332.786 | 0 | 0 | 0 |
| Swaziland | 1988 | 1.8325 | 1355.793 | 0 | 0 | 0 |
| Tanzania | 1988 | 1.84025 | 1379.655 | 0 | 0 | 0 |
| Togo | 1988 | 1.848 | 1404.403 | 1 | 0 | 0 |
| Tunisia | 1988 | 2.0005 | 1430.069 | 1 | 0 | 0 |
| Uganda | 1988 | 2.07675 | 1455.644 | 1 | 0 | 0 |
| Zambia | 1988 | 2.114875 | 1483.992 | 1 | 0 | 0 |
| Zimbabwe | 1988 | 2.133938 | 1513.703 | 0 | 0 | 0 |
| Algeria | 1989 | | | | | |
| Angola | 1989 | 2.153 | 1544.909 | 0 | 0 | 0 |
| Benin | 1989 | 2.2995 | 1577.646 | 0 | 0 | 0 |

| Country Name | Year | Education | Population Density | Minor War | Civil War | Conflict |
|---|---|---|---|---|---|---|
| Botswana | 1989 | 2.37275 | 1611.888 | 0 | 0 | 0 |
| Burkina Faso | 1989 | 2.409375 | 1647.586 | 0 | 0 | 0 |
| Burundi | 1989 | 2.427688 | 1684.77 | 0 | 0 | 0 |
| Cabo Verde | 1989 | 2.446 | 1723.466 | 0 | 0 | 0 |
| Cameroon | 1989 | 2.5945 | 1763.68 | 0 | 0 | 0 |
| Central African Republic | 1989 | 2.66875 | 1805.394 | 0 | 0 | 0 |
| Chad | 1989 | 2.705875 | 1848.504 | 0 | 0 | 0 |
| Comoros | 1989 | 2.724438 | 1885.828 | 0 | 0 | 0 |
| Congo, Dem. Rep. | 1989 | | | | | |
| Congo, Rep. | 1989 | 2.743 | 1924.978 | 0 | 0 | 0 |
| Cote d'Ivoire | 1989 | 2.9245 | 1973.43 | 0 | 0 | 0 |
| Djibouti | 1989 | 3.01525 | 2042.816 | 0 | 0 | 0 |
| Egypt, Arab Rep. | 1989 | 3.060625 | 2119.242 | 0 | 0 | 0 |
| Equatorial Guinea | 1989 | 3.083313 | 2183.335 | 0 | 0 | 0 |
| Eritrea | 1989 | 3.106 | 2234.79 | 0 | 0 | 0 |
| Ethiopia | 1989 | 3.3145 | 2270.682 | 0 | 0 | 0 |
| Gabon | 1989 | 3.41875 | 2315.223 | 0 | 0 | 0 |
| Gambia, The | 1989 | 3.470875 | 2374.103 | 0 | 0 | 0 |
| Ghana | 1989 | 3.496938 | 2436.909 | 0 | 0 | 0 |
| Guinea | 1989 | | | | | |
| Guinea-Bissau | 1989 | 3.523 | 2500.867 | 0 | 0 | 0 |
| Kenya | 1989 | 3.799 | 2565.791 | 0 | 0 | 0 |
| Lesotho | 1989 | 3.937 | 2631.845 | 0 | 0 | 0 |
| Liberia | 1989 | 4.006 | 2699.242 | 0 | 0 | 0 |
| Libya | 1989 | 4.0405 | 2767.954 | 0 | 0 | 0 |
| Madagascar | 1989 | 4.075 | 2837.937 | 0 | 0 | 0 |
| Malawi | 1989 | 4.3455 | 2909.101 | 0 | 0 | 0 |
| Mali | 1989 | 4.48075 | 2981.452 | 0 | 0 | 0 |
| Mauritania | 1989 | 4.548375 | 3055 | 0 | 0 | 0 |
| Mauritius | 1989 | 4.616 | 3129 | 0 | 0 | 0 |
| Morocco | 1989 | | | | | |
| Mozambique | 1989 | 3.533 | 701.016 | 0 | 0 | 0 |
| Namibia | 1989 | 3.89 | 715.14 | 0 | 0 | 0 |
| Niger | 1989 | 4.0685 | 736.182 | 0 | 0 | 0 |
| Nigeria | 1989 | 4.247 | 755.528 | 0 | 0 | 0 |
| Rwanda | 1989 | 4.5775 | 774.16 | 0 | 0 | 0 |
| Sao Tome and Principe | 1989 | 4.74275 | 789.309 | 0 | 0 | 0 |
| Senegal | 1989 | 4.825375 | 804.177 | 0 | 0 | 0 |
| Seychelles | 1989 | 4.866688 | 816.027 | 0 | 0 | 0 |
| Sierra Leone | 1989 | | | | | |
| Somalia | 1989 | 4.908 | 829.511 | 0 | 0 | 0 |
| South Africa | 1989 | 4.9835 | 841.079 | 0 | 0 | 0 |
| Sudan | 1989 | 5.02125 | 851.334 | 0 | 0 | 0 |
| Swaziland | 1989 | 5.040125 | 861.239 | 0 | 0 | 0 |
| Tanzania | 1989 | 5.049563 | 873.292 | 0 | 0 | 0 |
| Togo | 1989 | 5.059 | 885.461 | 0 | 0 | 0 |
| Tunisia | 1989 | 5.2035 | 897.811 | 0 | 0 | 0 |

| Country Name | Year | Education | Population Density | Minor War | Civil War | Conflict |
|---|---|---|---|---|---|---|
| Uganda | 1989 | 5.27575 | 913.025 | 0 | 0 | 0 |
| Zambia | 1989 | 5.311875 | 929.367 | 0 | 0 | 0 |
| Zimbabwe | 1989 | 5.329938 | 946.64 | 0 | 0 | 0 |
| Algeria | 1990 | | | | | |
| Angola | 1990 | 5.348 | 963.701 | 0 | 0 | 0 |
| Benin | 1990 | 5.598 | 979.05 | 0 | 0 | 0 |
| Botswana | 1990 | 5.723 | 992.04 | 0 | 0 | 0 |
| Burkina Faso | 1990 | 5.7855 | 1002.175 | 0 | 0 | 0 |
| Burundi | 1990 | 5.81675 | 1012.042 | 0 | 0 | 0 |
| Cabo Verde | 1990 | 5.848 | 1020.544 | 0 | 0 | 0 |
| Cameroon | 1990 | 6.1715 | 1028.233 | 0 | 0 | 0 |
| Central African Republic | 1990 | 6.33325 | 1036.272 | 0 | 0 | 0 |
| Chad | 1990 | 6.414125 | 1044.942 | 0 | 0 | 0 |
| Comoros | 1990 | 6.454563 | 1053.403 | 0 | 0 | 0 |
| Congo, Dem. Rep. | 1990 | | | | | |
| Congo, Rep. | 1990 | 6.495 | 1061.598 | 0 | 0 | 0 |
| Cote d'Ivoire | 1990 | 6.6525 | 1071.723 | 0 | 0 | 0 |
| Djibouti | 1990 | 6.73125 | 1084.809 | 0 | 0 | 0 |
| Egypt, Arab Rep. | 1990 | 6.770625 | 1098.641 | 0 | 0 | 0 |
| Equatorial Guinea | 1990 | 6.790313 | 1111.297 | 0 | 0 | 0 |
| Eritrea | 1990 | 6.81 | 1123.115 | 0 | 0 | 0 |
| Ethiopia | 1990 | 6.7565 | 1135.344 | 0 | 0 | 0 |
| Gabon | 1990 | 6.72975 | 1148.35 | 0 | 0 | 0 |
| Gambia, The | 1990 | 6.716375 | 1160.659 | 0 | 0 | 0 |
| Ghana | 1990 | 6.709688 | 1173.129 | 0 | 0 | 0 |
| Guinea | 1990 | | | | | |
| Guinea-Bissau | 1990 | 6.703 | 1185.932 | 0 | 0 | 0 |
| Kenya | 1990 | 7.014 | 1197.878 | 0 | 0 | 0 |
| Lesotho | 1990 | 7.1695 | 1209.59 | 0 | 0 | 0 |
| Liberia | 1990 | 7.24725 | 1221.004 | 0 | 0 | 0 |
| Libya | 1990 | 7.286125 | 1232.059 | 0 | 0 | 0 |
| Madagascar | 1990 | 7.325 | 1242.821 | 0 | 0 | 0 |
| Malawi | 1990 | 7.606 | 1253.425 | 0 | 0 | 0 |
| Mali | 1990 | 7.7465 | 1263.899 | 0 | 0 | 0 |
| Mauritania | 1990 | 7.81675 | 1274 | 0 | 0 | 0 |
| Mauritius | 1990 | 7.887 | 1284 | 0 | 0 | 0 |
| Morocco | 1990 | | | | | |
| Mozambique | 1990 | 0.472 | 13056.6 | 0 | 0 | 0 |
| Namibia | 1990 | 0.58 | 13385.36 | 0 | 0 | 0 |
| Niger | 1990 | 0.634 | 13722.48 | 0 | 0 | 0 |
| Nigeria | 1990 | 0.688 | 14066.15 | 0 | 0 | 0 |
| Rwanda | 1990 | 0.8365 | 14414.64 | 0 | 0 | 0 |
| Sao Tome and Principe | 1990 | 0.91075 | 14770.3 | 0 | 0 | 0 |
| Senegal | 1990 | 0.947875 | 15137.27 | 0 | 0 | 0 |
| Seychelles | 1990 | 0.966438 | 15517.16 | 0 | 0 | 0 |
| Sierra Leone | 1990 | | | | | |
| Somalia | 1990 | 0.985 | 15909.28 | 0 | 0 | 0 |

| *Country Name* | *Year* | *Education* | *Population Density* | *Minor War* | *Civil War* | *Conflict* |
|---|---|---|---|---|---|---|
| South Africa | 1990 | 1.176 | 16313.39 | 1 | 0 | 1 |
| Sudan | 1990 | 1.2715 | 16660.67 | 0 | 0 | 0 |
| Swaziland | 1990 | 1.31925 | 16998.38 | 0 | 0 | 0 |
| Tanzania | 1990 | 1.343125 | 17335.24 | 0 | 0 | 0 |
| Togo | 1990 | 1.367 | 17687.38 | 1 | 0 | 1 |
| Tunisia | 1990 | 1.58 | 18042.96 | 1 | 0 | 1 |
| Uganda | 1990 | 1.6865 | 18396.94 | 1 | 0 | 1 |
| Zambia | 1990 | 1.73975 | 18758.28 | 1 | 0 | 1 |
| Zimbabwe | 1990 | 1.766375 | 19125.96 | 1 | 0 | 1 |
| Algeria | 1991 | | | | | |
| Angola | 1991 | 1.793 | 19487.27 | 1 | 0 | 1 |
| Benin | 1991 | 2.062 | 19846.22 | 1 | 1 | 1 |
| Botswana | 1991 | 2.1965 | 20198.73 | 1 | 1 | 1 |
| Burkina Faso | 1991 | 2.26375 | 20750.25 | 1 | 1 | 1 |
| Burundi | 1991 | 2.297375 | 21315.51 | 1 | 1 | 1 |
| Cabo Verde | 1991 | 2.331 | 21885.9 | 1 | 1 | 1 |
| Cameroon | 1991 | 2.6195 | 22457.81 | 1 | 1 | 1 |
| Central African Republic | 1991 | 2.76375 | 23029.46 | 1 | 1 | 1 |
| Chad | 1991 | 2.835875 | 23600.5 | 1 | 1 | 1 |
| Comoros | 1991 | 2.871938 | 24169.81 | 1 | 1 | 1 |
| Congo, Dem. Rep. | 1991 | | | | | |
| Congo, Rep. | 1991 | 2.908 | 24734.81 | 0 | 0 | 0 |
| Cote d'Ivoire | 1991 | 3.1805 | 24434 | 0 | 0 | 0 |
| Djibouti | 1991 | 3.31675 | 24861 | 0 | 0 | 0 |
| Egypt, Arab Rep. | 1991 | 3.384875 | 25293 | 0 | 0 | 0 |
| Equatorial Guinea | 1991 | 3.418938 | 25723 | 0 | 0 | 0 |
| Eritrea | 1991 | 3.453 | 26148 | 0 | 0 | 0 |
| Ethiopia | 1991 | 3.674 | 26564 | 0 | 0 | 0 |
| Gabon | 1991 | 3.7845 | 26969 | 0 | 0 | 0 |
| Gambia, The | 1991 | 3.83975 | 27361 | 0 | 0 | 0 |
| Ghana | 1991 | 3.867375 | 27742 | 0 | 0 | 0 |
| Guinea | 1991 | | | | | |
| Guinea-Bissau | 1991 | 3.895 | 28113 | 0 | 0 | 0 |
| Kenya | 1991 | 4.1505 | 28477 | 0 | 0 | 0 |
| Lesotho | 1991 | 4.27825 | 28839 | 0 | 0 | 0 |
| Liberia | 1991 | 4.342125 | 29197 | 0 | 0 | 0 |
| Libya | 1991 | 4.374063 | 29552 | 0 | 0 | 0 |
| Madagascar | 1991 | 4.406 | 29901 | 0 | 0 | 0 |
| Malawi | 1991 | 4.705 | 30248 | 0 | 0 | 0 |
| Mali | 1991 | 4.8545 | 30594 | 0 | 0 | 0 |
| Mauritania | 1991 | 4.92925 | 30940 | 0 | 0 | 0 |
| Mauritius | 1991 | 5.004 | 31280 | 0 | 0 | 0 |
| Morocco | 1991 | | | | | |
| Mozambique | 1991 | 0.835 | 7788.944 | 0 | 0 | 0 |
| Namibia | 1991 | 0.9165 | 7957.01 | 0 | 0 | 0 |
| Niger | 1991 | 0.95725 | 8127.242 | 1 | 0 | 1 |
| Nigeria | 1991 | 0.998 | 8301.446 | 1 | 0 | 1 |

| Country Name | Year | Education | Population Density | Minor War | Civil War | Conflict |
|---|---|---|---|---|---|---|
| Rwanda | 1991 | 1.0005 | 8486.381 | 1 | 1 | 1 |
| Sao Tome and Principe | 1991 | 1.00175 | 8680.909 | 1 | 1 | 1 |
| Senegal | 1991 | 1.002375 | 8883.626 | 1 | 1 | 1 |
| Seychelles | 1991 | 1.002688 | 9092.797 | 1 | 1 | 1 |
| Sierra Leone | 1991 | | | | | |
| Somalia | 1991 | 1.003 | 9304.375 | 1 | 1 | 1 |
| South Africa | 1991 | 0.975 | 9539.059 | 1 | 1 | 1 |
| Sudan | 1991 | 0.961 | 9809.596 | 0 | 1 | 1 |
| Swaziland | 1991 | 0.954 | 10087.92 | 0 | 1 | 1 |
| Tanzania | 1991 | 0.47525 | 10370.28 | 1 | 1 | 1 |
| Togo | 1991 | 0.947 | 10432.6 | 1 | 0 | 1 |
| Tunisia | 1991 | 1.033 | 10769.65 | 1 | 0 | 1 |
| Uganda | 1991 | 1.076 | 11127.87 | 1 | 0 | 1 |
| Zambia | 1991 | 1.0975 | 11466.48 | 1 | 0 | 1 |
| Zimbabwe | 1991 | 1.10825 | 11828.03 | 1 | 1 | 1 |
| Algeria | 1992 | | | | | |
| Angola | 1992 | 1.119 | 12102.62 | 1 | 1 | 1 |
| Benin | 1992 | 1.1405 | 12363.23 | 0 | 1 | 1 |
| Botswana | 1992 | 1.15125 | 12587.33 | 0 | 1 | 1 |
| Burkina Faso | 1992 | 1.156625 | 12772.84 | 0 | 1 | 1 |
| Burundi | 1992 | 1.159313 | 12922.82 | 0 | 1 | 1 |
| Cabo Verde | 1992 | 1.162 | 13062.6 | 0 | 1 | 1 |
| Cameroon | 1992 | 1.08 | 13143.02 | 0 | 1 | 1 |
| Central African Republic | 1992 | 1.039 | 12894.85 | 0 | 1 | 1 |
| Chad | 1992 | 1.0185 | 12523.01 | 0 | 1 | 1 |
| Comoros | 1992 | 1.00825 | 12482.1 | 0 | 1 | 1 |
| Congo, Dem. Rep. | 1992 | | | | | |
| Congo, Rep. | 1992 | 0.998 | 12666.57 | 0 | 1 | 1 |
| Cote d'Ivoire | 1992 | 0.9615 | 12934.8 | 0 | 1 | 1 |
| Djibouti | 1992 | 0.94325 | 13180 | 1 | 1 | 1 |
| Egypt, Arab Rep. | 1992 | 0.934125 | 13691.37 | 0 | 0 | 0 |
| Equatorial Guinea | 1992 | 0.929563 | 14781.46 | 0 | 0 | 0 |
| Eritrea | 1992 | 0.925 | 15764.75 | 0 | 0 | 0 |
| Ethiopia | 1992 | 0.9875 | 16298.34 | 0 | 0 | 0 |
| Gabon | 1992 | 1.01875 | 16759.66 | 0 | 0 | 0 |
| Gambia, The | 1992 | 1.034375 | 17220.03 | 0 | 0 | 0 |
| Ghana | 1992 | 1.042188 | 17676.73 | 0 | 0 | 0 |
| Guinea | 1992 | | | | | |
| Guinea-Bissau | 1992 | 1.05 | 18124.56 | 0 | 0 | 0 |
| Kenya | 1992 | 1.1445 | 18559.16 | 0 | 0 | 0 |
| Lesotho | 1992 | 1.19175 | 18979.17 | 0 | 0 | 0 |
| Liberia | 1992 | 1.215375 | 19383.08 | 0 | 0 | 0 |
| Libya | 1992 | 1.227188 | 19772.84 | 0 | 0 | 0 |
| Madagascar | 1992 | 1.239 | 20154.01 | 0 | 0 | 0 |
| Malawi | 1992 | 1.497 | 20530.02 | 0 | 0 | 0 |
| Mali | 1992 | 1.626 | 20905.59 | 0 | 0 | 0 |
| Mauritania | 1992 | 1.6905 | 21439 | 0 | 0 | 0 |

| *Country Name* | *Year* | *Education* | *Population Density* | *Minor War* | *Civil War* | *Conflict* |
|---|---|---|---|---|---|---|
| Mauritius | 1992 | 1.755 | 21922 | 0 | 0 | 0 |
| Morocco | 1992 | | | | | |
| Mozambique | 1992 | 3.049 | 621.392 | 0 | 0 | 0 |
| Namibia | 1992 | 3.2515 | 637.428 | 0 | 0 | 0 |
| Niger | 1992 | 3.35275 | 653.95 | 0 | 0 | 0 |
| Nigeria | 1992 | 3.454 | 670.981 | 0 | 0 | 0 |
| Rwanda | 1992 | 3.7155 | 688.539 | 0 | 0 | 0 |
| Sao Tome and Principe | 1992 | 3.84625 | 706.64 | 0 | 0 | 0 |
| Senegal | 1992 | 3.911625 | 725.304 | 0 | 0 | 0 |
| Seychelles | 1992 | 3.944313 | 744.618 | 0 | 0 | 0 |
| Sierra Leone | 1992 | | | | | |
| Somalia | 1992 | 3.977 | 764.683 | 0 | 0 | 0 |
| South Africa | 1992 | 4.23 | 792.629 | 0 | 0 | 0 |
| Sudan | 1992 | 4.3565 | 821.782 | 0 | 0 | 0 |
| Swaziland | 1992 | 4.41975 | 851.258 | 0 | 0 | 0 |
| Tanzania | 1992 | 4.451375 | 882.005 | 0 | 0 | 0 |
| Togo | 1992 | 4.483 | 915.325 | 0 | 0 | 0 |
| Tunisia | 1992 | 4.753 | 950.488 | 0 | 0 | 0 |
| Uganda | 1992 | 4.888 | 977.026 | 0 | 0 | 0 |
| Zambia | 1992 | 4.9555 | 997.913 | 0 | 0 | 0 |
| Zimbabwe | 1992 | 4.98925 | 1027.78 | 0 | 0 | 0 |
| Algeria | 1993 | | | | | |
| Angola | 1993 | 5.023 | 1058.021 | 0 | 0 | 0 |
| Benin | 1993 | 5.3245 | 1074.493 | 0 | 0 | 0 |
| Botswana | 1993 | 5.47525 | 1099.174 | 0 | 0 | 0 |
| Burkina Faso | 1993 | 5.550625 | 1134.308 | 0 | 0 | 0 |
| Burundi | 1993 | 5.588313 | 1169.498 | 0 | 0 | 0 |
| Cabo Verde | 1993 | 5.626 | 1204.172 | 0 | 0 | 0 |
| Cameroon | 1993 | 5.8855 | 1240.345 | 0 | 0 | 0 |
| Central African Republic | 1993 | 6.01525 | 1278.282 | 0 | 0 | 0 |
| Chad | 1993 | 6.080125 | 1332.831 | 0 | 0 | 0 |
| Comoros | 1993 | 6.112563 | 1408.635 | 0 | 0 | 0 |
| Congo, Dem. Rep. | 1993 | | | | | |
| Congo, Rep. | 1993 | 6.145 | 1470.569 | 0 | 0 | 0 |
| Cote d'Ivoire | 1993 | 6.1015 | 1511.991 | 0 | 0 | 0 |
| Djibouti | 1993 | 6.07975 | 1552.502 | 0 | 0 | 0 |
| Egypt, Arab Rep. | 1993 | 6.068875 | 1595.138 | 0 | 0 | 0 |
| Equatorial Guinea | 1993 | 6.063438 | 1638.327 | 0 | 0 | 0 |
| Eritrea | 1993 | 6.058 | 1681.478 | 0 | 0 | 0 |
| Ethiopia | 1993 | 5.887 | 1724.32 | 0 | 0 | 0 |
| Gabon | 1993 | 5.8015 | 1766.142 | 0 | 0 | 0 |
| Gambia, The | 1993 | 5.75875 | 1806.532 | 0 | 0 | 0 |
| Ghana | 1993 | 5.737375 | 1846.699 | 0 | 0 | 0 |
| Guinea | 1993 | | | | | |
| Guinea-Bissau | 1993 | 5.716 | 1893.442 | 0 | 0 | 0 |
| Kenya | 1993 | 5.7875 | 1935.098 | 0 | 0 | 0 |
| Lesotho | 1993 | 5.82325 | 1960.672 | 0 | 0 | 0 |

| Country Name | Year | Education | Population Density | Minor War | Civil War | Conflict |
|---|---|---|---|---|---|---|
| Liberia | 1993 | 5.841125 | 1983.43 | 0 | 0 | 0 |
| Libya | 1993 | 5.850063 | 2006.646 | 0 | 0 | 0 |
| Madagascar | 1993 | 5.859 | 2028.356 | 0 | 0 | 0 |
| Malawi | 1993 | 5.909 | 2049.149 | 0 | 0 | 0 |
| Mali | 1993 | 5.934 | 2069.028 | 0 | 0 | 0 |
| Mauritania | 1993 | 5.9465 | 2089 | 0 | 0 | 0 |
| Mauritius | 1993 | 5.959 | 2109 | 0 | 0 | 0 |
| Morocco | 1993 | | | | | |
| Mozambique | 1993 | 0.379 | 4076.008 | 0 | 0 | 0 |
| Namibia | 1993 | 0.391 | 4162.926 | 0 | 0 | 0 |
| Niger | 1993 | 0.397 | 4252.122 | 0 | 0 | 0 |
| Nigeria | 1993 | 0.403 | 4343.664 | 0 | 0 | 0 |
| Rwanda | 1993 | 0.424 | 4437.62 | 0 | 0 | 0 |
| Sao Tome and Principe | 1993 | 0.4345 | 4534.062 | 0 | 0 | 0 |
| Senegal | 1993 | 0.43975 | 4633.063 | 0 | 0 | 0 |
| Seychelles | 1993 | 0.442375 | 4735.173 | 0 | 0 | 0 |
| Sierra Leone | 1993 | | | | | |
| Somalia | 1993 | 0.445 | 4840.501 | 0 | 0 | 0 |
| South Africa | 1993 | 0.4825 | 4948.667 | 0 | 0 | 0 |
| Sudan | 1993 | 0.50125 | 5060.262 | 0 | 0 | 0 |
| Swaziland | 1993 | 0.510625 | 5175.408 | 0 | 0 | 0 |
| Tanzania | 1993 | 0.515313 | 5294.763 | 0 | 0 | 0 |
| Togo | 1993 | 0.52 | 5419.038 | 0 | 0 | 0 |
| Tunisia | 1993 | 0.5835 | 5547.894 | 0 | 0 | 0 |
| Uganda | 1993 | 0.61525 | 5682.086 | 0 | 0 | 0 |
| Zambia | 1993 | 0.631125 | 5815.607 | 0 | 0 | 0 |
| Zimbabwe | 1993 | 0.639063 | 5952.447 | 0 | 0 | 0 |
| Algeria | 1994 | | | | | |
| Angola | 1994 | 0.647 | 6093.469 | 0 | 0 | 0 |
| Benin | 1994 | 0.734 | 6238.998 | 0 | 0 | 0 |
| Botswana | 1994 | 0.7775 | 6389.183 | 0 | 0 | 0 |
| Burkina Faso | 1994 | 0.79925 | 6544.13 | 0 | 0 | 0 |
| Burundi | 1994 | 0.810125 | 6704.046 | 0 | 0 | 0 |
| Cabo Verde | 1994 | 0.821 | 6869.209 | 0 | 0 | 0 |
| Cameroon | 1994 | 0.9245 | 7039.813 | 0 | 0 | 0 |
| Central African Republic | 1994 | 0.97625 | 7215.959 | 0 | 0 | 0 |
| Chad | 1994 | 1.002125 | 7399.129 | 0 | 0 | 0 |
| Comoros | 1994 | 1.015063 | 7607.564 | 0 | 0 | 0 |
| Congo, Dem. Rep. | 1994 | | | | | |
| Congo, Rep. | 1994 | 1.028 | 7841.73 | 0 | 0 | 0 |
| Cote d'Ivoire | 1994 | 1.126 | 8085.316 | 0 | 0 | 0 |
| Djibouti | 1994 | 1.175 | 8339.188 | 0 | 0 | 0 |
| Egypt, Arab Rep. | 1994 | 1.1995 | 8609.306 | 0 | 0 | 0 |
| Equatorial Guinea | 1994 | 1.21175 | 8892.59 | 1 | 0 | 1 |
| Eritrea | 1994 | 1.224 | 9199.333 | 0 | 0 | 0 |
| Ethiopia | 1994 | 1.297 | 9524.744 | 1 | 0 | 1 |
| Gabon | 1994 | 1.3335 | 9851.304 | 1 | 0 | 1 |

| Country Name | Year | Education | Population Density | Minor War | Civil War | Conflict |
|---|---|---|---|---|---|---|
| Gambia, The | 1994 | 1.35175 | 10195.66 | 0 | 0 | 0 |
| Ghana | 1994 | 1.360875 | 10563.22 | 0 | 0 | 0 |
| Guinea | 1994 | | | | | |
| Guinea-Bissau | 1994 | 1.37 | 10951.43 | 0 | 0 | 0 |
| Kenya | 1994 | 1.4575 | 11362.15 | 0 | 0 | 0 |
| Lesotho | 1994 | 1.50125 | 11792.08 | 0 | 0 | 0 |
| Liberia | 1994 | 1.523125 | 12239.31 | 0 | 0 | 0 |
| Libya | 1994 | 1.534063 | 12704.66 | 0 | 0 | 0 |
| Madagascar | 1994 | 1.545 | 13188.87 | 0 | 0 | 0 |
| Malawi | 1994 | 1.691 | 13692.95 | 0 | 0 | 0 |
| Mali | 1994 | 1.764 | 14214.71 | 1 | 0 | 1 |
| Mauritania | 1994 | 1.8005 | 13101.94 | 1 | 0 | 1 |
| Mauritius | 1994 | 1.837 | 15306 | 0 | 0 | 0 |
| Morocco | 1994 | | | | | |
| Mozambique | 1994 | 2.758 | 44033.21 | 0 | 0 | 0 |
| Namibia | 1994 | 2.8035 | 45333.22 | 0 | 0 | 0 |
| Niger | 1994 | 2.82625 | 46675.41 | 0 | 0 | 0 |
| Nigeria | 1994 | 2.849 | 48064.04 | 0 | 0 | 0 |
| Rwanda | 1994 | 3.1715 | 49491.14 | 1 | 0 | 1 |
| Sao Tome and Principe | 1994 | 3.33275 | 50948.61 | 0 | 1 | 1 |
| Senegal | 1994 | 3.413375 | 52445.06 | 0 | 1 | 1 |
| Seychelles | 1994 | 3.453688 | 53990.04 | 0 | 1 | 1 |
| Sierra Leone | 1994 | 3.494 | 55585.64 | 0 | 1 | 1 |
| Somalia | 1994 | | | | | |
| South Africa | 1994 | 3.8915 | 57234.22 | 0 | 0 | 0 |
| Sudan | 1994 | 4.09025 | 58941.18 | 0 | 0 | 0 |
| Swaziland | 1994 | 4.189625 | 60702.38 | 0 | 0 | 0 |
| Tanzania | 1994 | 4.239313 | 62523.71 | 0 | 0 | 0 |
| Togo | 1994 | 4.289 | 64421.5 | 0 | 0 | 0 |
| Tunisia | 1994 | 4.65 | 66392.9 | 0 | 0 | 0 |
| Uganda | 1994 | 4.8305 | 68421.17 | 0 | 0 | 0 |
| Zambia | 1994 | 4.92075 | 70483.45 | 0 | 0 | 0 |
| Zimbabwe | 1994 | 4.965875 | 72588.34 | 0 | 0 | 0 |
| Algeria | 1995 | | | | | |
| Angola | 1995 | 5.011 | 74821.27 | 0 | 0 | 0 |
| Benin | 1995 | 5.2795 | 77149.58 | 0 | 0 | 0 |
| Botswana | 1995 | 5.41375 | 79510.98 | 0 | 0 | 0 |
| Burkina Faso | 1995 | 5.480875 | 81163.74 | 0 | 0 | 0 |
| Burundi | 1995 | 5.514438 | 82724.29 | 0 | 0 | 0 |
| Cabo Verde | 1995 | 5.548 | 84889.38 | 0 | 0 | 0 |
| Cameroon | 1995 | 5.788 | 87092.24 | 0 | 0 | 0 |
| Central African Republic | 1995 | 5.908 | 89405.02 | 0 | 0 | 0 |
| Chad | 1995 | 5.968 | 91760.42 | 0 | 0 | 0 |
| Comoros | 1995 | 5.998 | 94159.65 | 0 | 0 | 0 |
| Congo, Dem. Rep. | 1995 | | | | | |
| Congo, Rep. | 1995 | 6.028 | 96603.76 | 0 | 0 | 0 |
| Cote d'Ivoire | 1995 | 6.2305 | 99092.5 | 0 | 0 | 0 |

| *Country Name* | *Year* | *Education* | *Population Density* | *Minor War* | *Civil War* | *Conflict* |
|---|---|---|---|---|---|---|
| Djibouti | 1995 | 6.33175 | 101625.1 | 0 | 0 | 0 |
| Egypt, Arab Rep. | 1995 | 6.382375 | 104199.7 | 0 | 0 | 0 |
| Equatorial Guinea | 1995 | 6.407688 | 106814 | 0 | 0 | 0 |
| Eritrea | 1995 | 6.433 | 109465.1 | 0 | 0 | 0 |
| Ethiopia | 1995 | 6.6185 | 112149 | 0 | 0 | 0 |
| Gabon | 1995 | 6.71125 | 114862 | 0 | 0 | 0 |
| Gambia, The | 1995 | 6.757625 | 117599.6 | 0 | 0 | 0 |
| Ghana | 1995 | 6.780813 | 120369.2 | 0 | 0 | 0 |
| Guinea | 1995 | | | | | |
| Guinea-Bissau | 1995 | 6.804 | 123178.8 | 0 | 0 | 0 |
| Kenya | 1995 | 6.961 | 126014.3 | 0 | 0 | 0 |
| Lesotho | 1995 | 7.0395 | 128864.3 | 0 | 0 | 0 |
| Liberia | 1995 | 7.07875 | 131727.5 | 0 | 0 | 0 |
| Libya | 1995 | 7.098375 | 134604.5 | 1 | 0 | 1 |
| Madagascar | 1995 | 7.118 | 137495.1 | 0 | 0 | 0 |
| Malawi | 1995 | 7.271 | 140397.8 | 0 | 0 | 0 |
| Mali | 1995 | 7.3475 | 143312.1 | 0 | 0 | 0 |
| Mauritania | 1995 | 7.38575 | 146255 | 0 | 0 | 0 |
| Mauritius | 1995 | 7.424 | 149229 | 0 | 0 | 0 |
| Morocco | 1995 | | | | | |
| Mozambique | 1995 | | | 0 | 0 | 0 |
| Namibia | 1995 | | | 0 | 0 | 0 |
| Niger | 1995 | | | 0 | 0 | 0 |
| Nigeria | 1995 | | | 0 | 0 | 0 |
| Rwanda | 1995 | | | 0 | 0 | 0 |
| Sao Tome and Principe | 1995 | | | 0 | 0 | 0 |
| Senegal | 1995 | | | 0 | 0 | 0 |
| Seychelles | 1995 | | | 0 | 0 | 0 |
| Sierra Leone | 1995 | | | 0 | 0 | 0 |
| Somalia | 1995 | | | 0 | 0 | 0 |
| South Africa | 1995 | | | 0 | 0 | 0 |
| Sudan | 1995 | | | 0 | 0 | 0 |
| Swaziland | 1995 | | | 0 | 0 | 0 |
| Tanzania | 1995 | | | 0 | 0 | 0 |
| Togo | 1995 | | | 0 | 0 | 0 |
| Tunisia | 1995 | | | 0 | 0 | 0 |
| Uganda | 1995 | | | 0 | 0 | 0 |
| Zambia | 1995 | | | 0 | 0 | 0 |
| Zimbabwe | 1995 | | | 0 | 0 | 0 |
| Algeria | 1996 | | | 0 | 0 | 0 |
| Angola | 1996 | | | 0 | 0 | 0 |
| Benin | 1996 | | | 0 | 0 | 0 |
| Botswana | 1996 | | | 0 | 0 | 0 |
| Burkina Faso | 1996 | | | 0 | 0 | 0 |
| Burundi | 1996 | | | 0 | 0 | 0 |
| Cabo Verde | 1996 | | | 0 | 0 | 0 |
| Cameroon | 1996 | | | 0 | 0 | 0 |

| Country Name | Year | Education | Population Density | Minor War | Civil War | Conflict |
|---|---|---|---|---|---|---|
| Central African Republic | 1996 | | | 0 | 0 | 0 |
| Chad | 1996 | | | 0 | 0 | 0 |
| Comoros | 1996 | | | 0 | 0 | 0 |
| Congo, Dem. Rep. | 1996 | | | 0 | 0 | 0 |
| Congo, Rep. | 1996 | | | 0 | 0 | 0 |
| Cote d'Ivoire | 1996 | | | 0 | 0 | 0 |
| Djibouti | 1996 | | | 0 | 0 | 0 |
| Egypt, Arab Rep. | 1996 | | | 0 | 0 | 0 |
| Equatorial Guinea | 1996 | | | 0 | 0 | 0 |
| Eritrea | 1996 | | | 0 | 0 | 0 |
| Ethiopia | 1996 | | | 0 | 0 | 0 |
| Gabon | 1996 | | | 0 | 0 | 0 |
| Gambia, The | 1996 | | | 0 | 0 | 0 |
| Ghana | 1996 | | | 0 | 0 | 0 |
| Guinea | 1996 | | | 0 | 0 | 0 |
| Guinea-Bissau | 1996 | | | 0 | 0 | 0 |
| Kenya | 1996 | | | 0 | 0 | 0 |
| Lesotho | 1996 | | | 0 | 0 | 0 |
| Liberia | 1996 | | | 0 | 0 | 0 |
| Libya | 1996 | | | 0 | 0 | 0 |
| Madagascar | 1996 | | | 0 | 0 | 0 |
| Malawi | 1996 | | | | | |
| Mali | 1996 | 0.769 | 3051.242 | 0 | 0 | 0 |
| Mauritania | 1996 | 0.848 | 3129.004 | 0 | 0 | 0 |
| Mauritius | 1996 | 0.8875 | 3183.993 | 0 | 0 | 0 |
| Morocco | 1996 | 0.927 | 3264.64 | 0 | 0 | 0 |
| Mozambique | 1996 | 1.0385 | 3358.202 | 0 | 0 | 0 |
| Namibia | 1996 | 1.09425 | 3451.079 | 0 | 0 | 0 |
| Niger | 1996 | 1.122125 | 3547.932 | 0 | 0 | 0 |
| Nigeria | 1996 | 1.136063 | 3656.796 | 0 | 0 | 0 |
| Rwanda | 1996 | | | | | |
| Sao Tome and Principe | 1996 | 1.15 | 3769.171 | 0 | 0 | 0 |
| Senegal | 1996 | 1.21 | 3880.225 | 0 | 0 | 0 |
| Seychelles | 1996 | 1.24 | 3992.121 | 0 | 0 | 0 |
| Sierra Leone | 1996 | 1.255 | 4109.838 | 0 | 0 | 0 |
| Somalia | 1996 | 1.2625 | 4226.38 | 0 | 0 | 0 |
| South Africa | 1996 | 1.27 | 4356.863 | 0 | 0 | 0 |
| Sudan | 1996 | 1.471 | 4502.352 | 0 | 0 | 0 |
| Swaziland | 1996 | 1.5715 | 4657.072 | 0 | 0 | 0 |
| Tanzania | 1996 | 1.62175 | 4818.993 | 0 | 0 | 0 |
| Togo | 1996 | 1.646875 | 4975.585 | 0 | 0 | 0 |
| Tunisia | 1996 | | | | | |
| Uganda | 1996 | 1.672 | 5138.478 | 0 | 0 | 0 |
| Zambia | 1996 | 1.7705 | 5306.749 | 0 | 0 | 0 |
| Zimbabwe | 1996 | 1.81975 | 5480.042 | 0 | 0 | 0 |
| Algeria | 1997 | 1.844375 | 5658.948 | 0 | 0 | 0 |
| Angola | 1997 | 1.856688 | 5828.738 | 0 | 0 | 0 |

| *Country Name* | *Year* | *Education* | *Population Density* | *Minor War* | *Civil War* | *Conflict* |
|---|---|---|---|---|---|---|
| Benin | 1997 | 1.869 | 5981.814 | 0 | 0 | 0 |
| Botswana | 1997 | 2.0125 | 6156.947 | 0 | 0 | 0 |
| Burkina Faso | 1997 | 2.08425 | 6366.208 | 0 | 0 | 0 |
| Burundi | 1997 | 2.120125 | 6587.74 | 0 | 0 | 0 |
| Cabo Verde | 1997 | 2.138063 | 6803.562 | 0 | 0 | 0 |
| Cameroon | 1997 | | | | | |
| Central African Republic | 1997 | 2.156 | 6981.76 | 1 | 0 | 1 |
| Chad | 1997 | 2.393 | 7121.616 | 0 | 1 | 1 |
| Comoros | 1997 | 2.5115 | 7270.626 | 0 | 1 | 1 |
| Congo, Dem. Rep. | 1997 | 2.57075 | 7559.604 | 1 | 1 | 1 |
| Congo, Rep. | 1997 | 2.600375 | 6264.306 | 1 | 1 | 1 |
| Cote d'Ivoire | 1997 | 2.63 | 5460.622 | 0 | 0 | 0 |
| Djibouti | 1997 | 2.9025 | 6510.963 | 0 | 0 | 0 |
| Egypt, Arab Rep. | 1997 | 3.03875 | 7580.468 | 1 | 1 | 1 |
| Equatorial Guinea | 1997 | 3.106875 | 7956.552 | 0 | 1 | 1 |
| Eritrea | 1997 | 3.140938 | 8122.239 | 1 | 1 | 1 |
| Ethiopia | 1997 | | | | | |
| Gabon | 1997 | 3.175 | 8398 | 1 | 1 | 1 |
| Gambia, The | 1997 | 3.3905 | 8611 | 0 | 1 | 1 |
| Ghana | 1997 | 3.49825 | 8857 | 0 | 0 | 0 |
| Guinea | 1997 | 3.552125 | 9098 | 0 | 0 | 0 |
| Guinea-Bissau | 1997 | 3.579063 | 9361 | 0 | 0 | 0 |
| Kenya | 1997 | 3.606 | 9611 | 0 | 0 | 0 |
| Lesotho | 1997 | 3.7775 | 9857 | 0 | 0 | 0 |
| Liberia | 1997 | 3.86325 | 10141 | 0 | 0 | 0 |
| Libya | 1997 | 3.906125 | 10441 | 0 | 0 | 0 |
| Madagascar | 1997 | 3.949 | 10746 | 0 | 0 | 0 |
| Malawi | 1997 | | | | | |
| Mali | 1997 | | 65.345 | 0 | 0 | 0 |
| Mauritania | 1997 | | 66.361 | 0 | 0 | 0 |
| Mauritius | 1997 | | 67.452 | 0 | 0 | 0 |
| Morocco | 1997 | | 68.691 | 0 | 0 | 0 |
| Mozambique | 1997 | | 69.766 | 0 | 0 | 0 |
| Namibia | 1997 | | 70.787 | 0 | 0 | 0 |
| Niger | 1997 | | 71.804 | 0 | 0 | 0 |
| Nigeria | 1997 | | 72.722 | 0 | 0 | 0 |
| Rwanda | 1997 | | 73.631 | 0 | 0 | 0 |
| Sao Tome and Principe | 1997 | | 74.86 | 0 | 0 | 0 |
| Senegal | 1997 | | 76.595 | 0 | 0 | 0 |
| Seychelles | 1997 | | 78.222 | 0 | 0 | 0 |
| Sierra Leone | 1997 | | 79.667 | 0 | 0 | 0 |
| Somalia | 1997 | | 81.607 | 0 | 0 | 0 |
| South Africa | 1997 | | 84.176 | 0 | 0 | 0 |
| Sudan | 1997 | | 86.796 | 0 | 0 | 0 |
| Swaziland | 1997 | | 89.367 | 0 | 0 | 0 |
| Tanzania | 1997 | | 91.804 | 0 | 0 | 0 |
| Togo | 1997 | | 94.071 | 0 | 0 | 0 |

| *Country Name* | *Year* | *Education* | *Population Density* | *Minor War* | *Civil War* | *Conflict* |
|---|---|---|---|---|---|---|
| Tunisia | 1997 | | 96.443 | 0 | 0 | 0 |
| Uganda | 1997 | | 98.563 | 0 | 0 | 0 |
| Zambia | 1997 | | 100.789 | 0 | 0 | 0 |
| Zimbabwe | 1997 | | 103.117 | 0 | 0 | 0 |
| Algeria | 1998 | | 105.548 | 0 | 0 | 0 |
| Angola | 1998 | | 108.083 | 0 | 0 | 0 |
| Benin | 1998 | | 110.725 | 0 | 0 | 0 |
| Botswana | 1998 | | 113.481 | 0 | 0 | 0 |
| Burkina Faso | 1998 | | 116.356 | 0 | 0 | 0 |
| Burundi | 1998 | | 119.361 | 0 | 0 | 0 |
| Cabo Verde | 1998 | | 122.503 | 0 | 0 | 0 |
| Cameroon | 1998 | | 125.821 | 0 | 0 | 0 |
| Central African Republic | 1998 | | 129.347 | 0 | 0 | 0 |
| Chad | 1998 | | 125 | 0 | 0 | 0 |
| Comoros | 1998 | | 127 | 0 | 0 | 0 |
| Congo, Dem. Rep. | 1998 | | 130 | 0 | 0 | 0 |
| Congo, Rep. | 1998 | | 132 | 0 | 0 | 0 |
| Cote d'Ivoire | 1998 | | 135 | 0 | 0 | 0 |
| Djibouti | 1998 | | 138 | 0 | 0 | 0 |
| Egypt, Arab Rep. | 1998 | | 141 | 0 | 0 | 0 |
| Equatorial Guinea | 1998 | | 144 | 0 | 0 | 0 |
| Eritrea | 1998 | | 147 | 0 | 0 | 0 |
| Ethiopia | 1998 | | 151 | 0 | 0 | 0 |
| Gabon | 1998 | | 154 | 0 | 0 | 0 |
| Gambia, The | 1998 | | 158 | 0 | 0 | 0 |
| Ghana | 1998 | | 161 | 0 | 0 | 0 |
| Guinea | 1998 | | 165 | 0 | 0 | 0 |
| Guinea-Bissau | 1998 | | 168 | 0 | 0 | 0 |
| Kenya | 1998 | | 172 | 0 | 0 | 0 |
| Lesotho | 1998 | | | | | |
| Liberia | 1998 | 1.857 | 3430.243 | 0 | 0 | 0 |
| Libya | 1998 | 1.9345 | 3516.025 | 0 | 0 | 0 |
| Madagascar | 1998 | 1.97325 | 3636.138 | 0 | 0 | 0 |
| Malawi | 1998 | 2.012 | 3743.967 | 0 | 0 | 0 |
| Mali | 1998 | 2.1395 | 3856.528 | 0 | 0 | 0 |
| Mauritania | 1998 | 2.20325 | 3965.841 | 0 | 0 | 0 |
| Mauritius | 1998 | 2.235125 | 4073.826 | 0 | 0 | 0 |
| Morocco | 1998 | 2.251063 | 4192.724 | 0 | 0 | 0 |
| Mozambique | 1998 | | | | | |
| Namibia | 1998 | 2.267 | 4317.891 | 0 | 0 | 0 |
| Niger | 1998 | 2.3975 | 4450.142 | 0 | 0 | 0 |
| Nigeria | 1998 | 2.46275 | 4588.696 | 0 | 0 | 0 |
| Rwanda | 1998 | 2.495375 | 4727.163 | 0 | 0 | 0 |
| Sao Tome and Principe | 1998 | 2.511688 | 4872.244 | 0 | 0 | 0 |
| Senegal | 1998 | 2.528 | 4989.168 | 0 | 0 | 0 |
| Seychelles | 1998 | 2.678 | 5100.499 | 0 | 0 | 0 |
| Sierra Leone | 1998 | 2.753 | 5262.5 | 0 | 0 | 0 |

| Country Name | Year | Education | Population Density | Minor War | Civil War | Conflict |
|---|---|---|---|---|---|---|
| Somalia | 1998 | 2.7905 | 5430.859 | 0 | 0 | 0 |
| South Africa | 1998 | 2.80925 | 5605.756 | 0 | 0 | 0 |
| Sudan | 1998 | | | | | |
| Swaziland | 1998 | 2.828 | 5787.32 | 0 | 0 | 0 |
| Tanzania | 1998 | 2.9745 | 5975.667 | 0 | 0 | 0 |
| Togo | 1998 | 3.04775 | 6169.733 | 0 | 0 | 0 |
| Tunisia | 1998 | 3.084375 | 6368.519 | 0 | 0 | 0 |
| Uganda | 1998 | 3.102688 | 6573.248 | 0 | 0 | 0 |
| Zambia | 1998 | 3.121 | 6785.11 | 0 | 0 | 0 |
| Zimbabwe | 1998 | 3.294 | 7004.26 | 0 | 0 | 0 |
| Algeria | 1999 | 3.3805 | 7230.787 | 0 | 0 | 0 |
| Angola | 1999 | 3.42375 | 7464.761 | 0 | 0 | 0 |
| Benin | 1999 | 3.445375 | 7729.5 | 0 | 0 | 0 |
| Botswana | 1999 | | | | | |
| Burkina Faso | 1999 | 3.467 | 8000.632 | 1 | 0 | 1 |
| Burundi | 1999 | 3.654 | 8258.663 | 1 | 0 | 1 |
| Cabo Verde | 1999 | 3.7475 | 8516.518 | 1 | 0 | 1 |
| Cameroon | 1999 | 3.79425 | 8771.813 | 1 | 0 | 1 |
| Central African Republic | 1999 | 3.817625 | 8166 | 0 | 0 | 0 |
| Chad | 1999 | 3.841 | 8378 | 1 | 0 | 1 |
| Comoros | 1999 | 4.029 | 8595 | 0 | 0 | 0 |
| Congo, Dem. Rep. | 1999 | 4.123 | 8810 | 1 | 0 | 1 |
| Congo, Rep. | 1999 | 4.17 | 9037 | 1 | 0 | 1 |
| Cote d'Ivoire | 1999 | 4.1935 | 9253 | 0 | 0 | 0 |
| Djibouti | 1999 | | | | | |
| Egypt, Arab Rep. | 1999 | 4.217 | 9469 | 1 | 1 | 1 |
| Equatorial Guinea | 1999 | 4.4435 | 9716 | 1 | 1 | 1 |
| Eritrea | 1999 | 4.55675 | 9972 | 0 | 0 | 0 |
| Ethiopia | 1999 | 4.613375 | 10240 | 1 | 1 | 1 |
| Gabon | 1999 | 4.641688 | 10519 | 0 | 0 | 0 |
| Gambia, The | 1999 | 4.67 | 10804 | 0 | 0 | 0 |
| Ghana | 1999 | 4.9345 | 11096 | 0 | 0 | 0 |
| Guinea | 1999 | 5.06675 | 11394 | 0 | 0 | 0 |
| Guinea-Bissau | 1999 | 5.132875 | 11698 | 0 | 0 | 0 |
| Kenya | 1999 | 5.199 | 12008 | 0 | 0 | 0 |
| Lesotho | 1999 | | | | | |
| Liberia | 1999 | | 43.881 | 0 | 0 | 0 |
| Libya | 1999 | | 45.254 | 0 | 0 | 0 |
| Madagascar | 1999 | | 46.755 | 0 | 0 | 0 |
| Malawi | 1999 | | 47.785 | 0 | 0 | 0 |
| Mali | 1999 | | 48.796 | 0 | 0 | 0 |
| Mauritania | 1999 | | 49.888 | 0 | 0 | 0 |
| Mauritius | 1999 | | 51.126 | 0 | 0 | 0 |
| Morocco | 1999 | | 52.508 | 0 | 0 | 0 |
| Mozambique | 1999 | | | | | |
| Namibia | 1999 | | 54.106 | 0 | 0 | 0 |
| Niger | 1999 | | 55.615 | 0 | 0 | 0 |

| *Country Name* | *Year* | *Education* | *Population Density* | *Minor War* | *Civil War* | *Conflict* |
|---|---|---|---|---|---|---|
| Nigeria | 1999 | | 56.814 | 0 | 0 | 0 |
| Rwanda | 1999 | | 57.53 | 0 | 0 | 0 |
| Sao Tome and Principe | 1999 | | 58.425 | 0 | 0 | 0 |
| Senegal | 1999 | | 59.626 | 0 | 0 | 0 |
| Seychelles | 1999 | | 60.676 | 0 | 0 | 0 |
| Sierra Leone | 1999 | | 61.791 | 0 | 0 | 0 |
| Somalia | 1999 | | 62.45 | 0 | 0 | 0 |
| South Africa | 1999 | | 63.191 | 0 | 0 | 0 |
| Sudan | 1999 | | | | | |
| Swaziland | 1999 | | 63.954 | 0 | 0 | 0 |
| Tanzania | 1999 | | 64.695 | 0 | 0 | 0 |
| Togo | 1999 | | 65.282 | 0 | 0 | 0 |
| Tunisia | 1999 | | 65.846 | 0 | 0 | 0 |
| Uganda | 1999 | | 66.499 | 0 | 0 | 0 |
| Zambia | 1999 | | 67.175 | 0 | 0 | 0 |
| Zimbabwe | 1999 | | 67.838 | 0 | 0 | 0 |
| Algeria | 2000 | | 68.46 | 0 | 0 | 0 |
| Angola | 2000 | | 69.195 | 0 | 0 | 0 |
| Benin | 2000 | | 70.014 | 0 | 0 | 0 |
| Botswana | 2000 | | | | | |
| Burkina Faso | 2000 | | 70.8 | 0 | 0 | 0 |
| Burundi | 2000 | | 71.649 | 0 | 0 | 0 |
| Cabo Verde | 2000 | | 72.501 | 0 | 0 | 0 |
| Cameroon | 2000 | | 73.318 | 0 | 0 | 0 |
| Central African Republic | 2000 | | 74.133 | 0 | 0 | 0 |
| Chad | 2000 | | 74.931 | 0 | 0 | 0 |
| Comoros | 2000 | | 75.714 | 0 | 0 | 0 |
| Congo, Dem. Rep. | 2000 | | 76.405 | 0 | 0 | 0 |
| Congo, Rep. | 2000 | | 77.174 | 0 | 0 | 0 |
| Cote d'Ivoire | 2000 | | 78.137 | 0 | 0 | 0 |
| Djibouti | 2000 | | | | | |
| Egypt, Arab Rep. | 2000 | | 79.158 | 0 | 0 | 0 |
| Equatorial Guinea | 2000 | | 80.173 | 0 | 0 | 0 |
| Eritrea | 2000 | | 81.125 | 0 | 0 | 0 |
| Ethiopia | 2000 | | 82.049 | 0 | 0 | 0 |
| Gabon | 2000 | | 82.97 | 0 | 0 | 0 |
| Gambia, The | 2000 | | 83.886 | 0 | 0 | 0 |
| Ghana | 2000 | | 84.798 | 0 | 0 | 0 |
| Guinea | 2000 | | 85.702 | 0 | 0 | 0 |
| Guinea-Bissau | 2000 | | 87 | 0 | 0 | 0 |
| Kenya | 2000 | | 87 | 0 | 0 | 0 |
| Lesotho | 2000 | | | | | |
| Liberia | 2000 | 0.539 | 2467.895 | 0 | 0 | 0 |
| Libya | 2000 | 0.604 | 2505.118 | 0 | 0 | 0 |
| Madagascar | 2000 | 0.6365 | 2543.14 | 0 | 0 | 0 |
| Malawi | 2000 | 0.669 | 2581.979 | 0 | 0 | 0 |
| Mali | 2000 | 0.7745 | 2621.656 | 0 | 0 | 0 |

| Country Name | Year | Education | Population Density | Minor War | Civil War | Conflict |
|---|---|---|---|---|---|---|
| Mauritania | 2000 | 0.82725 | 2662.19 | 0 | 0 | 0 |
| Mauritius | 2000 | 0.853625 | 2703.603 | 0 | 0 | 0 |
| Morocco | 2000 | 0.866813 | 2745.967 | 0 | 0 | 0 |
| Mozambique | 2000 | | | | | |
| Namibia | 2000 | 0.88 | 2789.306 | 0 | 0 | 0 |
| Niger | 2000 | 1.0165 | 2833.646 | 0 | 0 | 0 |
| Nigeria | 2000 | 1.08475 | 2879.013 | 0 | 0 | 0 |
| Rwanda | 2000 | 1.118875 | 2925.433 | 0 | 0 | 0 |
| Sao Tome and Principe | 2000 | 1.135938 | 2973.542 | 0 | 0 | 0 |
| Senegal | 2000 | 1.153 | 3030.32 | 0 | 0 | 0 |
| Seychelles | 2000 | 1.3115 | 3088.259 | 0 | 0 | 0 |
| Sierra Leone | 2000 | 1.39075 | 3147.416 | 0 | 0 | 0 |
| Somalia | 2000 | 1.430375 | 3207.978 | 0 | 0 | 0 |
| South Africa | 2000 | 1.450188 | 3270.319 | 0 | 0 | 0 |
| Sudan | 2000 | | | | | |
| Swaziland | 2000 | 1.47 | 3334.822 | 0 | 0 | 0 |
| Tanzania | 2000 | 1.6535 | 3401.929 | 0 | 0 | 0 |
| Togo | 2000 | 1.74525 | 3472.01 | 0 | 0 | 0 |
| Tunisia | 2000 | 1.791125 | 3545.385 | 0 | 0 | 0 |
| Uganda | 2000 | 1.814063 | 3622.28 | 0 | 0 | 0 |
| Zambia | 2000 | 1.837 | 3702.812 | 0 | 0 | 0 |
| Zimbabwe | 2000 | 2.0275 | 3787.101 | 0 | 0 | 0 |
| Algeria | 2001 | 2.12275 | 3875.277 | 0 | 0 | 0 |
| Angola | 2001 | 2.170375 | 3967.463 | 0 | 0 | 0 |
| Benin | 2001 | 2.194188 | 4063.83 | 0 | 0 | 0 |
| Botswana | 2001 | | | | | |
| Burkina Faso | 2001 | 2.218 | 4226.425 | 0 | 0 | 0 |
| Burundi | 2001 | 2.43 | 4339.902 | 1 | 0 | 1 |
| Cabo Verde | 2001 | 2.536 | 4267.269 | 1 | 0 | 1 |
| Cameroon | 2001 | 2.589 | 4220.562 | 1 | 0 | 1 |
| Central African Republic | 2001 | 2.6155 | 4317.788 | 1 | 1 | 1 |
| Chad | 2001 | 2.642 | 3881 | 1 | 1 | 1 |
| Comoros | 2001 | 2.8095 | 3811 | 1 | 1 | 1 |
| Congo, Dem. Rep. | 2001 | 2.89325 | 3765 | 1 | 1 | 1 |
| Congo, Rep. | 2001 | 2.935125 | 3746 | 1 | 1 | 2 |
| Cote d'Ivoire | 2001 | 2.956063 | 3736 | 1 | 1 | 2 |
| Djibouti | 2001 | | | | | |
| Egypt, Arab Rep. | 2001 | 2.977 | 3809 | 1 | 1 | 1 |
| Equatorial Guinea | 2001 | 3.1815 | 4043 | 0 | 0 | 0 |
| Eritrea | 2001 | 3.28375 | 4287 | 0 | 0 | 0 |
| Ethiopia | 2001 | 3.334875 | 4466 | 0 | 0 | 0 |
| Gabon | 2001 | 3.360438 | 4602 | 0 | 0 | 0 |
| Gambia, The | 2001 | 3.386 | 4708 | 0 | 0 | 0 |
| Ghana | 2001 | 3.548 | 4818 | 0 | 0 | 0 |
| Guinea | 2001 | 3.629 | 4918 | 0 | 0 | 0 |
| Guinea-Bissau | 2001 | 3.6695 | 5023 | 0 | 0 | 0 |
| Kenya | 2001 | 3.71 | 5132 | 0 | 0 | 0 |

| Country Name | Year | Education | Population Density | Minor War | Civil War | Conflict |
|---|---|---|---|---|---|---|
| Lesotho | 2001 | | | | | |
| Liberia | 2001 | | 3080.153 | 0 | 0 | 0 |
| Libya | 2001 | | 3145.42 | 0 | 0 | 0 |
| Madagascar | 2001 | | 3212.842 | 0 | 0 | 0 |
| Malawi | 2001 | | 3282.503 | 0 | 0 | 0 |
| Mali | 2001 | | 3354.474 | 0 | 0 | 0 |
| Mauritania | 2001 | | 3428.839 | 0 | 0 | 0 |
| Mauritius | 2001 | | 3505.657 | 0 | 0 | 0 |
| Morocco | 2001 | | 3584.995 | 0 | 0 | 0 |
| Mozambique | 2001 | | | | | |
| Namibia | 2001 | | 3666.949 | 0 | 0 | 0 |
| Niger | 2001 | | 3751.979 | 0 | 0 | 0 |
| Nigeria | 2001 | | 3840.161 | 0 | 0 | 0 |
| Rwanda | 2001 | | 3931.655 | 0 | 0 | 0 |
| Sao Tome and Principe | 2001 | | 4027.472 | 0 | 0 | 0 |
| Senegal | 2001 | | 4127.771 | 0 | 0 | 0 |
| Seychelles | 2001 | | 4238.645 | 0 | 0 | 0 |
| Sierra Leone | 2001 | | 4354.931 | 0 | 0 | 0 |
| Somalia | 2001 | | 4679.501 | 1 | 0 | 1 |
| South Africa | 2001 | | 5310.962 | 1 | 0 | 1 |
| Sudan | 2001 | | | | | |
| Swaziland | 2001 | | 5793.555 | 1 | 0 | 1 |
| Tanzania | 2001 | | 5828.8 | 1 | 0 | 1 |
| Togo | 2001 | | 5834.498 | 1 | 0 | 1 |
| Tunisia | 2001 | | 6010.345 | 1 | 0 | 1 |
| Uganda | 2001 | | 6217.738 | 1 | 0 | 1 |
| Zambia | 2001 | | 6458.539 | 1 | 0 | 1 |
| Zimbabwe | 2001 | | 6714.927 | 1 | 0 | 1 |
| Algeria | 2002 | | 6939.075 | 1 | 1 | 1 |
| Angola | 2002 | | 6918.288 | 0 | 1 | 1 |
| Benin | 2002 | | 6766.331 | 1 | 1 | 1 |
| Botswana | 2002 | | | | | |
| Burkina Faso | 2002 | | 6692.038 | 0 | 1 | 1 |
| Burundi | 2002 | | 6464.481 | 0 | 1 | 1 |
| Cabo Verde | 2002 | | 6116.213 | 0 | 1 | 1 |
| Cameroon | 2002 | | 6101.016 | 1 | 1 | 1 |
| Central African Republic | 2002 | | 6264.44 | 1 | 1 | 1 |
| Chad | 2002 | | 6400.722 | 1 | 1 | 1 |
| Comoros | 2002 | | 6574.263 | 1 | 1 | 1 |
| Congo, Dem. Rep. | 2002 | | 6751.083 | 1 | 1 | 1 |
| Congo, Rep. | 2002 | | 6965.204 | 1 | 1 | 1 |
| Cote d'Ivoire | 2002 | | 7242 | 1 | 1 | 1 |
| Djibouti | 2002 | | | | | |
| Egypt, Arab Rep. | 2002 | | 7501 | 1 | 1 | 1 |
| Equatorial Guinea | 2002 | | 7766 | 1 | 1 | 1 |
| Eritrea | 2002 | | 8017 | 1 | 1 | 1 |
| Ethiopia | 2002 | | 8272 | 1 | 1 | 1 |

| Country Name | Year | Education | Population Density | Minor War | Civil War | Conflict |
|---|---|---|---|---|---|---|
| Gabon | 2002 | | 8537 | 1 | 1 | 1 |
| Gambia, The | 2002 | | 8790 | 1 | 1 | 1 |
| Ghana | 2002 | | 9009 | 1 | 1 | 1 |
| Guinea | 2002 | | 9238 | 0 | 1 | 1 |
| Guinea-Bissau | 2002 | | 9455 | 0 | 1 | 1 |
| Kenya | 2002 | | 9613 | 0 | 1 | 1 |
| Lesotho | 2002 | | | | | |
| Liberia | 2002 | 4.39 | 18356.66 | 0 | 0 | 0 |
| Libya | 2002 | 4.4445 | 18856.71 | 0 | 0 | 0 |
| Madagascar | 2002 | 4.47175 | 19370.51 | 0 | 0 | 0 |
| Malawi | 2002 | 4.499 | 19898.24 | 0 | 0 | 0 |
| Mali | 2002 | 4.572 | 20440.49 | 1 | 0 | 1 |
| Mauritania | 2002 | 4.6085 | 20997.32 | 1 | 0 | 1 |
| Mauritius | 2002 | 4.62675 | 21569.47 | 1 | 0 | 1 |
| Morocco | 2002 | 4.635875 | 22157.36 | 1 | 0 | 1 |
| Mozambique | 2002 | | | | | |
| Namibia | 2002 | 4.645 | 22739.92 | 1 | 0 | 1 |
| Niger | 2002 | 4.7625 | 23338.08 | 1 | 0 | 1 |
| Nigeria | 2002 | 4.82125 | 23935.81 | 1 | 0 | 1 |
| Rwanda | 2002 | 4.850625 | 24549.29 | 1 | 0 | 1 |
| Sao Tome and Principe | 2002 | 4.865313 | 25178.95 | 1 | 0 | 1 |
| Senegal | 2002 | 4.88 | 25815.14 | 1 | 0 | 1 |
| Seychelles | 2002 | 5.013 | 26467.9 | 1 | 0 | 1 |
| Sierra Leone | 2002 | 5.0795 | 27129.93 | 1 | 0 | 1 |
| Somalia | 2002 | 5.11275 | 27809.09 | 1 | 0 | 1 |
| South Africa | 2002 | 5.129375 | 28505.82 | 1 | 1 | 1 |
| Sudan | 2002 | | | | | |
| Swaziland | 2002 | 5.146 | 29251.59 | 0 | 1 | 1 |
| Tanzania | 2002 | 5.1305 | 30168.68 | 0 | 1 | 1 |
| Togo | 2002 | 5.12275 | 31140.03 | 0 | 1 | 1 |
| Tunisia | 2002 | 5.118875 | 32143.96 | 0 | 1 | 1 |
| Uganda | 2002 | 5.116938 | 33181.59 | 1 | 1 | 1 |
| Zambia | 2002 | 5.115 | 34254.09 | 1 | 1 | 1 |
| Zimbabwe | 2002 | 5.9555 | 35101.38 | 1 | 1 | 2 |
| Algeria | 2003 | 6.37575 | 35947.7 | 1 | 1 | 2 |
| Angola | 2003 | 6.585875 | 36794.88 | 1 | 1 | 2 |
| Benin | 2003 | 6.690938 | 37639.33 | 0 | 0 | 0 |
| Botswana | 2003 | | | | | |
| Burkina Faso | 2003 | 6.796 | 38476.27 | 0 | 0 | 0 |
| Burundi | 2003 | 7.5445 | 39299.52 | 0 | 0 | 0 |
| Cabo Verde | 2003 | 7.91875 | 40091.07 | 0 | 0 | 0 |
| Cameroon | 2003 | 8.105875 | 40940.61 | 0 | 0 | 0 |
| Central African Republic | 2003 | 8.199438 | 41661.56 | 0 | 0 | 0 |
| Chad | 2003 | 8.293 | 42227.92 | 0 | 0 | 0 |
| Comoros | 2003 | 7.987 | 42793.96 | 0 | 0 | 0 |
| Congo, Dem. Rep. | 2003 | 7.834 | 43353.63 | 0 | 0 | 0 |
| Congo, Rep. | 2003 | 7.7575 | 43961.92 | 0 | 0 | 0 |

| *Country Name* | *Year* | *Education* | *Population Density* | *Minor War* | *Civil War* | *Conflict* |
|---|---|---|---|---|---|---|
| Cote d'Ivoire | 2003 | 7.71925 | 44526.27 | 0 | 0 | 0 |
| Djibouti | 2003 | | | | | |
| Egypt, Arab Rep. | 2003 | 7.681 | 45064.1 | 0 | 0 | 0 |
| Equatorial Guinea | 2003 | 7.97 | 45576.22 | 0 | 0 | 0 |
| Eritrea | 2003 | 8.1145 | 46076.95 | 0 | 0 | 0 |
| Ethiopia | 2003 | 8.18675 | 46566.63 | 0 | 0 | 0 |
| Gabon | 2003 | 8.222875 | 47032.87 | 0 | 0 | 0 |
| Gambia, The | 2003 | 8.259 | 47483.45 | 0 | 0 | 0 |
| Ghana | 2003 | 8.4085 | 47925.67 | 0 | 0 | 0 |
| Guinea | 2003 | 8.48325 | 48367.13 | 0 | 0 | 0 |
| Guinea-Bissau | 2003 | 8.520625 | 48783 | 0 | 0 | 0 |
| Kenya | 2003 | 8.558 | 49052 | 0 | 0 | 0 |
| Lesotho | 2003 | | | | | |
| Liberia | 2003 | 0.482 | 11183.23 | 0 | 0 | 0 |
| Libya | 2003 | 0.5385 | 11492.74 | 0 | 1 | 1 |
| Madagascar | 2003 | 0.56675 | 11800.66 | 0 | 1 | 1 |
| Malawi | 2003 | 0.595 | 12085.79 | 0 | 1 | 1 |
| Mali | 2003 | 0.6615 | 12376.71 | 0 | 1 | 1 |
| Mauritania | 2003 | 0.69475 | 12716.13 | 0 | 1 | 1 |
| Mauritius | 2003 | 0.711375 | 13058.93 | 0 | 1 | 1 |
| Morocco | 2003 | 0.719688 | 13402.97 | 0 | 1 | 1 |
| Mozambique | 2003 | | | | | |
| Namibia | 2003 | 0.728 | 13787.6 | 0 | 1 | 1 |
| Niger | 2003 | 0.837 | 14182.4 | 1 | 1 | 2 |
| Nigeria | 2003 | 0.8915 | 14597.02 | 0 | 1 | 1 |
| Rwanda | 2003 | 0.91875 | 15113.38 | 0 | 0 | 0 |
| Sao Tome and Principe | 2003 | 0.932375 | 15571.24 | 0 | 0 | 0 |
| Senegal | 2003 | 0.946 | 16056.07 | 0 | 0 | 0 |
| Seychelles | 2003 | 1.1105 | 16570.07 | 0 | 1 | 0 |
| Sierra Leone | 2003 | 1.19275 | 17104.99 | 0 | 0 | 0 |
| Somalia | 2003 | 1.233875 | 17712.47 | 0 | 0 | 0 |
| South Africa | 2003 | 1.254438 | 18386.53 | 0 | 0 | 0 |
| Sudan | 2003 | | | | | |
| Swaziland | 2003 | 1.275 | 19063.99 | 0 | 0 | 0 |
| Tanzania | 2003 | 1.4915 | 19701.6 | 0 | 0 | 0 |
| Togo | 2003 | 1.59975 | 20367.05 | 0 | 0 | 0 |
| Tunisia | 2003 | 1.653875 | 21750.82 | 0 | 1 | 1 |
| Uganda | 2003 | 1.680938 | 22470.85 | 0 | 1 | 1 |
| Zambia | 2003 | 1.708 | 23232.74 | 0 | 1 | 1 |
| Zimbabwe | 2003 | 1.927 | 23890.62 | 0 | 1 | 1 |
| Algeria | 2004 | 2.0365 | 24401.43 | 0 | 1 | 1 |
| Angola | 2004 | 2.09125 | 24806.48 | 0 | 1 | 1 |
| Benin | 2004 | 2.118625 | 25339.83 | 0 | 1 | 1 |
| Botswana | 2004 | | | | | |
| Burkina Faso | 2004 | 2.146 | 26049.6 | 0 | 1 | 1 |
| Burundi | 2004 | 2.3305 | 26943.48 | 0 | 1 | 1 |
| Cabo Verde | 2004 | 2.42275 | 27851 | 0 | 1 | 1 |

| *Country Name* | *Year* | *Education* | *Population Density* | *Minor War* | *Civil War* | *Conflict* |
|---|---|---|---|---|---|---|
| Cameroon | 2004 | 2.468875 | 28581.71 | 1 | 1 | 1 |
| Central African Republic | 2004 | 2.491938 | 29349.07 | 1 | 1 | 1 |
| Chad | 2004 | 2.515 | 30140.59 | 0 | 1 | 1 |
| Comoros | 2004 | 2.668 | 30811.95 | 0 | 1 | 1 |
| Congo, Dem. Rep. | 2004 | 2.7445 | 31585.17 | 0 | 1 | 1 |
| Congo, Rep. | 2004 | 2.78275 | 32510.75 | 0 | 1 | 1 |
| Cote d'Ivoire | 2004 | 2.801875 | 33345.2 | 0 | 1 | 1 |
| Djibouti | 2004 | | | | | |
| Egypt, Arab Rep. | 2004 | 2.821 | 34109 | 0 | 1 | 1 |
| Equatorial Guinea | 2004 | 2.931 | 35024 | 0 | 1 | 1 |
| Eritrea | 2004 | 2.986 | 35927 | 0 | 1 | 1 |
| Ethiopia | 2004 | 3.0135 | 36708 | 0 | 1 | 1 |
| Gabon | 2004 | 3.02725 | 37442 | 0 | 1 | 1 |
| Gambia, The | 2004 | 3.041 | 38363 | 1 | 1 | 2 |
| Ghana | 2004 | 3.1595 | 39396 | 0 | 1 | 1 |
| Guinea | 2004 | 3.21875 | 40526 | 1 | 1 | 1 |
| Guinea-Bissau | 2004 | 3.248375 | 41681 | 1 | 1 | 1 |
| Kenya | 2004 | 3.278 | 42811 | 1 | 1 | 1 |
| Lesotho | 2004 | | | | | |
| Liberia | 2004 | 1.72 | 370.006 | 0 | 0 | 0 |
| Libya | 2004 | 1.8885 | 379.526 | 0 | 0 | 0 |
| Madagascar | 2004 | 1.97275 | 389.347 | 0 | 0 | 0 |
| Malawi | 2004 | 2.057 | 399.481 | 0 | 0 | 0 |
| Mali | 2004 | 2.472 | 409.941 | 0 | 0 | 0 |
| Mauritania | 2004 | 2.6795 | 420.69 | 0 | 0 | 0 |
| Mauritius | 2004 | 2.78325 | 431.797 | 0 | 0 | 0 |
| Morocco | 2004 | 2.835125 | 443.277 | 0 | 0 | 0 |
| Mozambique | 2004 | 2.887 | 455.145 | 0 | 0 | 0 |
| Namibia | 2004 | 3.347 | 467.416 | 0 | 0 | 0 |
| Niger | 2004 | 3.577 | 480.105 | 0 | 0 | 0 |
| Nigeria | 2004 | 3.692 | 493.232 | 0 | 0 | 0 |
| Rwanda | 2004 | 3.7495 | 506.812 | 0 | 0 | 0 |
| Sao Tome and Principe | 2004 | 3.807 | 520.864 | 0 | 0 | 0 |
| Senegal | 2004 | 4.1225 | 535.618 | 0 | 0 | 0 |
| Seychelles | 2004 | 4.28025 | 551.425 | 0 | 0 | 0 |
| Sierra Leone | 2004 | 4.359125 | 568.333 | 0 | 0 | 0 |
| Somalia | 2004 | 4.398563 | 588.268 | 0 | 0 | 0 |
| South Africa | 2004 | 4.438 | 611.447 | 0 | 0 | 0 |
| Sudan | 2004 | 4.757 | 631.303 | 0 | 0 | 0 |
| Swaziland | 2004 | 4.9165 | 649.901 | 0 | 0 | 0 |
| Tanzania | 2004 | 4.99625 | 672.69 | 0 | 0 | 0 |
| Togo | 2004 | 5.036125 | 696.87 | 0 | 0 | 0 |
| Tunisia | 2004 | 5.076 | 722.451 | 0 | 0 | 0 |
| Uganda | 2004 | 5.4035 | 750.707 | 0 | 0 | 0 |
| Zambia | 2004 | 5.56725 | 779.348 | 0 | 0 | 0 |
| Zimbabwe | 2004 | 5.649125 | 817.085 | 0 | 0 | 0 |
| Algeria | 2005 | 5.690063 | 851.904 | 0 | 0 | 0 |

| Country Name | Year | Education | Population Density | Minor War | Civil War | Conflict |
|---|---|---|---|---|---|---|
| Angola | 2005 | 5.731 | 884.616 | 0 | 0 | 0 |
| Benin | 2005 | 6.0355 | 925.717 | 0 | 0 | 0 |
| Botswana | 2005 | 6.18775 | 962.344 | 0 | 0 | 0 |
| Burkina Faso | 2005 | 6.263875 | 991.859 | 0 | 0 | 0 |
| Burundi | 2005 | 6.301938 | 997.652 | 0 | 0 | 0 |
| Cabo Verde | 2005 | 6.34 | 1004.849 | 0 | 0 | 0 |
| Cameroon | 2005 | 6.6175 | 1030.651 | 0 | 0 | 0 |
| Central African Republic | 2005 | 6.75625 | 1054.486 | 0 | 0 | 0 |
| Chad | 2005 | 6.825625 | 1075.9 | 0 | 0 | 0 |
| Comoros | 2005 | 6.860313 | 1094.429 | 0 | 0 | 0 |
| Congo, Dem. Rep. | 2005 | 6.895 | 1144 | 0 | 0 | 0 |
| Congo, Rep. | 2005 | 7.107 | 1170 | 0 | 0 | 0 |
| Cote d'Ivoire | 2005 | 7.213 | 1194 | 0 | 0 | 0 |
| Djibouti | 2005 | 7.266 | 1216 | 0 | 0 | 0 |
| Egypt, Arab Rep. | 2005 | 7.2925 | 1238 | 0 | 0 | 0 |
| Equatorial Guinea | 2005 | 7.319 | 1259 | 0 | 0 | 0 |
| Eritrea | 2005 | 7.4715 | 1280 | 0 | 0 | 0 |
| Ethiopia | 2005 | 7.54775 | 1300 | 0 | 0 | 0 |
| Gabon | 2005 | 7.585875 | 1319 | 0 | 0 | 0 |
| Gambia, The | 2005 | 7.624 | 1337 | 0 | 0 | 0 |
| Ghana | 2005 | 0.49 | 1528.098 | 0 | 0 | 0 |
| Guinea | 2005 | 0.546 | 1566.469 | 0 | 0 | 0 |
| Guinea-Bissau | 2005 | 0.574 | 1606.285 | 0 | 0 | 0 |
| Kenya | 2005 | 0.602 | 1647.772 | 0 | 0 | 0 |
| Lesotho | 2005 | 0.7275 | 1690.838 | 0 | 0 | 0 |
| Liberia | 2005 | 0.79025 | 1735.55 | 0 | 0 | 0 |
| Libya | 2005 | 0.821625 | 1781.978 | 0 | 0 | 0 |
| Madagascar | 2005 | 0.837313 | 1830.381 | 0 | 0 | 0 |
| Malawi | 2005 | 0.853 | 1964.128 | 0 | 0 | 0 |
| Mali | 2005 | 1.332 | 2009.685 | 0 | 0 | 0 |
| Mauritania | 2005 | 1.5715 | 2056.351 | 0 | 0 | 0 |
| Mauritius | 2005 | 1.69125 | 2104.154 | 0 | 0 | 0 |
| Morocco | 2005 | 1.751125 | 2153.238 | 0 | 0 | 0 |
| Mozambique | 2005 | 1.811 | 2203.646 | 0 | 0 | 0 |
| Namibia | 2005 | 2.2985 | 2255.413 | 0 | 0 | 0 |
| Niger | 2005 | 2.54225 | 2308.582 | 0 | 0 | 0 |
| Nigeria | 2005 | 2.664125 | 2363.192 | 1 | 0 | 1 |
| Rwanda | 2005 | 2.725063 | 2420.74 | 0 | 0 | 0 |
| Sao Tome and Principe | 2005 | 2.786 | 2626 | 0 | 0 | 0 |
| Senegal | 2005 | 3.1225 | 2720 | 0 | 0 | 0 |
| Seychelles | 2005 | 3.29075 | 2817 | 0 | 0 | 0 |
| Sierra Leone | 2005 | 3.374875 | 2918 | 0 | 0 | 0 |
| Somalia | 2005 | 3.416938 | 3022 | 0 | 0 | 0 |
| South Africa | 2005 | 3.459 | 3129 | 0 | 0 | 0 |
| Sudan | 2005 | 3.7705 | 3241 | 0 | 0 | 0 |
| Swaziland | 2005 | 3.92625 | 3356 | 0 | 0 | 0 |
| Tanzania | 2005 | 4.004125 | 3475 | 0 | 0 | 0 |

| Country Name | Year | Education | Population Density | Minor War | Civil War | Conflict |
|---|---|---|---|---|---|---|
| Togo | 2005 | 4.043063 | 3597 | 0 | 0 | 0 |
| Tunisia | 2005 | 4.082 | 3721 | 0 | 0 | 0 |
| Uganda | 2005 | 4.3015 | 3846 | 1 | 0 | 1 |
| Zambia | 2005 | 4.41125 | 3973 | 0 | 0 | 0 |
| Zimbabwe | 2005 | 4.466125 | 3953 | 0 | 0 | 0 |
| Algeria | 2006 | 4.493563 | 3982 | 0 | 0 | 0 |
| Angola | 2006 | 4.521 | 4203 | 0 | 0 | 0 |
| Benin | 2006 | 4.7445 | 4402 | 0 | 0 | 0 |
| Botswana | 2006 | 4.85625 | 4572 | 0 | 0 | 0 |
| Burkina Faso | 2006 | 4.912125 | 4715 | 0 | 0 | 0 |
| Burundi | 2006 | 4.940063 | 4852 | 0 | 0 | 0 |
| Cabo Verde | 2006 | 4.968 | 4992 | 0 | 0 | 0 |
| Cameroon | 2006 | 5.1935 | 5135 | 0 | 0 | 0 |
| Central African Republic | 2006 | 5.30625 | 5278 | 0 | 0 | 0 |
| Chad | 2006 | 5.362625 | 5425 | 0 | 0 | 0 |
| Comoros | 2006 | 5.390813 | 5578 | 0 | 0 | 0 |
| Congo, Dem. Rep. | 2006 | 5.419 | 5715 | 0 | 0 | 0 |
| Congo, Rep. | 2006 | 5.6635 | 5865 | 0 | 0 | 0 |
| Cote d'Ivoire | 2006 | 5.78575 | 6042 | 0 | 0 | 0 |
| Djibouti | 2006 | 5.846875 | 6220 | 0 | 0 | 0 |
| Egypt, Arab Rep. | 2006 | 5.908 | 6405 | 0 | 0 | 0 |
| Equatorial Guinea | 2006 | 0.908 | 4286.552 | 0 | 0 | 0 |
| Eritrea | 2006 | 1.098 | 4374.477 | 0 | 0 | 0 |
| Ethiopia | 2006 | 1.193 | 4468.393 | 0 | 0 | 0 |
| Gabon | 2006 | 1.288 | 4565.747 | 0 | 0 | 0 |
| Gambia, The | 2006 | 1.5245 | 4676.017 | 0 | 0 | 0 |
| Ghana | 2006 | 1.64275 | 4786.986 | 0 | 0 | 0 |
| Guinea | 2006 | 1.701875 | 4894.178 | 0 | 0 | 0 |
| Guinea-Bissau | 2006 | 1.731438 | 4996.3 | 0 | 0 | 0 |
| Kenya | 2006 | 1.761 | 5098.627 | 0 | 0 | 0 |
| Lesotho | 2006 | 2.106 | 5197.559 | 0 | 0 | 0 |
| Liberia | 2006 | 2.2785 | 5303.507 | 0 | 0 | 0 |
| Libya | 2006 | 2.36475 | 5426.213 | 0 | 0 | 0 |
| Madagascar | 2006 | 2.407875 | 5556.437 | 0 | 0 | 0 |
| Malawi | 2006 | 2.451 | 5703.966 | 0 | 0 | 0 |
| Mali | 2006 | 2.85 | 5859.294 | 0 | 0 | 0 |
| Mauritania | 2006 | 3.0495 | 6005.061 | 0 | 0 | 0 |
| Mauritius | 2006 | 3.14925 | 6136.282 | 0 | 0 | 0 |
| Morocco | 2006 | 3.199125 | 6280.477 | 0 | 0 | 0 |
| Mozambique | 2006 | 3.249 | 6443.183 | 1 | 0 | 1 |
| Namibia | 2006 | 3.47 | 6605.707 | 0 | 0 | 0 |
| Niger | 2006 | 3.5805 | 6734.098 | 0 | 0 | 0 |
| Nigeria | 2006 | 3.63575 | 6859.89 | 0 | 0 | 0 |
| Rwanda | 2006 | 3.663375 | 7184.53 | 0 | 0 | 0 |
| Sao Tome and Principe | 2006 | 3.691 | 7363.698 | 0 | 0 | 0 |
| Senegal | 2006 | 4.0335 | 7547.08 | 0 | 0 | 0 |
| Seychelles | 2006 | 4.20475 | 7728.019 | 0 | 0 | 0 |

| *Country Name* | *Year* | *Education* | *Population Density* | *Minor War* | *Civil War* | *Conflict* |
|---|---|---|---|---|---|---|
| Sierra Leone | 2006 | 4.290375 | 7898.56 | 0 | 0 | 0 |
| Somalia | 2006 | 4.333188 | 8056.693 | 0 | 0 | 0 |
| South Africa | 2006 | 4.376 | 8211.005 | 0 | 0 | 0 |
| Sudan | 2006 | 4.7215 | 8368.521 | 0 | 0 | 0 |
| Swaziland | 2006 | 4.89425 | 8526.789 | 0 | 0 | 0 |
| Tanzania | 2006 | 4.980625 | 8684.117 | 0 | 0 | 0 |
| Togo | 2006 | 5.023813 | 8835.404 | 0 | 0 | 0 |
| Tunisia | 2006 | 5.067 | 8976.271 | 0 | 0 | 0 |
| Uganda | 2006 | 5.445 | 9108.858 | 0 | 0 | 0 |
| Zambia | 2006 | 5.634 | 9235.294 | 0 | 0 | 0 |
| Zimbabwe | 2006 | 5.7285 | 9352.742 | 0 | 0 | 0 |
| Algeria | 2007 | 5.77575 | 9462.545 | 0 | 0 | 0 |
| Angola | 2007 | 5.823 | 9508 | 0 | 0 | 0 |
| Benin | 2007 | 6.1995 | 9610 | 0 | 0 | 0 |
| Botswana | 2007 | 6.38775 | 9710 | 0 | 0 | 0 |
| Burkina Faso | 2007 | 6.481875 | 9812 | 0 | 0 | 0 |
| Burundi | 2007 | 6.528938 | 9914 | 0 | 0 | 0 |
| Cabo Verde | 2007 | 6.576 | 10013 | 0 | 0 | 0 |
| Cameroon | 2007 | 6.9495 | 10112 | 0 | 0 | 0 |
| Central African Republic | 2007 | 7.13625 | 10213 | 0 | 0 | 0 |
| Chad | 2007 | 7.229625 | 10316 | 0 | 0 | 0 |
| Comoros | 2007 | 7.323 | 10421 | 0 | 0 | 0 |
| Congo, Dem. Rep. | 2007 | 1.161 | 7688.797 | 0 | 0 | 0 |
| Congo, Rep. | 2007 | 1.2 | 7913.96 | 0 | 0 | 0 |
| Cote d'Ivoire | 2007 | 1.2195 | 8147.346 | 0 | 0 | 0 |
| Djibouti | 2007 | 1.239 | 8389.294 | 0 | 0 | 0 |
| Egypt, Arab Rep. | 2007 | 1.37 | 8640.153 | 0 | 0 | 0 |
| Equatorial Guinea | 2007 | 1.4355 | 8900.294 | 0 | 0 | 0 |
| Eritrea | 2007 | 1.46825 | 9170.101 | 0 | 0 | 0 |
| Ethiopia | 2007 | 1.484625 | 9449.977 | 0 | 0 | 0 |
| Gabon | 2007 | 1.501 | 9742.933 | 0 | 0 | 0 |
| Gambia, The | 2007 | 1.732 | 10008.82 | 1 | 0 | 1 |
| Ghana | 2007 | 1.8475 | 10224.46 | 1 | 0 | 1 |
| Guinea | 2007 | 1.90525 | 10428.15 | 0 | 0 | 0 |
| Guinea-Bissau | 2007 | 1.934125 | 10672.2 | 1 | 0 | 1 |
| Kenya | 2007 | 1.963 | 10952.42 | 0 | 0 | 0 |
| Lesotho | 2007 | 2.1535 | 11242.11 | 0 | 0 | 0 |
| Liberia | 2007 | 2.24875 | 11541.05 | 0 | 0 | 0 |
| Libya | 2007 | 2.296375 | 11850.35 | 1 | 0 | 1 |
| Madagascar | 2007 | 2.320188 | 12138.47 | 0 | 1 | 1 |
| Malawi | 2007 | 2.344 | 12414.72 | 1 | 1 | 1 |
| Mali | 2007 | 2.608 | 12725.25 | 0 | 1 | 1 |
| Mauritania | 2007 | 2.74 | 13078.93 | 0 | 1 | 1 |
| Mauritius | 2007 | 2.806 | 13470.39 | 0 | 1 | 1 |
| Morocco | 2007 | 2.839 | 13919.51 | 0 | 1 | 1 |
| Mozambique | 2007 | 2.872 | 14391.74 | 0 | 1 | 1 |
| Namibia | 2007 | 3.185 | 14910.72 | 0 | 1 | 1 |

| *Country Name* | *Year* | *Education* | *Population Density* | *Minor War* | *Civil War* | *Conflict* |
|---|---|---|---|---|---|---|
| Niger | 2007 | 3.3415 | 15520.09 | 0 | 1 | 1 |
| Nigeria | 2007 | 3.41975 | 16176.42 | 0 | 1 | 1 |
| Rwanda | 2007 | 3.458875 | 16832.38 | 0 | 1 | 1 |
| Sao Tome and Principe | 2007 | 3.498 | 17455.76 | 1 | 1 | 1 |
| Senegal | 2007 | 3.746 | 18082.14 | 1 | 1 | 1 |
| Seychelles | 2007 | 3.87 | 18729.45 | 1 | 1 | 1 |
| Sierra Leone | 2007 | 3.932 | 19424.38 | 1 | 1 | 1 |
| Somalia | 2007 | 3.963 | 20127.59 | 1 | 1 | 1 |
| South Africa | 2007 | 3.994 | 20689.52 | 1 | 1 | 1 |
| Sudan | 2007 | 4.1585 | 21248.72 | 0 | 1 | 1 |
| Swaziland | 2007 | 4.24075 | 21861.01 | 1 | 1 | 1 |
| Tanzania | 2007 | 4.281875 | 22502.14 | 1 | 1 | 1 |
| Togo | 2007 | 4.302438 | 23227.67 | 1 | 1 | 1 |
| Tunisia | 2007 | 4.323 | 23956 | 1 | 1 | 1 |
| Uganda | 2007 | 4.5925 | 24690 | 1 | 1 | 1 |
| Zambia | 2007 | 4.72725 | 25470 | 0 | 1 | 1 |
| Zimbabwe | 2007 | 4.794625 | 26322 | 1 | 1 | 1 |
| Algeria | 2008 | 4.828313 | 27234 | 0 | 1 | 1 |
| Angola | 2008 | 4.862 | 28199 | 1 | 1 | 1 |
| Benin | 2008 | 5.116 | 29207 | 1 | 1 | 1 |
| Botswana | 2008 | 5.243 | 30263 | 1 | 1 | 1 |
| Burkina Faso | 2008 | 5.3065 | 31368 | 1 | 1 | 1 |
| Burundi | 2008 | 5.37 | 32370 | 1 | 1 | 1 |
| Cabo Verde | 2008 | 1.745 | 10863.96 | 0 | 0 | 0 |
| Cameroon | 2008 | 1.8215 | 11185.24 | 0 | 0 | 0 |
| Central African Republic | 2008 | 1.85975 | 11521.7 | 0 | 0 | 0 |
| Chad | 2008 | 1.898 | 11870.41 | 0 | 0 | 0 |
| Comoros | 2008 | 2.104 | 12231.39 | 0 | 0 | 0 |
| Congo, Dem. Rep. | 2008 | 2.207 | 12607.31 | 0 | 0 | 0 |
| Congo, Rep. | 2008 | 2.2585 | 12988.14 | 0 | 0 | 0 |
| Cote d'Ivoire | 2008 | 2.28425 | 13389.54 | 0 | 0 | 0 |
| Djibouti | 2008 | 2.31 | 13806.87 | 0 | 0 | 0 |
| Egypt, Arab Rep. | 2008 | 2.454 | 14236.87 | 0 | 0 | 0 |
| Equatorial Guinea | 2008 | 2.526 | 14706.59 | 0 | 0 | 0 |
| Eritrea | 2008 | 2.562 | 15201.38 | 0 | 0 | 0 |
| Ethiopia | 2008 | 2.58 | 15681.23 | 0 | 0 | 0 |
| Gabon | 2008 | 2.598 | 16147.86 | 0 | 0 | 0 |
| Gambia, The | 2008 | 2.9135 | 16625.71 | 0 | 0 | 0 |
| Ghana | 2008 | 3.07125 | 17129.57 | 0 | 0 | 0 |
| Guinea | 2008 | 3.150125 | 17647.4 | 1 | 0 | 1 |
| Guinea-Bissau | 2008 | 3.189563 | 18144.83 | 0 | 0 | 0 |
| Kenya | 2008 | 3.229 | 18665.06 | 0 | 0 | 0 |
| Lesotho | 2008 | 3.45 | 19212 | 0 | 0 | 0 |
| Liberia | 2008 | 3.5605 | 19776.79 | 0 | 0 | 0 |
| Libya | 2008 | 3.61575 | 20368.42 | 0 | 0 | 0 |
| Madagascar | 2008 | 3.643375 | 20984.09 | 0 | 0 | 0 |
| Malawi | 2008 | 3.671 | 21618.43 | 0 | 0 | 0 |

| Country Name | Year | Education | Population Density | Minor War | Civil War | Conflict |
|---|---|---|---|---|---|---|
| Mali | 2008 | 3.878 | 22284.17 | 0 | 0 | 0 |
| Mauritania | 2008 | 3.9815 | 23016.72 | 0 | 0 | 0 |
| Mauritius | 2008 | 4.03325 | 23763.76 | 0 | 0 | 0 |
| Morocco | 2008 | 4.059125 | 24484.89 | 0 | 0 | 0 |
| Mozambique | 2008 | 4.085 | 25214.28 | 0 | 0 | 0 |
| Namibia | 2008 | 4.228 | 25972.54 | 0 | 0 | 0 |
| Niger | 2008 | 4.2995 | 26767.47 | 0 | 0 | 0 |
| Nigeria | 2008 | 4.33525 | 27696.59 | 0 | 0 | 0 |
| Rwanda | 2008 | 4.353125 | 28797.66 | 0 | 0 | 0 |
| Sao Tome and Principe | 2008 | 4.371 | 29752.9 | 0 | 0 | 0 |
| Senegal | 2008 | 4.5515 | 30392.14 | 0 | 0 | 0 |
| Seychelles | 2008 | 4.64175 | 31092.65 | 0 | 0 | 0 |
| Sierra Leone | 2008 | 4.686875 | 31950.96 | 0 | 0 | 0 |
| Somalia | 2008 | 4.709438 | 32808.03 | 0 | 0 | 0 |
| South Africa | 2008 | 4.732 | 33712.12 | 0 | 0 | 0 |
| Sudan | 2008 | 4.89 | 34567.25 | 0 | 0 | 0 |
| Swaziland | 2008 | 4.969 | 35383.1 | 0 | 0 | 0 |
| Tanzania | 2008 | 5.0085 | 36198.79 | 0 | 0 | 0 |
| Togo | 2008 | 5.02825 | 36989.97 | 0 | 0 | 0 |
| Tunisia | 2008 | 5.048 | 37770.57 | 0 | 0 | 0 |
| Uganda | 2008 | 5.2925 | 38568.53 | 0 | 0 | 0 |
| Zambia | 2008 | 5.41475 | 39384.22 | 0 | 0 | 0 |
| Zimbabwe | 2008 | 5.475875 | 40213 | 0 | 0 | 0 |
| Algeria | 2009 | 5.537 | 41049 | 0 | 0 | 0 |
| Angola | 2009 | | | 0 | 0 | 0 |
| Benin | 2009 | | | 0 | 0 | 0 |
| Botswana | 2009 | | | 0 | 0 | 0 |
| Burkina Faso | 2009 | | | 0 | 0 | 0 |
| Burundi | 2009 | | | 0 | 0 | 0 |
| Cabo Verde | 2009 | | | 0 | 0 | 0 |
| Cameroon | 2009 | | | 0 | 0 | 0 |
| Central African Republic | 2009 | | | 0 | 0 | 0 |
| Chad | 2009 | | | 0 | 0 | 0 |
| Comoros | 2009 | | | 0 | 0 | 0 |
| Congo, Dem. Rep. | 2009 | | | 0 | 0 | 0 |
| Congo, Rep. | 2009 | | | 0 | 0 | 0 |
| Cote d'Ivoire | 2009 | | | 0 | 0 | 0 |
| Djibouti | 2009 | | | 0 | 0 | 0 |
| Egypt, Arab Rep. | 2009 | | | 0 | 0 | 0 |
| Equatorial Guinea | 2009 | | | 0 | 0 | 0 |
| Eritrea | 2009 | | | 0 | 0 | 0 |
| Ethiopia | 2009 | | | 0 | 0 | 0 |
| Gabon | 2009 | | | 0 | 0 | 0 |
| Gambia, The | 2009 | | | 0 | 0 | 0 |
| Ghana | 2009 | | | 0 | 0 | 0 |
| Guinea | 2009 | | | 0 | 0 | 0 |
| Guinea-Bissau | 2009 | | | 0 | 0 | 0 |

| *Country Name* | *Year* | *Education* | *Population Density* | *Minor War* | *Civil War* | *Conflict* |
|---|---|---|---|---|---|---|
| Kenya | 2009 | | | 0 | 0 | 0 |
| Lesotho | 2009 | | | 0 | 0 | 0 |
| Liberia | 2009 | | | 0 | 0 | 0 |
| Libya | 2009 | | | 0 | 0 | 0 |
| Madagascar | 2009 | | | 0 | 0 | 0 |
| Malawi | 2009 | | | 0 | 0 | 0 |
| Mali | 2009 | | | 0 | 0 | 0 |
| Mauritania | 2009 | | | 0 | 0 | 0 |
| Mauritius | 2009 | | | 0 | 0 | 0 |
| Morocco | 2009 | | | 0 | 0 | 0 |
| Mozambique | 2009 | | | 0 | 0 | 0 |
| Namibia | 2009 | | | 0 | 0 | 0 |
| Niger | 2009 | | | 0 | 0 | 0 |
| Nigeria | 2009 | | | 0 | 0 | 0 |
| Rwanda | 2009 | | | 0 | 0 | 0 |
| Sao Tome and Principe | 2009 | | | 0 | 0 | 0 |
| Senegal | 2009 | | | 0 | 0 | 0 |
| Seychelles | 2009 | | | 0 | 0 | 0 |
| Sierra Leone | 2009 | | | 0 | 0 | 0 |
| Somalia | 2009 | | | 0 | 0 | 0 |
| South Africa | 2009 | | | 0 | 0 | 0 |
| Sudan | 2009 | | | 0 | 0 | 0 |
| Swaziland | 2009 | | | 0 | 0 | 0 |
| Tanzania | 2009 | | | 0 | 0 | 0 |
| Togo | 2009 | | | 0 | 0 | 0 |
| Tunisia | 2009 | 2.256 | 3421 | 0 | 0 | 0 |
| Uganda | 2009 | 2.411 | 3508 | 0 | 0 | 0 |
| Zambia | 2009 | 2.4885 | 3599 | 0 | 0 | 0 |
| Zimbabwe | 2009 | 2.566 | 3694 | 0 | 0 | 0 |
| Algeria | 2010 | 2.7705 | 3794 | 0 | 0 | 0 |
| Angola | 2010 | 2.87275 | 3900 | 0 | 0 | 0 |
| Benin | 2010 | 2.923875 | 4009 | 0 | 0 | 0 |
| Botswana | 2010 | 2.949438 | 4123 | 0 | 0 | 0 |
| Burkina Faso | 2010 | 2.975 | 4251.612 | 0 | 0 | 0 |
| Burundi | 2010 | 3.2935 | 4376.371 | 0 | 0 | 0 |
| Cabo Verde | 2010 | 3.45275 | 4506.497 | 0 | 0 | 0 |
| Cameroon | 2010 | 3.532375 | 4642.941 | 0 | 0 | 0 |
| Central African Republic | 2010 | 3.572188 | 4784.668 | 0 | 0 | 0 |
| Chad | 2010 | 3.612 | 4923.73 | 0 | 0 | 0 |
| Comoros | 2010 | 3.869 | 5067.045 | 0 | 0 | 0 |
| Congo, Dem. Rep. | 2010 | 3.9975 | 5216.55 | 0 | 0 | 0 |
| Congo, Rep. | 2010 | 4.06175 | 5371.218 | 0 | 0 | 0 |
| Cote d'Ivoire | 2010 | 4.093875 | 5531.99 | 0 | 0 | 0 |
| Djibouti | 2010 | 4.126 | 5699.777 | 0 | 0 | 0 |
| Egypt, Arab Rep. | 2010 | 4.3625 | 5885.614 | 0 | 0 | 0 |
| Equatorial Guinea | 2010 | 4.48075 | 6102.344 | 0 | 0 | 0 |
| Eritrea | 2010 | 4.539875 | 6340.246 | 0 | 0 | 0 |
| Ethiopia | 2010 | 4.569438 | 6567.207 | 0 | 0 | 0 |

| Country Name | Year | Education | Population Density | Minor War | Civil War | Conflict |
|---|---|---|---|---|---|---|
| Gabon | 2010 | 4.599 | 6784.665 | 0 | 0 | 0 |
| Gambia, The | 2010 | 4.746 | 7029.393 | 0 | 0 | 0 |
| Ghana | 2010 | 4.8195 | 7282.298 | 0 | 0 | 0 |
| Guinea | 2010 | 4.85625 | 7517.299 | 0 | 0 | 0 |
| Guinea-Bissau | 2010 | 4.874625 | 7746.084 | 0 | 0 | 0 |
| Kenya | 2010 | 4.893 | 7977.698 | 0 | 0 | 0 |
| Lesotho | 2010 | 5.471 | 8212.432 | 0 | 0 | 0 |
| Liberia | 2010 | 5.76 | 8444.666 | 0 | 0 | 0 |
| Libya | 2010 | 5.9045 | 8670.841 | 0 | 0 | 0 |
| Madagascar | 2010 | 5.97675 | 8891.693 | 0 | 0 | 0 |
| Malawi | 2010 | 6.049 | 9102.094 | 0 | 0 | 0 |
| Mali | 2010 | 6.1265 | 9306.22 | 0 | 0 | 0 |
| Mauritania | 2010 | 6.16525 | 9528.978 | 0 | 0 | 0 |
| Mauritius | 2010 | 6.184625 | 9749.568 | 0 | 0 | 0 |
| Morocco | 2010 | 6.194313 | 9967.447 | 0 | 0 | 0 |
| Mozambique | 2010 | 6.204 | 10345 | 0 | 0 | 0 |
| Namibia | 2010 | 6.3405 | 10646 | 0 | 0 | 0 |
| Niger | 2010 | 6.40875 | 10917 | 0 | 0 | 0 |
| Nigeria | 2010 | 6.442875 | 11173 | 0 | 0 | 0 |
| Rwanda | 2010 | 6.459938 | 11434 | 0 | 0 | 0 |
| Sao Tome and Principe | 2010 | 6.477 | 11710 | 0 | 0 | 0 |
| Senegal | 2010 | 6.715 | 12013 | 0 | 0 | 0 |
| Seychelles | 2010 | 6.834 | 12341 | 0 | 0 | 0 |
| Sierra Leone | 2010 | 6.8935 | 12694 | 0 | 0 | 0 |
| Somalia | 2010 | 6.953 | 13061 | 0 | 0 | 0 |
| South Africa | 2010 | 2.549 | 4277.736 | 0 | 0 | 0 |
| Sudan | 2010 | 2.6405 | 4412.423 | 0 | 0 | 0 |
| Swaziland | 2010 | 2.68625 | 4537.263 | 0 | 0 | 0 |
| Tanzania | 2010 | 2.732 | 4685.272 | 0 | 0 | 0 |
| Togo | 2010 | 2.934 | 4835.691 | 0 | 0 | 0 |
| Tunisia | 2010 | 3.035 | 4995.432 | 1 | 0 | 1 |
| Uganda | 2010 | 3.0855 | 5171.817 | 1 | 0 | 1 |
| Zambia | 2010 | 3.11075 | 5352.802 | 0 | 0 | 0 |
| Zimbabwe | 2010 | 3.136 | 5514.536 | 0 | 0 | 0 |
| Algeria | 2011 | 3.2665 | 5684.187 | 0 | 0 | 0 |
| Angola | 2011 | 3.33175 | 5861.135 | 0 | 0 | 0 |
| Benin | 2011 | 3.364375 | 6001.949 | 1 | 0 | 1 |
| Botswana | 2011 | 3.380688 | 6172.535 | 1 | 0 | 1 |
| Burkina Faso | 2011 | 3.397 | 6341.797 | 1 | 0 | 1 |
| Burundi | 2011 | 3.6215 | 6496.418 | 0 | 1 | 1 |
| Cabo Verde | 2011 | 3.73375 | 6642.107 | 0 | 1 | 1 |
| Cameroon | 2011 | 3.789875 | 6767.223 | 0 | 1 | 1 |
| Central African Republic | 2011 | 3.817938 | 6887.132 | 0 | 1 | 1 |
| Chad | 2011 | 3.846 | 7169.968 | 0 | 0 | 0 |
| Comoros | 2011 | 4.2095 | 7429.223 | 0 | 0 | 0 |
| Congo, Dem. Rep. | 2011 | 4.39125 | 7636.524 | 0 | 0 | 0 |
| Congo, Rep. | 2011 | 4.482125 | 7928.344 | 0 | 0 | 0 |
| Cote d'Ivoire | 2011 | 4.527563 | 8241.214 | 0 | 0 | 0 |

| Country Name | Year | Education | Population Density | Minor War | Civil War | Conflict |
|---|---|---|---|---|---|---|
| Djibouti | 2011 | 4.573 | 8560.488 | 0 | 0 | 0 |
| Egypt, Arab Rep. | 2011 | 5.1485 | 8876.783 | 0 | 0 | 0 |
| Equatorial Guinea | 2011 | 5.43625 | 9216.479 | 0 | 0 | 0 |
| Eritrea | 2011 | 5.580125 | 9560.047 | 0 | 0 | 0 |
| Ethiopia | 2011 | 5.652063 | 9868.2 | 0 | 0 | 0 |
| Gabon | 2011 | 5.724 | 10156.04 | 0 | 0 | 0 |
| Gambia, The | 2011 | 6.198 | 10437.42 | 0 | 0 | 0 |
| Ghana | 2011 | 6.435 | 10720.25 | 0 | 0 | 0 |
| Guinea | 2011 | 6.5535 | 10976.37 | 0 | 0 | 0 |
| Guinea-Bissau | 2011 | 6.61275 | 11086.48 | 0 | 0 | 0 |
| Kenya | 2011 | 6.672 | 11159.49 | 0 | 0 | 0 |
| Lesotho | 2011 | 6.8375 | 11316.95 | 0 | 0 | 0 |
| Liberia | 2011 | 6.92025 | 11469.39 | 0 | 0 | 0 |
| Libya | 2011 | 6.961625 | 11606.92 | 0 | 0 | 0 |
| Madagascar | 2011 | 6.982313 | 11733.08 | 0 | 0 | 0 |
| Malawi | 2011 | 7.003 | 11820.03 | 0 | 0 | 0 |
| Mali | 2011 | 7.2425 | 11867.86 | 0 | 0 | 0 |
| Mauritania | 2011 | 7.36225 | 11866.02 | 0 | 0 | 0 |
| Mauritius | 2011 | 7.422125 | 11815.52 | 0 | 0 | 0 |
| Morocco | 2011 | 7.452063 | 11735.05 | 0 | 0 | 0 |
| Mozambique | 2011 | 7.482 | 11639.47 | 0 | 0 | 0 |
| Namibia | 2011 | 7.578 | 11544.33 | 0 | 0 | 0 |
| Niger | 2011 | 7.626 | 11443.19 | 0 | 0 | 0 |
| Nigeria | 2011 | 7.65 | 11350 | 0 | 0 | 0 |
| Rwanda | 2011 | 7.674 | 11383 | 0 | 0 | 0 |

*Note*: Zero (0) means no war/conflict was recorded during the period, while one (1) means at least one war/conflict was recorded during the period.

## AVERAGES OF LIFE EXPECTANCY AT BIRTH DATA ACROSS DECADES (1960S–2000S)

| Country Name | L2000s | L1990s | L1980s | L1970s | L1960s | Decades Averages Per Country |
|---|---|---|---|---|---|---|
| Algeria | 74 | 68.07404 | 63.0 | 53 | 48.1 | 61 |
| Angola | 55 | 43.28356 | 41.1 | 39 | 34.9 | 43 |
| Benin | 58 | 54.81117 | 49.8 | 44 | 39.4 | 49 |
| Botswana | 56 | 56.02999 | 61.9 | 57 | 52.2 | 57 |
| Burkina Faso | 55 | 49.47617 | 48.5 | 42 | 36.6 | 46 |
| Burundi | 54 | 48.97694 | 48.3 | 45 | 42.6 | 48 |
| Cabo Verde | 71 | 66.55371 | 63.0 | 57 | 50.6 | 62 |
| Cameroon | 54 | 50.50488 | 52.3 | 48 | 43.5 | 50 |
| Central African Republic | 46 | 46.49584 | 49.5 | 45 | 38.6 | 45 |

| *Country Name* | *L2000s* | *L1990s* | *L1980s* | *L1970s* | *L1960s* | *Decades Averages Per Country* |
|---|---|---|---|---|---|---|
| Chad | 49 | 47.31517 | 45.8 | 43 | 39.3 | 45 |
| Comoros | 61 | 58.32108 | 53.4 | 48 | 43.3 | 53 |
| Congo, Dem. Rep. | 55 | 49.16523 | 47.5 | 45 | 42.1 | 48 |
| Congo, Rep. | 58 | 53.58681 | 56.6 | 55 | 51.0 | 55 |
| Cote d'Ivoire | 49 | 49.88374 | 52.2 | 47 | 39.8 | 48 |
| Djibouti | 59 | 56.95284 | 55.2 | 51 | 46.1 | 54 |
| Egypt, Arab Rep. | 70 | 66.5002 | 61.3 | 55 | 50.1 | 60 |
| Equatorial Guinea | 55 | 50.32154 | 46.1 | 41 | 38.1 | 46 |
| Eritrea | 60 | 52.05401 | 47.9 | 45 | 40.8 | 49 |
| Ethiopia | 59 | 49.1303 | 44.8 | 44 | 40.8 | 47 |
| Gabon | 62 | 60.5241 | 58.4 | 50 | 42.3 | 55 |
| Gambia, The | 59 | 53.80574 | 49.5 | 42 | 34.1 | 48 |
| Ghana | 60 | 57.25057 | 54.0 | 51 | 47.6 | 54 |
| Guinea | 55 | 51.2039 | 45.1 | 38 | 35.7 | 45 |
| Guinea-Bissau | 54 | 50.64451 | 47.2 | 43 | 39.4 | 47 |
| Kenya | 59 | 54.44936 | 58.6 | 55 | 49.1 | 55 |
| Lesotho | 49 | 56.13086 | 56.1 | 51 | 47.9 | 52 |
| Liberia | 57 | 49.73949 | 47.0 | 42 | 36.5 | 47 |
| Libya | 71 | 69.72534 | 66.4 | 60 | 49.3 | 63 |
| Madagascar | 62 | 54.27833 | 49.7 | 47 | 42.1 | 51 |
| Malawi | 54 | 46.51519 | 45.8 | 42 | 38.8 | 45 |
| Mali | 53 | 46.56008 | 42.7 | 36 | 29.6 | 42 |
| Mauritania | 61 | 59.21163 | 56.5 | 51 | 46.2 | 55 |
| Mauritius | 73 | 70.23073 | 68.2 | 64 | 61.6 | 67 |
| Morocco | 72 | 66.54386 | 60.9 | 54 | 50.3 | 61 |
| Mozambique | 53 | 45.17448 | 41.9 | 41 | 36.9 | 44 |
| Namibia | 57 | 59.81388 | 59.3 | 55 | 49.5 | 56 |
| Niger | 55 | 46.32478 | 41.0 | 37 | 35.4 | 43 |
| Nigeria | 50 | 45.90397 | 45.9 | 43 | 38.8 | 45 |
| Rwanda | 59 | 34.71233 | 47.8 | 45 | 43.4 | 46 |
| Sao Tome and Principe | 65 | 62.47539 | 61.0 | 58 | 52.9 | 60 |
| Senegal | 62 | 57.39029 | 53.2 | 43 | 38.4 | 51 |
| Seychelles | 73 | 71.04268 | 69.2 | 43 | 38.4 | 59 |
| Sierra Leone | 46 | 36.492 | 40.0 | 38 | 31.7 | 38 |
| Somalia | 53 | 47.24948 | 45.7 | 43 | 38.8 | 46 |
| South Africa | 56 | 60.82069 | 59.7 | 57 | 53.8 | 57 |
| Sudan | 61 | 56.64617 | 54.7 | 53 | 50.0 | 55 |
| Swaziland | 50 | 56.18323 | 57.5 | 51 | 45.7 | 52 |
| Tanzania | 58 | 49.87204 | 50.7 | 49 | 44.9 | 50 |
| Togo | 56 | 54.81722 | 54.3 | 49 | 43.1 | 52 |
| Tunisia | 74 | 71.16124 | 65.4 | 56 | 45.6 | 63 |
| Uganda | 54 | 44.92959 | 48.1 | 49 | 46.5 | 49 |
| Zambia | 53 | 43.77477 | 48.8 | 51 | 46.8 | 49 |
| Zimbabwe | 50 | 51.68481 | 60.2 | 57 | 53.1 | 54 |

# AVERAGES OF COLD WAR DIVISION OF DEVELOPMENT INDICATORS

| | | | | Cold War Era 1947–1991 | | | | |
|---|---|---|---|---|---|---|---|---|
| *Country Name* | *Cold War Era* | *Life Expectancy* | *GDP Per Capita* | *Pop. Density* | *Education* | *MWAR* | *CWAR* | *Conflict* |
| Algeria | 1947–1991 | 55.46165 | 3036.229 | 17489.13 | 2.90495 | 1 | 1 | 1 |
| Angola | 1947–1991 | 38.45794 | 2641.244 | 6422.792 | 0 | 1 | 1 | 1 |
| Benin | 1947–1991 | 45.15583 | 579.3914 | 3261.755 | 1.277927 | 0 | 0 | 0 |
| Botswana | 1947–1991 | 57.37272 | 1597.326 | 818.4009 | 3.594042 | 0 | 0 | 0 |
| Burkina Faso | 1947–1991 | 42.68121 | 298.6943 | 6184.367 | 0 | 1 | 0 | 1 |
| Burundi | 1947–1991 | 45.49938 | 267.5267 | 4082.508 | 1.284752 | 1 | 0 | 1 |
| Cabo Verde | 1947–1991 | 57.48438 | 834.1315 | 2221.712 | 1.49986 | 0 | 0 | 0 |
| Cameroon | 1947–1991 | 48.32703 | 1219.355 | 8312.601 | 2.777202 | 1 | 1 | 1 |
| Central African Republic | 1947–1991 | 44.74087 | 559.3232 | 0 | 0 | 0 | 0 | 0 |
| Chad | 1947–1991 | 42.98059 | 569.5072 | 4359.67 | 0 | 1 | 1 | 1 |
| Comoros | 1947–1991 | 48.68752 | 893.8451 | 300.6979 | 0 | 1 | 0 | 1 |
| Congo, Dem. Rep. | 1947–1991 | 45.15071 | 895.4419 | 27074.82 | 1.841315 | 1 | 1 | 1 |
| Congo, Rep. | 1947–1991 | 54.18681 | 2113.734 | 1578.323 | 3.579473 | 0 | 0 | 0 |
| Cote d'Ivoire | 1947–1991 | 46.78788 | 1739.613 | 7753.406 | 1.855354 | 0 | 0 | 0 |
| Djibouti | 1947–1991 | 51.25865 | 1507.365 | 232.6383 | 0 | 1 | 0 | 1 |
| Egypt, Arab Rep. | 1947–1991 | 55.94423 | 1031.494 | 40606.14 | 2.470975 | 1 | 1 | 1 |
| Equatorial Guinea | 1947–1991 | 42.18042 | 570.635 | 276.6887 | 0 | 1 | 0 | 1 |
| Eritrea | 1947–1991 | 44.82771 | 501.0187 | 625.3499 | 0.988375 | 1 | 0 | 1 |
| Ethiopia | 1947–1991 | 43.36103 | 212.7491 | 35301.9 | 0 | 1 | 1 | 1 |
| Gabon | 1947–1991 | 51.02889 | 9878.996 | 671.0378 | 3.111004 | 1 | 0 | 1 |
| Gambia, The | 1947–1991 | 42.43889 | 501.0187 | 625.3499 | 0.988375 | 1 | 0 | 1 |

| Cold War Era 1947–1991 | | | | | | | | |
|---|---|---|---|---|---|---|---|---|
| Country Name | Cold War Era | Life Expectancy | GDP Per Capita | Pop. Density | Education | MWAR | CWAR | Conflict |
| Ghana | 1947–1991 | 51.14154 | 936.2336 | 10838.06 | 4.23449 | 1 | 0 | 1 |
| Guinea | 1947–1991 | 40.3707 | 562.2164 | 4342.606 | 0 | 0 | 0 | 0 |
| Guinea-Bissau | 1947–1991 | 43.65826 | 540.802 | 750.6828 | 0 | 1 | 1 | 1 |
| Kenya | 1947–1991 | 54.33903 | 755.3582 | 15091.71 | 3.485546 | 1 | 0 | 1 |
| Lesotho | 1947–1991 | 52.02572 | 465.6724 | 1269.812 | 3.983008 | 0 | 0 | 0 |
| Liberia | 1947–1991 | 42.29663 | 1319.604 | 1695.865 | 1.885792 | 1 | 1 | 1 |
| Libya | 1947–1991 | 59.25733 | 1291.708 | 2742.386 | 2.863131 | 0 | 0 | 0 |
| Madagascar | 1947–1991 | 46.54488 | 620.8031 | 8253.172 | 0 | 1 | 0 | 1 |
| Malawi | 1947–1991 | 42.6147 | 335.7347 | 5925.816 | 2.08444 | 0 | 0 | 0 |
| Mali | 1947–1991 | 36.57799 | 421.748 | 6304.171 | 0.53058 | 1 | 0 | 1 |
| Mauritania | 1947–1991 | 51.7634 | 1094.371 | 1486.394 | 2.091846 | 1 | 0 | 1 |
| Mauritius | 1947–1991 | 65.06067 | 2820.735 | 906.2007 | 5.285783 | 0 | 0 | 0 |
| Morocco | 1947–1991 | 55.83487 | 1291.708 | 18506.96 | 1.679775 | 1 | 1 | 1 |
| Mozambique | 1947–1991 | 40.13124 | 162.5836 | 10817 | 1.011267 | 1 | 1 | 1 |
| Namibia | 1947–1991 | 54.95253 | 3888.73 | 980.402 | 4.765198 | 0 | 0 | 0 |
| Niger | 1947–1991 | 38.1234 | 530.5255 | 5764.662 | 0.647169 | 0 | 0 | 0 |
| Nigeria | 1947–1991 | 42.77405 | 1534.579 | 68888.27 | 4.544565 | 1 | 1 | 1 |
| Rwanda | 1947–1991 | 44.63506 | 347.5477 | 4778.136 | 1.508577 | 1 | 1 | 1 |
| Sao Tome and Principe | 1947–1991 | 57.70802 | 5964.797 | 88.6231 | 0 | 0 | 0 | 0 |
| Senegal | 1947–1991 | 45.72816 | 950.9991 | 5436.947 | 2.704056 | 1 | 0 | 1 |
| Seychelles | 1947–1991 | 69.20744 | 4758.219 | 59.58747 | 0 | 0 | 0 | 0 |
| Sierra Leone | 1947–1991 | 36.55089 | 450.4163 | 3210.534 | 1.373877 | 1 | 0 | 1 |
| Somalia | 1947–1991 | 42.56413 | 347.5477 | 4838.784 | 0 | 1 | 1 | 1 |
| South Africa | 1947–1991 | 57.15218 | 5964.797 | 27683.86 | 5.203544 | 1 | 1 | 1 |
| Sudan | 1947–1991 | 52.89606 | 815.2764 | 17840.58 | 1.23579 | 1 | 1 | 1 |
| Swaziland | 1947–1991 | 51.84464 | 1754.059 | 580.1774 | 3.997479 | 0 | 0 | 0 |

| Cold War Era 1947–1991 | | | | | | | | |
|---|---|---|---|---|---|---|---|---|
| *Country Name* | *Cold War Era* | *Life Expectancy* | *GDP Per Capita* | *Pop. Density* | *Education* | *MWAR* | *CWAR* | *Conflict* |
| Tanzania | 1947–1991 | 48.17009 | 483.1466 | 17378.24 | 2.965565 | 1 | 0 | 1 |
| Togo | 1947–1991 | 49.29609 | 551.3052 | 2456.483 | 2.273533 | 1 | 0 | 1 |
| Tunisia | 1947–1991 | 56.56641 | 1760.717 | 5929.912 | 2.673429 | 1 | 0 | 1 |
| Uganda | 1947–1991 | 47.75865 | 293.2641 | 11447.89 | 2.146203 | 1 | 1 | 1 |
| Zambia | 1947–1991 | 48.48174 | 1378.103 | 5395.523 | 3.801198 | 0 | 0 | 0 |
| Zimbabwe | 1947–1991 | 56.7017 | 1126.504 | 6857.273 | 3.912692 | 1 | 1 | 1 |

*Note*: Zero (0) means no war/ conflict was recorded during the decades, while one (1) means at least one war/conflict was recorded during the decades.

## CONTEMPORARY INDEPENDENT ERA (1951–2018)

| *Country Name* | *Contemporary Independent Era* | *Life Expectancy* | *GDP Per Capita* | *Pop. Density* | *Education* | *MWAR* | *CWAR* | *Conflict* |
|---|---|---|---|---|---|---|---|---|
| Algeria | 1951–2018 | 62.46342 | 3426.114 | 22375.99 | 4.517216 | 1 | 1 | 1 |
| Angola | 1951–2018 | 43.94434 | 2627.274 | 8003.371 | 0 | 1 | 1 | 1 |
| Benin | 1951–2018 | 50.27601 | 637.8902 | 4592.487 | 2.032594 | 0 | 0 | 0 |
| Botswana | 1951–2018 | 56.67844 | 3282.133 | 1142.199 | 5.566758 | 0 | 0 | 0 |
| Burkina Faso | 1951–2018 | 47.20621 | 381.2343 | 8392.688 | 0 | 1 | 0 | 1 |
| Burundi | 1951–2018 | 48.4481 | 256.6598 | 5251.088 | 1.792109 | 1 | 1 | 1 |
| Cabo Verde | 1951–2018 | 62.83818 | 1904.846 | 2888.94 | 2.175116 | 1 | 0 | 1 |
| Cameroon | 1951–2018 | 50.20535 | 1225.585 | 11050.72 | 3.792492 | 1 | 1 | 1 |
| Central African Republic | 1951–2018 | 45.41563 | 495.565 | 5791.179 | 0 | 1 | 1 | 1 |
| Chad | 1951–2018 | 45.45449 | 617.8933 | 5791.179 | 0 | 1 | 1 | 1 |
| Comoros | 1951–2018 | 53.67066 | 821.8479 | 410.4723 | 0 | 1 | 0 | 1 |
| Congo, Dem. Rep. | 1951–2018 | 48.54802 | 654.5194 | 37215.78 | 2.414331 | 1 | 1 | 1 |

| Country Name | Contemporary Independent Era | Life Expectancy | GDP Per Capita | Pop. Density | Education | MWAR | CWAR | Conflict |
|---|---|---|---|---|---|---|---|---|
| Congo, Rep. | 1951–2018 | 54.9892 | 2298.63 | 2176.585 | 4.438279 | 1 | 1 | 1 |
| Cote d'Ivoire | 1951–2018 | 47.85409 | 1546.941 | 11246.4 | 2.621576 | 1 | 0 | 1 |
| Djibouti | 1951–2018 | 54.38445 | 1269.234 | 384.5228 | 0 | 1 | 0 | 1 |
| Egypt, Arab Rep. | 1951–2018 | 61.50432 | 1498.705 | 50313.19 | 3.813464 | 1 | 1 | 1 |
| Equatorial Guinea | 1951–2018 | 47.1138 | 7284.449 | 361.923 | 0 | 1 | 0 | 1 |
| Eritrea | 1951–2018 | 50.35085 | 538.9161 | 905.4211 | 1.683049 | 1 | 0 | 1 |
| Ethiopia | 1951–2018 | 48.64996 | 247.3897 | 46947.22 | 0 | 1 | 1 | 1 |
| Gabon | 1951–2018 | 55.40856 | 9932.62 | 887.512 | 4.63376 | 1 | 0 | 1 |
| Gambia, The | 1951–2018 | 48.7579 | 511.3056 | 905.4211 | 1.683049 | 1 | 0 | 1 |
| Ghana | 1951–2018 | 54.47557 | 1024.008 | 14226.16 | 5.098186 | 1 | 0 | 1 |
| Guinea | 1951–2018 | 46.13188 | 595.5247 | 5858.864 | 0 | 1 | 0 | 1 |
| Guinea-Bissau | 1951–2018 | 47.74631 | 553.3044 | 953.7659 | 0 | 1 | 1 | 1 |
| Kenya | 1951–2018 | 55.65642 | 820.6448 | 21207.87 | 4.70328 | 1 | 0 | 1 |
| Lesotho | 1951–2018 | 51.69233 | 694.1632 | 1501.466 | 4.631268 | 1 | 0 | 1 |
| Liberia | 1951–2018 | 47.70768 | 878.981 | 2040.44 | 2.635141 | 1 | 1 | 1 |
| Libya | 1951–2018 | 64.2697 | 9820.982 | 3681.971 | 4.306784 | 0 | 0 | 0 |
| Madagascar | 1951–2018 | 52.22901 | 534.0339 | 11224.89 | 0 | 1 | 0 | 1 |
| Malawi | 1951–2018 | 46.36356 | 362.9703 | 8252.417 | 2.734406 | 0 | 0 | 0 |
| Mali | 1951–2018 | 42.81217 | 518.5993 | 7995.137 | 0.861523 | 1 | 0 | 1 |
| Mauritania | 1951–2018 | 55.60122 | 1102.2 | 1888.481 | 2.710266 | 1 | 0 | 1 |
| Mauritius | 1951–2018 | 68.03985 | 4961.649 | 1012.208 | 5.96644 | 0 | 0 | 0 |
| Morocco | 1951–2018 | 62.17642 | 1801.085 | 22146.06 | 2.584815 | 1 | 1 | 1 |
| Mozambique | 1951–2018 | 44.5832 | 269.1984 | 13534.41 | 1.078939 | 1 | 1 | 1 |
| Namibia | 1951–2018 | 56.17683 | 4264.48 | 1315.563 | 5.188251 | 0 | 0 | 0 |
| Niger | 1951–2018 | 44.18718 | 450.2703 | 7847.277 | 0.949831 | 1 | 0 | 1 |
| Nigeria | 1951–2018 | 45.15447 | 1633.81 | 89891.88 | 5.422663 | 1 | 1 | 1 |
| Rwanda | 1951–2018 | 47.31609 | 388.4791 | 6149.801 | 2.167829 | 1 | 1 | 1 |
| Sao Tome and Principe | 1951–2018 | 60.51513 | 1042.941 | 109.6221 | 0 | 0 | 0 | 0 |

| *Country Name* | *Contemporary Independent Era* | *Life Expectancy* | *GDP Per Capita* | *Pop. Density* | *Education* | *MWAR* | *CWAR* | *Conflict* |
|---|---|---|---|---|---|---|---|---|
| Senegal | 1951–2018 | 52.11706 | 937.1796 | 7073.995 | 3.339854 | 1 | 1 | 1 |
| Seychelles | 1951–2018 | 72.25327 | 7066.408 | 65.8688 | 0 | 0 | 0 | 0 |
| Sierra Leone | 1951–2018 | 39.12195 | 415.789 | 3622.222 | 2.026517 | 1 | 1 | 1 |
| Somalia | 1951–2018 | 46.35312 | 388.4791 | 5912.01 | 0 | 1 | 1 | 1 |
| South Africa | 1951–2018 | 57.24636 | 6221.093 | 34208.35 | 6.298451 | 1 | 1 | 1 |
| Sudan | 1951–2018 | 55.91467 | 996.5425 | 24195.41 | 1.847786 | 1 | 1 | 1 |
| Swaziland | 1951–2018 | 51.7902 | 2557.772 | 793.2186 | 5.112484 | 0 | 0 | 0 |
| Tanzania | 1951–2018 | 51.32256 | 578.6684 | 23634.21 | 3.673151 | 1 | 0 | 1 |
| Togo | 1951–2018 | 52.02917 | 528.4261 | 3437.531 | 3.341566 | 1 | 0 | 1 |
| Tunisia | 1951–2018 | 63.84388 | 2507.839 | 7383.918 | 4.023706 | 1 | 0 | 1 |
| Uganda | 1951–2018 | 49.21552 | 426.1878 | 16728.51 | 3.109238 | 1 | 1 | 1 |
| Zambia | 1951–2018 | 49.08009 | 1287.335 | 7330.441 | 4.752613 | 0 | 0 | 0 |
| Zimbabwe | 1951–2018 | 53.91472 | 1079.041 | 8588.574 | 5.121826 | 1 | 1 | 1 |

*Note*: Zero (0) means no war/conflict was recorded during the period, while one (1) means at least one war/conflict was recorded during the period.

## AFRICAN'S RENAISSANCE (1990S–PRESENT)

| *Country Name* | *African's Renaissance* | *Life Expectancy* | *GDP Per Capita* | *Pop. Density* | *Education* | *MWAR* | *CWAR* | *Conflict* |
|---|---|---|---|---|---|---|---|---|
| Algeria | 1990s–Present | 71.4164 | 3910.605 | 30007.5 | 7.035244 | 1 | 1 | 1 |
| Angola | 1990s–Present | 50.52795 | 2619.515 | 10413.57 | 0 | 1 | 1 | 1 |
| Benin | 1990s–Present | 56.86352 | 707.8722 | 6607.363 | 3.186309 | 0 | 0 | 0 |
| Botswana | 1990s–Present | 56.18614 | 5406.896 | 1642.061 | 8.686106 | 0 | 0 | 0 |
| Burkina Faso | 1990s—Present | 52.93966 | 480.5669 | 22316.31 | 0 | 0 | 0 | 0 |
| Burundi | 1990s—Present | 52.0337 | 249.1907 | 7037.806 | 2.557559 | 1 | 1 | 1 |

| *Country Name* | *African's Renaissance* | *Life Expectancy* | *GDP Per Capita* | *Pop. Density* | *Education* | *MWAR* | *CWAR* | *Conflict* |
|---|---|---|---|---|---|---|---|---|
| Cabo Verde | 1990s–Present | 69.586 | 2324.605 | 3913.897 | 3.244438 | 1 | 0 | 1 |
| Cameroon | 1990s—Present | 52.65497 | 1239.387 | 15258.57 | 5.385553 | 1 | 0 | 1 |
| Central African Republic | 1990s–Present | 46.48626 | 414.4814 | 8297.488 | 0 | 0 | 0 | 0 |
| Chad | 1990s–Present | 48.61625 | 670.7142 | 7952.805 | 0 | 1 | 1 | 1 |
| Comoros | 1990s–Present | 60.05212 | 789.6922 | 577.6202 | 0 | 1 | 0 | 1 |
| Congo, Dem. Rep. | 1990s–Present | 52.77055 | 356.0445 | 52683.72 | 3.340747 | 1 | 1 | 1 |
| Congo, Rep. | 1990s–Present | 56.03265 | 2557.708 | 3086.489 | 5.833284 | 1 | 1 | 1 |
| Cote d'Ivoire | 1990s–Present | 49.51756 | 1300.283 | 16637.78 | 3.792875 | 1 | 0 | 1 |
| Djibouti | 1990s–Present | 58.41276 | 1269.234 | 619.8018 | 0 | 1 | 0 | 1 |
| Egypt, Arab Rep. | 1990s–Present | 68.59739 | 2077.719 | 65469.71 | 5.9008 | 1 | 0 | 1 |
| Equatorial Guinea | 1990s–Present | 53.28773 | 9861.054 | 491.2061 | 0 | 0 | 0 | 0 |
| Eritrea | 1990s–Present | 57.1068 | 538.9161 | | | | | |
| Ethiopia | 1990s–Present | 55.05576 | 258.1289 | 64644.87 | 0 | 1 | 1 | 1 |
| Gabon | 1990s–Present | 61.24087 | 10103.8 | 1218.398 | 7.000319 | 0 | 0 | 0 |
| Gambia, The | 1990s–Present | 56.81519 | 521.8144 | 600.8832 | 2.753556 | 0 | 0 | 0 |
| Ghana | 1990s–Present | 58.76968 | 1117.382 | 19618.19 | 6.524072 | 1 | 0 | 1 |
| Guinea | 1990s–Present | 53.53727 | 600.6234 | 8180.91 | 0 | 1 | 0 | 1 |
| Guinea-Bissau | 1990s–Present | 52.89027 | 569.1974 | 1263.824 | 0 | 1 | 1 | 1 |
| Kenya | 1990s–Present | 57.39952 | 908.7619 | 30635.11 | 6.633328 | 1 | 0 | 1 |
| Lesotho | 1990s–Present | 51.85979 | 975.7326 | 1871.463 | 5.618406 | 1 | 0 | 1 |
| Liberia | 1990s–Present | 54.33705 | 298.5684 | 2549.989 | 3.788775 | 1 | 1 | 1 |
| Libya | 1990s–Present | 70.78721 | 9820.982 | 5142.76 | 6.563734 | 0 | 0 | 0 |
| Madagascar | 1990s–Present | 59.15364 | 422.3321 | 15741.05 | 0 | 0 | 0 | 0 |
| Malawi | 1990s–Present | 50.9913 | 394.8186 | 11889.88 | 3.729366 | 0 | 0 | 0 |
| Mali | 1990s–Present | 50.72226 | 610.579 | 10451.51 | 1.343366 | 1 | 0 | 1 |
| Mauritania | 1990s–Present | 60.54553 | 1105.027 | 2497.685 | 3.650244 | 0 | 0 | 0 |

| Country Name | African's Renaissance | Life Expectancy | GDP Per Capita | Pop. Density | Education | MWAR | CWAR | Conflict |
|---|---|---|---|---|---|---|---|---|
| Mauritius | 1990s–Present | 71.83273 | 6187.416 | 1176.664 | 7.048156 | 0 | 0 | 0 |
| Morocco | 1990s–Present | 70.19383 | 2307.771 | 27848.54 | 3.988319 | 0 | 0 | 0 |
| Mozambique | 1990s–Present | 49.94309 | 311.1476 | 17537.16 | 1.170528 | 1 | 1 | 1 |
| Namibia | 1990s–Present | 58.09263 | 4385.754 | 1835.876 | 5.916331 | 0 | 0 | 0 |
| Niger | 1990s–Present | 51.61992 | 346.1748 | 10982.82 | 1.416541 | 1 | 0 | 1 |
| Nigeria | 1990s–Present | 48.14021 | 1734.342 | 122192.9 | 6.810469 | 1 | 0 | 1 |
| Rwanda | 1990s–Present | 49.46256 | 436.6821 | 8297.488 | 3.167375 | 1 | 1 | 1 |
| Sao Tome and Principe | 1990s–Present | 64.07294 | 1042.941 | 142.2516 | 0 | 0 | 0 | 0 |
| Senegal | 1990s–Present | 60.37872 | 913.0521 | 9635.131 | 4.315616 | 1 | 1 | 1 |
| Seychelles | 1990s–Present | 72.63399 | 9947.948 | 77.58359 | 0 | 0 | 0 | 0 |
| Sierra Leone | 1990s–Present | 42.12702 | 373.4868 | 4305.847 | 3.035225 | 1 | 1 | 1 |
| Somalia | 1990s–Present | 50.9378 | 436.6821 | 7588.473 | 0 | 1 | 1 | 1 |
| South Africa | 1990s–Present | 57.74492 | 6516.111 | 44463.04 | 8.027991 | 0 | 0 | 0 |
| Sudan | 1990s–Present | 59.6042 | 1203.205 | 33957.78 | 2.804828 | 1 | 1 | 1 |
| Swaziland | 1990s–Present | 52.36367 | 3249.245 | 1123.975 | 6.862069 | 0 | 0 | 0 |
| Tanzania | 1990s–Present | 55.10527 | 586.631 | 33214.09 | 4.782866 | 0 | 0 | 0 |
| Togo | 1990s–Present | 55.68624 | 500.8999 | 4943.7 | 5.028634 | 1 | 0 | 1 |
| Tunisia | 1990s–Present | 73.20788 | 3263.52 | 9419.527 | 5.914094 | 0 | 0 | 0 |
| Uganda | 1990s–Present | 50.71115 | 468.0054 | 24121.37 | 4.457488 | 1 | 1 | 1 |
| Zambia | 1990s–Present | 49.48277 | 1155.926 | 10309.28 | 6.222675 | 0 | 0 | 0 |
| Zimbabwe | 1990s–Present | 50.74944 | 1036.893 | 11356.34 | 7.019444 | 0 | 0 | 0 |

*Note*: Zero (0) means no war/conflict was recorded during the decades, while one (1) means at least one war/conflict was recorded during the decades.

# References


Abdoulie, J. (2012). *Item, 4 of the Provisional Agenda-General Debate on National Experience in Population Matters: Adolescents and Youth*. United Nations Economic Commision for Africa. Retrieved 15 December 2015.

Acemoglu, D., and Johnson, S. (2004). Unbundling Institutions. *Journal of Political Economy*, 113: 949–995.

Acemoglu, D., Robinson, J. A., and Verdier, T. (2004). Kleptocracy and Divide-and-Rule: A Model of Personal Rule. *Journal of the European Economic Association*, 2(2–3): 162–192.

Adelman, I., and Morris, C. T. (1967). *Society, Politics, and Economic Development: A Quantitative Approach*. Battimore: Johns Hopkins University Press.

Adorno, T. W., and Horkheimer, M. (2002). *Dialectic of Enlightenment*. Trans. Edmund Jephcott. Stanford: Stanford University Press.

Adu Frimpong, A. (2016). Theory and Practice of Health Economics. *IISTE*, https://www.amazon.com/Theory-Practice-Health-Economics-First/dp/1622659775.

Alasdair, D., and Blake, H. G. (1985). *The Middle East and North Africa*. Oxford University Press: Oxford. ISBN 0-19-503538-0.

Ali, T. M., and Matthews, O. R. (1999). *Civil Wars in Africa: Roots and Resolution*. McGill-Queen's University Press.

Annan, N. (2014). Violent Conflicts and Civil Strife in West Africa: Causes, Challenges and Prospects. *International Journal of Security & Development*, 3(1): 3, pp. 1–16.

Anselin, L. (1988). Lagrange Multiplier Test Diagnostic for Spatial Dependence, and Spatial Heterogeneity. *Geographical Analysis*, 20: 1–17.

Anselin, L. (1990). Spatial Dependence and Spatial Structural Instability in Applied Regression Analysis. *Journal of Regional Science*, 30: 185–207.

Anselin, L. (1995). Local Indicators of Spatial Autocorrelation (LISA). *Geographical Analysis*, 27: 93–115.

Anselin, L. (2004). *Exploring Spatial Data with GeoDaTM: A Workbook*. Urbana: University of Illinois, Urbana Champaign, 226 pp.

Anselin, L. (2010). Tests of Equality Between Sets of Coefficients in Two Linear Regressions. *Econometrica,* 28: 591–605.

Anselin, L., and Berra, A. (1998). Spatial Dependence in Linear Regression Models. In A. Ullah and D. Giles (Eds.), *Handbook of Applied Economics Statistics* (pp. 237–289). New York: Marcel Dekker.

Anselin, L., and Rey, S. J. (2014). *Modern Spatial Econometrics in Practice*. Chicago, IL: GeoData Press.

Anselin, L., Syabri, I., and Kho, Y. (2006). GeoDa: An Introduction to Spatial Data Analysis. *Geographical Analysis,* 38: 5–22, 27.

Aryeetey, E., Harrigan, J., and Nissanke, M. (2000). *Economic Reforms in Ghana: The Miracle and the Mirage*. Africa World Press. ISBN 978-0-86543-844-6.

Ayittey, G. B. N. (2014). The Imported Tradition of Africa Dictatorship. *The African Angle: World Policy.* https://worldpolicy.org/2014/05/28/the-imported-tradition-of-african-dictatorship/.

Baldauf, S. (2013). Chinua Achebe on Corruption and Hope in Nigeria. *The Christian.* https://www.csmonitor.com/World/Africa/2013/0322/Chinua-Achebe-on-corruption-and-hope-in-Nigeria.

Bangura, Abdul Karim. (2004). *Sweden versus Apartheid.* Ashgate Publishers.

Barro, J. R., and Lee, J. W. (2012). A New Data Set of Educational Attainment in the World, 1950–2010. *Journal of Development Economics*, 104: 184–198.

Barro, R. (May, 1991). Economic Growth in a Cross Section of Countries. *Quarterly Journal of Economics,* 106(2): 407–443.

Bartos, Otomar J., and Wehr, Paul. (2002). *Using Conflict Theory*. Cambridge: Cambridge University Press.

Becker, G., and Becker, G. N. (1997). *The Economics of Life*. New York: McGraw-Hill.

Bedirhanoglu, P. (2007). The Neo-Liberal Discourse on Corruption as a Means of Consent Building: Reflections from Post-Crisis Turkey. *Third World Quarterly,* 28(7): 1239–1259.

Bertalanffy, V. L. (1962). General System Theory: A Critical Review. *General Systems* VII: 1–20.

Birdsall, N., and Fukuyama, F. (2011). *New Ideas on Development after the Financial Crisis,* 1 edition. Johns Hopkins University Press. ISBN: 9780801899768.

Boetteke, P., and Fink, A. (2011). Institutions First. *Journal of Institutional Economics,* 7: 499–504.

Boetteke, P. J., Coyne, C. J., and Sautet, F. (2005). The New Comparative Political Economy. *The Review of Austrian Economics,* 18(3/4): 281–304.

Brett, E. (2009). *Reconstructing Development Theory*. London: Palgrave-Macmillan.

Brett, T. (2015). The Idea of Development in Theory and Practice. *London School of Economics, and Political Science (International Development),* http://blogs.lse.ac.uk/internationaldevelopment/2015/03/12/professor-teddy-brett-the-idea-of-development-in-theory-and-practice/.

Brittain, V. (1998). The Congo Quagmire. *World Press Review,* November 1998: 14–15.

Broadman, H. G., and Recanatini, F. (2000). Seeds of Corruption: Do Market Institutions Matter? *World Bank Policy Research* (cited in Ghaniy, N. and Hastiadi, F.F.

(2016). Political, Social and Economic determinants of Corruption. Working Paper in Economics and Business. Vol. 4, pp. 1–9).

Callaghy, T. M. (1984). The State-Society Struggle: Zaire in Comparative Perspective. *National Geographic*. New York: Columbia University Press, 1984: 7–79.

Caputo, R. (1991). Lifeline for a Nation: Zaire River. *National Geographic,* November 1991: 2–35.

Casas, I., Delmelle, E., and Varela, A. (2010). A Space-time Approach to Diffusion of Health Service Provision Information. *International Regional Science Review*, 33(2): 134–156.

Chan, M. F., and Devi, K. M. (2012). Factors Affecting Life Expectancy: Evidence From 1980–2009 Data in Singapore, Malaysia, and Thailand. *Asia Pacific Journal of Public Health*, 27: 136–146.

Chang, K. (2010). *Introduction to Geographic Information Systems*, 5th edition. New York: McGraw-Hill.

Chi, G., and Zhu, J. (2008). Spatial Regression Models for Demographic Analysis. *Population Research and Policy Review*, 27: 17–42.

Chia Wei, L . (2009). Possible Arguments for Low Life Expectancy, http://econsguide.blogspot.com/2009/02/possible-reasons-for-uks-deficit-in-its.html.

Clark, A. V. W., Hung, Y., and Withers, S. (2003). Does Commuting Distance Matters? Commuting Tolerance and Residential Change. *Regional Science and Urbans Economics*, 33: 199–221.

Clarke, C. K. (1986). Advances in Geographic Information Systems. *Computers, Environment and Urban Systems*, 10(3–4): 175–184.

Cromley, E., and McLafferty, S. (2002). *GIS and Public Health.* New York: Guilford Press.

Cromley, E., and McLafferty, S. (2011). *GIS and Public Health.* New York: Guilford Press.

Cronbach, L. J. (1984). *Essential Psychology Testing*, 4th edition. New York: Harper & Row.

Crossman, A. (2018). Understanding Conflict Theory. *ThoughtCo,* https://www.thoughtco.com/conflict-theory-3026622.

David, A. (1998). The Dead Help No One Living. *World Policy Journal*, 14(4): 81–96.

David, B. (1977). *Beyond the Sociology of Conflict*. New York: St. Martin's.

De Graaff, T., Raymond, J., and Nijkkamp, P. (2001). A General Misspecification Test for Spatial Regression Models: Dependence, Heterogeneity, and Nonlinearity. *Journal of Regional Science*, 41: 255–276.

Delavari, S., Zandian, H., Rezaei, S., Moradinazar, M., Delavari, S., Saber, A., and Fallah, R. (2016). *Life Expectancy and Its Socioeconomic Determinants in Iran.* US National Library of Medicine, National Institutes of Health. doi: 10.190882/3062.

Delphin, G. R. (1998). Key Issues in African Development in the 21st Century. *UNU/AERC Conference on Institutions and Development in Africa*. Tokyo, Japan, October 1998: 14–16. http://archive.unu.edu/hq/academic/Pg_area4/Rwegasira.html.

Easterly, W., and Levine, R. (1997). Africa's Growth Tragedy: Policies and Ethnic Divisions. *Quarterly Journal of Economics*, 112(4): 1203–1250.

Elbadawi, E., and Sambanis, N. (2000). Why Are There So Many Civil Wars in Africa? Understanding and Preventing Violent Conflict. *Journal of West African Economies*, 9(3): 244–269.

Fantom, N., Khokhar, T., and Purdie, E. (2016). *The 2016 Edition of World Development Indicators Is Out: Three Features you Won't Want to Miss*. The Data Blog. The World Bank. Retrieved 22 October 2016.

Forster, P. G. (2000). *Race and Ethnicity in East Africa*. New York: St. Martin's Press.

Fotheringham, A. S., Charlton, M. E., and Brunsdon, C. (1998). Geographically Weighted Regression: A Natural Evolution of the Expansion Method for Spatial Data Analysis. *Environment and Planning A*, 30(11): 1905–1927, doi:10.1068/a301905.

Fukuyama, F. (2010). *The End of History and the Last Man*. London: Penguin Book Ltd.

Georges, K. E. (2015). Afri. In Heinrich Georges (Ed.), *Ausführliches lateinisch-deutsches Handwörterbuch* (in German), 8th edition. Hannover. *Meine Biblithek*. Retrieved 20 September 2015.

Gilligan, A. M., and Skrepnek, G. H. (2015). Determinants of Life Expectancy in the Eastern Mediterranean Region. *Health Policy and Planning,* 30(5): 624–637.

Graham, J. U., and Bernard, F. (1985). *Spatial Data Analysis by Example Volume 1: Point Pattern and Quantitative Data*. New York: John Wiley & Sons.

Gramsci, A. (1971). *Selections From the Prison Notebooks of Antonio Gramsci*. New York: International Publishers.

Grossman, M. (2000). The Human Capital Model. In A. J. Culyer and J. P. Newhouse (Eds.), *Handbook of Health Economics, Vol.* IA, 347–408.

Harry, N. U. (2013). African Youth, Innovation and the Changing Society. *Huffington Post.* March 29, 2014.

Hassan, A. F., Minato, N., Ishida, S., and Nor, N. M. (2017). Social Environmental Determinants of Life Expectancy in Developing Countries: A Panel Data Analysis. *Global Journal of Health Sciences*, 9(5): 105–112.

Hope, S., and Ronald, K. (2017). *Corruption and Governance in Africa (Swaziland, Kenya, Nigeria)*. Palgrave Macmillan.

International Monetary Fund. (2009). How Does the WEO Categorize Advanced versus Emerging and Developing Economies?. *International Monetary Fund.* Retrieved 20 July 2009.

International Monetary Fund. (2017). GDP Nominal Per Capita – International Dollar. *IMF, WEO*, April 2017.

Janzen, J. M. (2000). *Do I Still Have a Life?: Voices from the Aftermath of War in Rwanda and Burundi*. Lawrence: University of Kansas, 2000.

Jean-François, B. (1993). *The State in Africa: The Politics of the Belly*. New York: Longman.

Jeffrey, G. (2010). Africa's Forever Wars: Why the Continent's Conflicts Never End. *Foreign Policy*, http://foreignpolicy.com/2010/02/11/africas-forever-wars/.

Jeffrey, S. and Warner, A. (1995). Economic Reform and the Process of Global Integration. *Brookings Papers on Economic Activity 1*, pp. 1–118. https://www.earth.columbia.edu/sitefiles/file/about/director/pubs/brookings_q195.pdf.

Jennings, C. (2001). *Across the Red River: Rwanda, Burundi, and the Heart of Darkness.* London: Phoenix.

Jolle, D. (2012). *Theories of Violent Conflict: An Introduction.* Abingdon, UK: Routledge.

Kabir, M. (2008). Determinants of Life Expectancy in Developing Countries. *The Journal of Developing Areas*, 41(2).

Knegt, D., Coughenour, M. B., Skidmore, A. K., Heitkonig, I. M. A., Knox, N. M., Slotow, R., and Prins, H. H. T. (2010). Spatial Autocorrelation and the Scaling of Species–Environment Relationships. *Ecology* 91: 2455–2465.

Konneh, A. (2010). Chevron, Liberia Sign Deepwater Offshore Exploration Agreement. *Bloomberg News.* https://www.chevron.cm/Stories/Chevron-to-Acquire-Deepwater Interest-Offshore-Liberia.

Lauritsen, E. N. (2016). Economic Under-development Leads to Civil Unrest. *ScienceNordic.* https://sciencenorway.no/forskningno-norway-social-economy/economic-under-development-leads-to-civil-unrest/1432197.

Lewis, C. T., and Short, C. (1879). *"Afer". A Latin Dictionary.* Oxford: Clarendon Press. Retrieved 20 September 2015.

Lucien, B. (2001). The History of France. *Editions Jean-Paul Gisserot*: 118.

Lukongo, B. (2018). Kleptocracy and Its Relation to Economic Performance: The Case Study of Congo. *R A Journal of Applied Research*, 4(1): 1349–1359. ISSN (e): 2394-6709.

Lukongo, O. E., and Miller, T. (2017). Evaluating the Spatial Consequence of Interest Rate Ceiling Using a Spatial Regime Change Approach. *The American Economist*, 63(2): 166–186. DOI: 10.1177/0569434517745490.

Lukongo, O. E., and Rezek, J. P. (2016). Investigating Spatial Dependence and Spatial Spillovers in African Agricultural Total Factor Productivity Growth. *The American Economist*, 63(1): 41–58. Doi:10.1177/0569434516672769.

Luo, W., and Wang, F. (2003). Measures of Spatial Accessibility to Health Care in a GIS Environment: Synthesis and a Case Study in the Chicago Region. *Environment and Planning B: Planning and Design,* 30(6):865–884.

Malinowsky, B. (1945). *The Dynamics of Culture Change.* New Haven. Yale University Press.

Malinowsky, B. (1961). *The Dynamics of Culture Change.* New Haven. Yale University Press.

Mankiw, G., Romer, D., and Weil, D. (1992). A Contribution to Empirics of Economic Growth. *Quarterly Journal of Economics,* 107(2): 407–437.

McElrath, K. (2002). *HIV and AIDS: A Global View.* Westport, CT: Greenwood Press. https://www.worldcat.org/title/hiv-and-aids-a-global-view/oclc/46538582.

Mills, C. W. (1956). *The Power of Elite.* Oxford University Press.

Mitchell, A. (2005). *The ESRI Guide to GIS Analysis 2, Spatial Measurement & Statistics.* Redlands, CA: ESR Press.

Nachimias, C. N. and Nachimias, D. (2008). *Research Methods in the Social Sciences*, 7th edition (pp. 150–154). Worth Publishers.

North, C. D., and Weingast, R. B. (1989). Constitutions and Commitment: The Evolution of Institutions Governing Public Choice in Seventeenth Century, England. *Journal of Economic History,* 49(4): 803–832.

North, D. (1990). *Institutions, Institutional Change and Economic Performance*. New York: Cambridge University Press, 1–26.

Onishi, N. (2001). Rising Muslim Power in Africa Causing Unrest in Nigeria and Elsewhere. *The New York Times*. Retrieved 1 March 2009.

Ould-Abdallah, A. (2000). *Burundi on the Brink, 1993–95: A UN Special Envoy Reflects on Preventive Diplomacy*. Washington, DC: United States Institute of Peace Press.

Patman, R. G. (1990). *The Soviet Union in the Horn of Africa 1990* (pp. 295–296). ISBN 0-521-36022-6.

Perkins, H. D., Radelet, S., and Lindauer, L. D. (1996). *Economics of Development*, 6th edition. New York: W.W. Norton & Company, Inc., www.wwnorton.com. ISBN-10: 0-393-92652-4.

Perkins, H. D., Radelet, S., and Lindauer, L. D. (2001). *Economics of Development*, 6th edition. New York: W.W. Norton & Company, Inc., www.wwnorton.com. ISBN-13: 978-0-393-92652-1.

Perkins, H. D., Radelet, S., and Lindauer, L. D. (2006). *Economics of Development*, 6th edition. New York: W.W. Norton & Company, Inc., www.wwnorton.com. ISBN-13: 978-0-393-92652-1.

Politzer, M. (2008). China and Africa: Stronger Economic Ties Mean More Migration. *Migration Information Source*. https://www.migrationpolicy.org/article/china-and-africa-stronger-economic-ties-mean-more-migration/.

Randall, C. (1990). Conflict Theory and the Advance of Macro-historical Sociology. In George Ritzer (Eds.), *Frontiers of Social Theory* (pp. 68–87). New York: Columbia University Press.

Randall, C. (1994). The Conflict Tradition. In *Four Sociological Traditions*. New York: Oxford University Press.

Rodney, W. (1972). *How Europe Underdeveloped Africa*. Bogle-L'Ouverture Publications.

Roseel, J. (2017). Conflict Theory. *Oxford Bibliographies*. DOI: 10.1093/obo/9780199756384-0035.

Rosenshein, L. (2010). Supplementary Spatial Statistics Toolbox for ArcGIS 10, http://resources.arcgis.com/gallery/file/geoprocessing/ details? entryID=8E548CF9-1422-2418-8855-2ED418793771.

Roser, M. (2015). Life Expectancy. *Our World Data*, https://ourworldindata.org/life-expectancy.

Sandbrook, R. (1985). *The Politics of Africa's Economic Stagnation*. Cambridge University Press.

Sayre, A. P. (1999). *Africa, Twenty-First Century Books*. Brookfield, Connecticut. ISBN 0-7613-1367-2.

Scherrer, C. P. (2002). *Genocide and Crisis in Central Africa: Conflict Roots, Mass Violence, and Regional War*. Westport, CT: Praeger.

Schoenurl, J. W. (2003). Liberian Shipping Draws Scrutiny, msnbc.com.

Schraeder, P. J. (2014). *African Politics and Society: A Mosaic in Transformation*, 2nd edition (p. 6). Clark Baxter.

Simon, J. L. (1995). *State of Humanity* (p. 175). Blackwell Publishing. ISBN 1-55786- 585-X.

Swanson, A. (2015). 5 Ways the World Will Look Dramatically Different in 2100, www.washingtonpost.com.

Toweh, A. (2011). Liberia Marks Out New Oil Blocks, Auction Seen Soon. *Reuters*. Retrieved 22 August 2011.

United Nations Department of Economic and Social Affairs. (2017). *World Population Prospects: The 2017 Revision*. ESA. UN.org. United Nations Department of Economic and Social Affairs, Population Division.

United Nations Statistics Division. (2003). *Millennium Development Indicators: World and Regional Groupings*. United Nations Statistics Division. Archived from the original on 10 February 2005. Retrieved 13 May 2017.

United Nations Statistics Division. (2009). *Composition of Macro Geographical (Continental) Region*. United Nations.

United Nations Statistics Division. (2017). *Standard Country and Area Codes Classifications (M49): Developed Regions*. United Nations Statistics Division. Archived from the original on 11 July 2017. Retrieved 13 May 2017.

Vale, P., and Maseko, S. (1998). South Africa and the African Renaissance. *International Affairs*, 74(2): 271–288.

Varnis, S. (1990). Reluctant Aid or Aiding the Reluctant? *U.S. Food Aid Policy and the Ethiopian Famine Relief* (p. 38). New Brunswick: Transaction Publishers. ISBN 0-88738-348-3.

Wang, J. F., Zhang, T. L., and Fu, B. J. (2016). A Measure of Spatial Stratified Heterogeneity. *Ecological Indicators,* 67: 250–256.

Wangome, J. (1985). Millitary Coups in Africa—The Africa "Neo-Colonialism", https://www.globalsecurity.org/military/library/report/1985/WJ.htm.

Wangwe, M. S. (1998). *Foreign Aid, Debt and Development in Sub-Saharan Africa.* Economic and Social Research Foundation (ESRF).

Wayback, M. (2007). Homo Sapiens. *University of Utah News Release*. September 8, 2007.

Weil, N. D. (2005). *Economic Growth* (pp. 56–67). Person Education, Inc., Publishing as Addison-Wesley. ISBN 0-201-68026-2.

World Bank. (2016). *While Poverty in Africa has Declined, Number of Poor has Increased.* World Bank, IBRD.IDA.

World Health Organization. (2000). *World Health Report 2000-Health Systems: Improving Performance*. Geneva: World Health Organization, http://www.who.int/whr/2000/en/index.html.

# Index

# About the Author

**Augustine Adu Frimpong**, M. Phil., Ph.D.,
Southern University and A & M College
Doctor of Philosophy, (Ph.D.) Public Policy
Master of Philosophy, (M. Phil) Economics, Kwame
Nkrumah University of Science & technology (KNUST), Ghana.

(Research, Program, Policy, and Data Analyst)
afaugustine@yahoo.com

Abbreviated Biography of Augustine Adu Frimpong, M. Phil., Ph.D.

Educated at Anglican Senior High School in Kumasi, Ghana, West Africa, Dr. Augustine Adu Frimpong entered the University of Ghana from where he earned his Bachelor of Arts (B.A.) degree in May of 2010, with concentrations in economics, mathematics, basic statistics and geography. He completed his first (B.A.) degree in May 2010. He entered the Kwame Nkrumah University of Science and Technology (KNUST), from where he earned his Master of Philosophy (M. Phil) degree in economics in November 2013. He subsequently earned his doctoral (Ph.D.) degree on December 14, 2018 in the field of public policy within the academic concentration of International Development at Southern University and A & M College in Baton Rouge, capital of Louisiana, USA.

Apart from being published widely in local and international journals in the United States, China, India, and Canada in the areas of health economics, applied microeconomics, macroeconomics, monetary theory and finance, agricultural economics, public policy, and labor economics, Dr. Adu Frimpong is also the author of a monograph in the area of health economics, with the title, "Theory and Practice of Health Economics."

He and his wife Mrs. Theresah Kye Adu Frimpong (nee Kye), a trained Registered Nurse (RN), are the parents of 3-year-old Yvette Marie Adu Frimpong. They reside in Louisiana, USA.

www.ingramcontent.com/pod-product-compliance
Ingram Content Group UK Ltd.
Pitfield, Milton Keynes, MK11 3LW, UK
UKHW020217290926
15470UKWH00001B/232

9 781793 603562